Cash's Textbook of General Medical and Surgical Conditions for Physiotherapists

CASH'S TEXTBOOK OF GENERAL MEDICAL AND SURGICAL CONDITIONS FOR PHYSIOTHERAPISTS

edited by
PATRICIA A. DOWNIE FCSP

faber and faber LONDON·BOSTON

First published under this title in 1984
by Faber and Faber Limited
3 Queen Square London WC1N 3AU
Photoset by Wilmaset Birkenhead Merseyside
Printed in Great Britain by
Redwood Burn Ltd Trowbridge Wiltshire
All rights reserved

Previously published as part of *Cash's Textbook of Medical Conditions
for Physiotherapists* 1951, 1957, 1965, 1971, 1976, 1979 and *Cash's
Textbook of Physiotherapy in Some Surgical Conditions* 1955, 1958,
1966, 1971, 1977, 1979

British Library Cataloguing in Publication Data

Cash, Joan E.
Cash's textbook of general medical and
surgical conditions for physiotherapists
1. Pathology   2. Physical therapy
I. Title   II. Downie, Patricia A.
616'. 0024616   RB111

ISBN 0-571-13161-1

Contents

Contributors

MISS S. BOARDMAN MCSP
Superintendent Physiotherapist, Orthopaedic Unit and Regional Plastic Surgery Centre
Mount Vernon Hospital, Northwood HA6 2RN

MISS P. A. DOWNIE FCSP
Medical and Nursing Editor, Faber and Faber
3 Queen Square, London WC1N 3AU

D. M. D. EVANS MD, FRCP, FRCPath
Consultant Pathologist, South Glamorgan Health Authority
Llandough Hospital, Penarth CF6 1XX

MRS S. M. HARRISON MCSP
Superintendent Physiotherapist
John Radcliffe Maternity Hospital, Oxford OX3 9DU

MISS B. V. JONES MA, MCSP, DipTP
Director, School of Physiotherapy
University College and Mater Misericordiae Hospital, Dublin 7

MISS B. KENNEDY MCSP
Superintendent Physiotherapist, Paediatric Department
St George's Hospital, London SW17 0QT

MRS K. M. KESSON MCSP
Physiotherapist, Ashford and William Harvey Hospitals
Ashford, Kent

MISS M. LIGHTBODY MCSP
Senior Physiotherapist, Neurosurgical Unit
The Radcliffe Infirmary, Oxford OX2 6HE

D. B. McHUTCHISON BPharm, MPS
Staff Pharmacist
Addenbrooke's Hospital, Cambridge CB2 2QQ

MISS J. MCKENNA MCSP
Senior Obstetric Physiotherapist
The Royal Free Hospital, London NW3 2QG

MISS L. MITCHELL MCSP, DipTP
8 Gainsborough Gardens
Well Walk, London NW3 1BJ

JAMES PARTRIDGE BA (Oxon), MSc
Maison de Bas
St Andrews, Guernsey

J. R. PEPPER MChir, FRCS
Consultant Cardiothoracic Surgeon
St George's Hospital, London SW17 0QT

MISS S. SAYWELL FCSP
Superintendent Physiotherapist
Winford Orthopaedic Hospital, Bristol BS18 8AO

D. W. C. STEWART BA, ALA
Librarian, The Royal Society of Medicine
London W1M 8AE

MISS C. VAN DE VEN MCSP
Superintendent Physiotherapist, DHSS Limb Fitting Centre
Queen Mary's Hospital, Roehampton, London SW15 5PN

MISS P. M. WALKER MCSP
Superintendent Physiotherapist
Harefield Hospital and Mount Vernon Hospital

Editor's Preface

More than 30 years have passed since Joan Cash wrote *Physiotherapy in Medical Conditions*. This was one of the first textbooks to be produced by a physiotherapist for physiotherapists, and was an immediate success. It was followed by *Physiotherapy in Some Surgical Conditions*. At first Joan Cash wrote these books herself, seeking advice and information from both medical and physiotherapy colleagues at the Queen Elizabeth Hospital, Birmingham. As medicine and surgery became more specialised, as well as technical, she invited additional contributors to share their expertise in these two books. In the intervening years physiotherapy has developed, and widened its horizons, so that now it is indeed true to say that it embraces the needs of patients from the cradle to the grave.

Joan Cash herself recognised the growth of specialisation when she removed first the neurology chapters and developed them into *Neurology for Physiotherapists*, and then the cardiovascular chapters to become *Chest, Heart and Vascular Disorders for Physiotherapists*. Now I, too, have felt the need to rationalise the present medical and surgical textbooks. They have both continued to grow in a haphazard manner, with overlap and idiosyncratic division. It seemed reasonable that the orthopaedic, fracture and rheumatology chapters could come together logically, and so *Cash's Textbook of Orthopaedics and Rheumatology for Physiotherapists* has been born, and joins the other specialist volumes.

The remains of the two original textbooks relating to important areas of the physiotherapist's work, together with other aspects that I have wanted to introduce, now become this particular volume: *Cash's Textbook of General Medical and Surgical Conditions for Physiotherapists*.

If I was asked to define the common theme of this new title I would be tempted to say it was the direct practical care and concern for the individual patient. That might, at first sight, be doing an injustice to the other three volumes; it is certainly not meant to be. Yet, somehow, this volume does reflect the very personal concern of physiotherapists for their patients. The chapter from James Partridge, remarkable by any standard, pays tribute to 'his physios' for their ability to 'always have time to visit, listen, and understand'. That chapter (17) should be compulsory reading for *every* physiotherapist, whether student or trained throughout the world, for it provides the *raison d'être* of so much of our work.

In this day of specialisation, research and the questioning of so much, it is salutary to stand aside and consider the message of James Partridge. He remembers his 'physio' not for her practical skills, oh yes he is grateful for that aspect, but he remembers her because of her humanity, compassion and understanding.

Then there is the fascinating chapter on riding for the disabled from Stella Saywell FCSP. As far back as 1953 I can recall seeing a truly magnificent display of dressage by the Danish rider Lise Hartel, an Olympic silver medallist. Nothing remarkable about that, you may think – but, she had suffered a severe attack of poliomyelitis and had to be lifted into the saddle. Then I think of a distinguished polo player with a split-hook arm prosthesis (he had lost an arm in the war), and recently there was certainly one member of the House of Lords – a paraplegic – who hunted. Not only then is riding for the disabled a tangible reality, it is also something which disabled persons can share as equals with the able.

It is interesting to note that riding for the disabled was born out of adversity – those polio epidemics of the 1940s and '50s. Stella Saywell does not tell us (for she is too modest) that it actually began at Winford Orthopaedic Hospital as a definite part of the official rehabilitation programme for those polio victims. From small beginnings this has grown to its present acceptance, with a national association and a royal patron. The mutual trust and affection between man and horse is well known; somehow, the fact that the rider is disabled seems to be transmitted to the horse, who in turn transmits a greater confidence to the rider. This is an interesting chapter which gives the lie to the misconception (sometimes expressed) that riding for the disabled bears little resemblance to actual treatment techniques in the department.

Dr David Evans has rewritten the pathology chapters. Mr McHutchison, a staff pharmacist, has provided an explanatory chapter on drugs, particularly those which may be encountered by the physiotherapist. Miss Laura Mitchell MCSP allowed herself to be persuaded to write a chapter on relaxation and stress: I do commend it as a very useful basis to many aspects of physiotherapy. Once again she echoes James Partridge about the need and ability to 'listen'. Miss Barbara Kennedy MCSP has rewritten the paediatric section and expanded the section on handicap. Miss Julie McKenna MCSP has provided a much needed chapter on obstetrics.

While some of these aspects have allowed physiotherapists to become specialists, and in a number of areas to come together in specific interest groups, it still remains the norm for the majority of physiotherapists to be able to turn their hands to many conditions. The importance of specialists should not be overlooked, but their greatest contribution must ever be the sharing of knowledge so that patients continue to receive the very best that the individual therapist can offer.

To all the contributors, old and new, I do express my very warm thanks and gratitude. As I have said before, it is they who make the book – I only edit it!

Once again Audrey Besterman has risen to the occasion – Could she draw horses? I asked with trepidation. The result in Chapter 24 is plain to see – yes, she can! On behalf of all the contributors, and myself, I extend thanks and appreciation to Audrey Besterman for her continued illustrative talent.

P.A.D.
London, 1983

Chapter 1

Using Medical Libraries

by D. W. C. STEWART, BA, ALA

Medical libraries vary considerably in size and scope of coverage and run from what may be little more than a shelf of books to collections of hundreds of thousands of volumes. All are doing essentially the same job – giving access to some of the considerable body of literature on medical matters which has been building up over many centuries. Medical workers have always been ready to make public their findings though the pattern of publication has changed and continues to change. In 1628 William Harvey (1578–1657) published what some regard as the most important medical book of all time his *De Motu Cordis*, on the circulation of the blood. Harvey's work had been done over a number of years but he did not feel under any pressure to publish any earlier than he did. In contrast, a 20th century Harvey would first have published a preliminary communication in a letter to the *British Medical Journal* or the *Lancet* and followed it up with perhaps a series of papers in specialised journals. He might then have delivered papers on the subject to various international conferences whose proceedings would be published as monographs or journal supplements emanating from publishers in Prague, London, Amsterdam and Buenos Aires.

In the days of Harvey it was not impossible to be aware of what most other researchers were doing through personal contact but even 200 years ago this was becoming impossible and more and more reliance had to be placed on the published record of research. Today, medical libraries play a vital role in controlling, through cataloguing and indexing, the output of literature and making it available to potential users.

The average medical library forms part of an institution such as a hospital or research institute and as such will endeavour to identify a readership whose needs it can reasonably try to meet. A teaching hospital library, for example, will be concerned primarily with the needs of medical students, teaching staff, consultants and researchers. It will also cover the needs of other health professionals such as physiotherapists, radiographers and pharmacists and it may also aim to provide for administrative and technical staff not directly concerned with patient care. Provision of nursing literature may also be made but that often depends on whether there is a school of nursing in which case there will probably be a separate nursing library.

It is important to define which is your primary library, that is to say, the one to which you belong and on whose services you have a right to call. It may be the library of a hospital, an authority, a public library system or a professional society. The more libraries to which you can have access the better, as it can be more useful to visit another library if you are working on a subject in which it specialises rather than trying to gather a lot of material by inter-library loan. A visit will also give access to specialised material such as dictionaries and bibliographies which would not normally be made available on loan.

Most libraries produce some kind of printed guide; it may be a lavishly produced booklet or a single duplicated sheet. In addition to digesting this, try to make yourself known to the library staff and get an individual introduction to the library; explain also what you are working on so that the librarian can help you get the most out of the library. Larger libraries such as those of universities have formal introductory procedures for new readers while some have audio-visual presentations on how they work or on the use of some specific types of material such as government publications.

The catalogue

Make the acquaintance of the catalogue; this is all the more important if it seems daunting in its complexity. It is the key to the library and it is designed both to act as a list of what is held and to provide an alternative approach to the stock from that of the arrangement of books and journals on the shelves. Catalogues are constructed according to fairly elaborate rules to ensure conformity of entry; they deal with how one files a name such as Van Winkle (under 'Van' if he's American, under 'Winkle' if he's Dutch) and how the publications of organisations – as opposed to individuals – should be treated and so on. Unhappily not all libraries use the same rules and large older libraries may have rather old-fashioned styles of entry. Regular use of the catalogue should make the reader familiar with the peculiarities of the system.

Traditional catalogues are on cards filed in cabinets but increasingly common are catalogues on microfilm; they may be on cassettes which can be slipped into a reader and wound on to the appropriate entry or on a series of sheets of microfilm – microfiche – also viewed through a reader. The physical format of the catalogue does not affect the internal arrangement of entries. It is important to know what is in the catalogue and what is not; for example, very few library catalogues aim to list individual articles in periodicals or chapters in books, though a highly specialised library may maintain such an index possibly as a file separate from the catalogue itself.

Most libraries regard the author entry as the 'main entry' so that some catalogues may expect the reader to refer to the author card for the fullest details of the publication in question. While the author of a book is usually an individual the term 'author' is used to cover editors, compilers, sponsoring bodies, government departments and so forth. The name of a publisher is not normally used, so it is rarely any use going to a catalogue knowing that a report was published by the government and expecting to find it under Her Majesty's Stationery Office as it will have its entry under the name of the government department responsible for it. However, a publication such as the *Faber Medical Dictionary* would have an entry under publisher as the publisher's name is an integral part of the title. A good catalogue will try to cover some of the possible headings a reader might approach and there should be a good system of cross references. These consist of '*see*' references which direct from a heading not used, to one which is, such as 'Petrograd *see* Leningrad', and '*see also*' references which refer to a related heading, for example 'Music Therapy *see also* Art Therapy'.

Dictionary catalogue

A subject approach may be provided by a separate subject catalogue but some libraries inter-file authors and subjects in a dictionary catalogue. Problems can arise here if a word can be used in different senses and a dictionary catalogue distinguishes between, say, 'Brain' as an individual's name (Lord Brain, the distinguished neurologist), the name of something (*Brain*, the neurology journal), the same word as the name of a place and the word as a common noun. A catalogue would file the entries in the order in which I have given them here. Dictionary catalogues should be used in rather the same way as one uses encyclopaedias.

Subject catalogue

A separate subject catalogue may be arranged by the names of subjects as in a dictionary catalogue or in classified order. A library classification is used mainly for ensuring that books on the same subject are together on the shelves and is based on the principle of analysing subjects into definable groups and assigning to these groups a notation in letters or numbers which places these subjects (and the books or catalogue entries) in correct relationship to each other. Most users of British or American public libraries will have a nodding acquaintance with the widely used Dewey Decimal Classification; this is used in medical libraries but more common is a development of Dewey known as the Universal Decimal Classification (UDC).

UNIVERSAL DECIMAL CLASSIFICATION

In medicine UDC takes as its starting point the discipline, in that its divisions are into anatomy, physiology and pathology to produce filing orders like:

6	Applied Sciences. Medicine. Technology
61	Medicine
611	Anatomy
611.1	Cardiovascular Anatomy
612	Physiology
612.1	Cardiovascular Physiology
616	Pathology
616.1	Cardiovascular Disease

The UDC class 615 covers therapy of all kinds including physiotherapy at 615.8 subdivided into headings such as massage at 615.82. However, the treatment of a disease is classified with material on the disease so that books on physiotherapy will also be filed at other places if they deal with physiotherapy of a specific disorder.

NATIONAL LIBRARY OF MEDICINE CLASSIFICATION

Another classification is that of the National Library of Medicine which takes the system (cardiovascular etc) as its basis of arrangement and subdivides by anatomy, physiology, pathology to produce:

WG	Cardiovascular System
WG 200	Heart, general works
WG 201	Cardiovascular Anatomy
WG 202	Cardiovascular Physiology

Physical Therapy is classified at WB 460.

Thus in the one scheme you will find all physiological material together while in the other all cardiological material is in one place. However good a classification may be it is impossible always to keep related material together as many topics have quite complex relationships. Most classifications give librarians some latitude within the rules to suit the needs of the individual library so it is possible to find the same book classified in different ways in two libraries which use the same classification. It is useful to be in the habit of using the catalogue rather than relying on physiotherapy books being on the third shelf down inside the door.

Having found the entry for a book you want in the catalogue it should not be too difficult to find it on the shelves. The information on the catalogue card should include the author, the title and the subtitle, the 'collation' which indicates size, number of pages and other details of physical form, and perhaps an annotation which may provide additional information about the title, e.g.:

MORTON, Leslie Thomas, Editor.

Use of Medical Literature. 2nd edition.
London, Butterworth, 1977

x, 462 p

(Information Sources for Research and Development)

In addition the entry will include information such as an accession number which identifies the book for library administrative purposes and a classification number or other indicator of where the book is shelved.

A library may have more than one sequence of books depending perhaps on whether they are earlier than a specific date, available for reference only or of unusual size, so it is important to read the catalogue entry carefully for any indication of this. The libraries of medical schools often have a 'reserve' collection of course reading and standard texts which may be issued for limited periods only.

Periodicals

Medical libraries spend a fairly large proportion of their book grants on periodicals and give this kind of material special treatment. Periodicals may be listed in the catalogue but more often there is a separate list arranged by title which gives an indication of the holdings available. It may also be available as a printed handlist for distribution to readers. In addition the library will maintain a detailed stock record which gives precise details about dates of receipt of issues, what parts have not arrived and so on.

INDEXING PERIODICALS

While the library catalogue lists the book stock in some detail the contents of periodical issues are not normally indexed though special issues of importance may be. Instead, reliance is placed on what are known as 'secondary' publications (usually themselves journals) which index the contents of the 'primary' journals which publish original work. Some secondary publications are designed to keep practitioners and researchers aware of new material appearing while others provide a means of making searches of the literature for information on specific subjects. Occasionally a secondary journal may carry one or two original papers, usually reviews of the literature on some aspect of a subject, while some primary journals may have an abstracting section which draws attention to papers in other periodicals.

The Institute for Scientific Information in the USA publishes a series of journals called *Current Contents* three of which relate closely to medicine, *Current Contents-Life Sciences*, *Current Contents-Clinical Practice* and *Current Contents-Social and Behavioral Sciences*. There is some overlap between the three. Each issue either details or reproduces the contents pages of the journals it covers and also provides a subject index and a list of authors' addresses. It is a useful means of keeping in touch with what is appearing in journals which your own library may not take and as it is air-freighted from the USA for rapid distribution in Europe it generally reproduces the contents pages of North American journals before the journals themselves get to this country.

THE INDEX MEDICUS

The *Index Medicus* (or the *Abridged Index Medicus*) is probably the most widely available of all medical indexing sources. It is a monthly index to the contents of some 2500 medical journals and to a small number of selected congresses, symposia etc, which arranges the papers it indexes according to a carefully compiled list of index terms (Medical Subject Headings or 'MeSH') while also indexing by author. *Index Medicus* has been published almost continuously since 1879 and in its present form it cumulates annually for ease of retrospective searching. It is selective but it covers all aspects of medicine and a good range of journals world-wide though there is a slight bias in favour of US material. Some time spent getting familiar with *Index Medicus* is well worth while.

Index Medicus places physiotherapy in its subject category E2 – PROCEDURES AND TECHNICS – THERAPEUTICS. The main specific heading is PHYSICAL THERAPY; other specific headings of interest to physiotherapists include EXERCISE THERAPY, HYDRO-THERAPY, MASSAGE, and ULTRAVIOLET THERAPY. A useful broader heading is REHABILITATION.

Sub-headings are used to assist in arranging entries and include: anatomy, adverse effects, diagnosis, etiology, education, instrumentation, methods, treatment, prevention and so on. An article will be indexed under three or so headings if appropriate and only under the most specific headings available. It is important to check the MeSH list before making a search to ensure that the most appropriate headings are being checked.

EXCERPTA MEDICA

The Excerpta Medica Foundation is the publisher of *Excerpta Medica*, an abstracting journal which appears in 44 sections covering different aspects of medicine from Anatomy to Virology and including a section *Rehabilitation and Physical Medicine*. Papers will be listed in as many sections as are necessary so that an article on the physical training of patients after mitral valve replacement appears in the Rehabilitation and Physical Medicine section as well as in Cardiovascular Diseases and Cardiovascular Surgery. The advantage of *Excerpta Medica* is that it publishes abstracts in English of the papers covered from which the reader may get enough information to make the reading of the original paper unnecessary. Each issue has an index by subject and author while the main part consists of abstracts arranged in subject groups so that an issue can be used as a current awareness source. The headings used in the Rehabilitation and Physical Medicine section include Anatomy, Function Tests, Rehabilitation of Somatic Disorders (subdivided by the site of the disorder), Physiotherapy (subdivided into exercise therapy, massage, electrotherapy, etc), Occupational Therapy, Technical Aids and so on. To assist in retrospective searching an annual index is published.

Only the largest libraries will subscribe to all sections of *Excerpta Medica* but most medical libraries will take enough to cover the main fields of interest of their readers. As the coverage and approach of no two indexing tools is the same there are advantages (though it is time consuming) in making searches in more than one. Index Medicus, Excerpta Medica and the Institute for Scientific Information also offer computerised information services.

Distinguishing references

In using secondary sources it is useful to be able to distinguish between book and periodical references as libraries usually treat them differently. An *Index Medicus* journal reference is presented:

Improvement in arm and hand function following head injury: a single case study. Kerley J. **Physiotherapy** 1982 Mar; 68(3):74–6.

If the article appears in a monograph it looks like this:

> The role of physiotherapy in the overall treatment programme for rheumatoid arthritis. pp 256–9 Gross D.
> In: Wagenhauser FJ, ed. Chronic forms of polyarthritis. Bern, Huber, 1976. WE 344 C559 1975

The last line includes the National Library of Medicine classification number. Chapters in monographs are no longer indexed, and will only be found in *Index Medicus* up to 1980.

An *Excerpta Medica* reference is cited before the abstract and includes the address of the author:

> Early feeding history of children with learning disorders-Menkes J.H. – Dept. Ped., Neurol. Psychiat., UCLA, Los Angeles, Calif. 90210 USA–DEV.MED. CHILD.NEUROL. 1977 19/2(169–171) summ in FREN,GERM

The title of the journal is less clear here but it is *Developmental Medicine and Child Neurology.*

Inter-lending systems

No library can aim to provide everything its readers could want so libraries co-operate through various inter-lending systems locally, nationally and internationally. Within the National Health Service several regions have well-developed library systems which effectively make available to library users the resources of all the libraries in the region. A library will have available a range of listings of the periodical holdings of other libraries though it is rather more difficult to locate books and monographs. The University of London, for example, publishes a microform list of the periodical holdings of all the libraries of the University including the medical schools and the specialist institutes which is extremely useful. Some individual libraries publish their own lists and there are other listings such as *British Books in Print* which act as means of confirming that a publication actually exists or that the details are correct.

The British Library Lending Division (BLLD) collects almost comprehensively in the field of medicine and is the first source on which many medical libraries call if they fail to supply material from their own stock. It aims to provide a rapid service and acts as a referral centre by passing requests it cannot meet to a group of 'back-up' libraries which includes several major university and medical libraries. If required requests will also be sent abroad. The BLLD can only be approached for loans through another library but its reading room at its site near Leeds is open to members of the public.

The Reference Division of the British Library is located at several sites in London and scientific material is housed in the two parts known as the Science Reference Library. Access is available to the general public without formality and a wide range of medical material is held.

Medical library provision in the United Kingdom has improved greatly in the last ten years, particularly outside London, though there is still a wealth of resources in the capital. The *Directory of Medical Libraries in the British Isles* (fourth edition, London, The Library Association, 1977) lists all the significant libraries and is arranged geographically with supporting indexes; it is an invaluable guide to the resources available in one's area and it also indicates who may use a particular library. The regulations governing access to libraries will vary from place to place and it is a good idea to make enquiries before paying a visit. Every library has its main group of readers to look after first of all and while most are happy to be of help there may be limits to what they can do.

References for publication

Having found the material which you wish to consult you may then find yourself in the position of writing a paper for publication. There are many books on the writing of scientific papers and publishers will also have their own rules and recommendations on format and presentation. Most medical papers have to supply references to the work of other people which may have been quoted in the text; editors are very hard on the author who produces unsupported statements. Not only must references be provided but they must also be checked for accuracy both in content and presentation. Badly presented or inaccurate references reflect on the general accuracy and diligence of the author and a good paper can be spoiled by inadequate references. Never quote something which you have not read; at the time you read a paper make an accurate and complete note of it avoiding the shorthand like APM&R 3/77 48 which you may be unable to reconstruct accurately when you need to. Note the titles of papers and the last as well as the first page number as some publishers require it. If you have used a variety of libraries in your researches it may help to note where you saw something that took you a while to find as you may want to use it again. Five-by-three-inch index cards in a small file are still the best physical means of organising reference lists.

The *Index Medicus* style of reference citation is increasingly being used as a standard and is known as the 'Vancouver' system (International Committee of Medical Journal Editors, 1982). Even if the project in hand is not destined to get into print the uniform requirements can be applied to essays to greatly improve the quality of the finished work from the point of view of appearance and presentation. Book publishers will advise as to their particular house style for listing references.

There are two systems for citing references in papers; either by the quoting of the author's name with a superior numeral, e.g. Smith[3] or the author's name and the date of the paper, e.g. Smith (1976). The second system, generally and inexplicably known as the Harvard system, is still preferred by many journals. In the bibliography references are arranged numerically by the first system and alphabetically by the second system. Some publishers prefer that journal titles be given in full while others recommend abbreviations; a good standard abbreviation list appears in the first issue of *Index Medicus* each year.

When checking the references after typing your paper always check them from the original publication; do not take the short cut of looking them up in the *Index Medicus* for it can make mistakes and it may not give you all the information you need. One of the longest running wrong references appeared off and on in the literature from 1887 to 1938 and was only sorted out when someone took the trouble to read the original paper referred to!

REFERENCE

International Committee of Medical Journal Editors (1982). Uniform requirements for manuscripts submitted to biomedical journals. *British Medical Journal*, **284**, 1766–70.

BIBLIOGRAPHY

Morton, L. T. (ed) (1977). *Use of Medical Literature*, 2nd edition. Butterworths, London.
Morton, L. T. (1980). *How to Use a Medical Library*, 6th edition. William Heinemann Medical Books Limited, London.
Morton, L. T. and Godbolt, S. (eds) (1984). *Information Sources in Medical Sciences*, 3rd edition. Butterworths, London.

Chapter 2

Inflammation and Healing

by D. M. D. EVANS, MD, FRCP, FRCPath

In Shakespeare's time most disease was ascribed to the four 'humours', used as a cloak to hide the almost complete ignorance of disease processes. Sometimes the relationship between a disease and its cause was dimly appreciated, as between the 'ague' (malaria) and marshland districts, but several hundred years elapsed before the relationship between marshland, the breeding of mosquitoes and their role in the transmission of malarial parasites to man was discovered.

Before its disorders could be understood, the normal human body had to be studied. This required international co-operation. An Englishman, William Harvey (1578–1657) paved the way by his work on the circulation of blood. A Dutchman, Anton Van Leeuwenhoek (1632–1723) developed microscopes with which he discovered the existence of red blood cells and the capillary circulation. With the aid of the microscope an Italian, Marcello Malpighi (1628–1694) investigated the cellular structure of normal organs, earning the title 'Father of Histology'. A German, Rudolf Virchow (1821–1901) used the microscope to study diseased tissues and became the founder of cellular pathology. A Frenchman, Louis Pasteur (1822–1895) demonstrated the existence of bacteria and their importance in causing disease. A Russian, Ilya Metchnikoff (1845–1916) elucidated the process of inflammation in living tissues. Workers from many other countries have advanced our knowledge to its present stage.

INFLAMMATION (Latin, *inflamare*, to burn)

Inflammation is the sequence of changes which take place in living tissue in response to damage. The termination '-itis' as in meningitis indicates inflammation of the relevant tissue, in this case the meninges.

Causes

The main causes of inflammation are injury, infection, infarction and immune reactions.

INJURY

This may be physical, thermal, radiational, electrical or chemical.

1. *Physical* injury (trauma) includes bruises, wounds, surgical intervention, fractures and crush injuries.
2. *Thermal* injury is produced by excessive heat or cold. Heat injury includes scalds from hot water bottles, wax baths and various types of burn. Cold injuries include chilblains and frostbite.
3. *Radiational* injury includes sunburn, ultraviolet irradiation burns and flash burns from nuclear explosions.
4. *Electrical* injury is the result of an electric current passing through the tissues, of sufficient power to damage them. Short wave diathermy may produce a similar type of burn injury.
5. *Chemical* injury includes burns from acids, alkalis and corrosive metal salts. There are other poisons which can damage various organs, such as cantharides (Spanish fly) which produces its aphrodisiac effect by causing inflammation of the urinary tract.

INFECTION

This may be due to viruses, rickettsiae, bacteria, fungi, protozoa and metazoa.

1. *Viruses* are organisms too small to be visible with the light microscope, but with the electron microscope they have been found to have a wide range of size and shape. Many of the infectious diseases are caused by viruses, including colds, influenza, measles, mumps, hepatitis and poliomyelitis. They can only multiply inside living cells which are often killed in the process, but the resting stage of a virus is able to survive outside the body for long periods.
2. *Rickettsiae* are slightly larger than viruses and are just visible with the highest magnification of the light microscope. They cause a number of severe diseases such as typhus and psittacosis. Like viruses they can survive for long periods outside the body and may be transmitted by mosquitoes, lice and, in the case of psittacosis, by birds.
3. *Bacteria* are larger than the viruses and rickettsiae: using the light microscope different groups of bacteria can be recognised by their shapes (Fig. 2/1) and staining properties. Organisms that stain with methyl violet (Gram's stain) and are not decolourised by alcohol are called Gram positive, and those which are decolourised are called

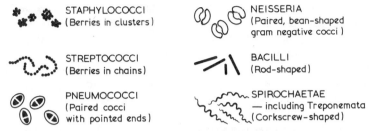

STAPHYLOCOCCI
(Berries in clusters)

NEISSERIA
(Paired, bean-shaped
gram negative cocci)

STREPTOCOCCI
(Berries in chains)

BACILLI
(Rod-shaped)

PNEUMOCOCCI
(Paired cocci
with pointed ends)

SPIROCHAETAE
— including Treponemata
(Corkscrew-shaped)

Fig. 2/1   Groups of bacteria with characteristic shapes and patterns

Gram negative. Small round organisms are called cocci (Latin, berries). Gram positive cocci include: staphylococci, causing boils, pustules and abscesses; streptococci, causing tonsillitis, cellulitis and septicaemia; and pneumococci, causing pneumonia and meningitis. Gram negative cocci (Neisseria) include *N. gonorrhoeae* causing gonorrhoea; and *N. meningitidis* causing meningitis. Rod-shaped organisms are called bacilli of which there are numerous different Gram positive and negative types, causing many varieties of infection from tuberculosis, Legionnaire's disease and gas gangrene to gastro-enteritis and typhoid. Some organisms are corkscrew-shaped, the best known probably being *Treponema pallidum*, causing syphilis.

Mycoplasmae have many of the characteristics of bacteria but have no definite shape. This is because they have no capsule and their outer skin is so thin that they can bend into any shape. An example is *Mycoplasma pneumoniae* which causes primary atypical pneumonia.

Actinomyces are generally considered as bacteria but they have branching threads, like fungi. Fortunately actinomycosis, the disease which they cause, is fairly rare. It has recently been found that contraceptive devices left in the uterus for a year or two may be associated with actinomyces or actinomyces-like organisms. Only occasionally are they involved in pelvic infections such as tubo-ovarian abscess.

4. *Fungi* are rather larger than bacteria. They have branching threads or hyphae and produce spores by which infection is spread. They cause superficial infections such as athlete's foot and ringworm. In debilitated patients they can cause internal infections such as aspergillosis of the lung or torulosis of the brain. Fungi can also produce inflammation as an immune reaction in sensitised subjects, e.g. farmer's lung.

5. *Protozoa* are small animals composed of a single cell. An example is the amoeba of which one variety, *Entamoeba histolytica*, causes a particularly unpleasant form of dysentery which can give rise to liver

abscesses. Protozoa include malarial parasites: *Trichomonas vaginalis* causing sexually transmitted vaginal infection; and trypanosomes causing sleeping sickness. Many protozoal infections are tropical diseases and are spread by mosquitoes or other insects.

6. *Metazoa* are larger multicellular animals. A major group causing human disease are the parasitic worms or helminths. They are encountered most frequently in hot countries. They include roundworms, tapeworms and flukes.

Many of these parasites also infect animals which usually act as an 'intermediate host'. In the case of hydatid disease man and sheep are the intermediate hosts, being infected by eggs from a tiny tapeworm living in the intestine of a dog.

INFARCTION

This is produced by blockage of the blood supply to an organ. An example is a heart attack due to a coronary artery being blocked by a blood clot. Deprivation of a blood supply causes tissue death which then gives rise to an inflammatory response. Infarction is considered in more detail on page 50.

IMMUNE REACTIONS

These are reactions which give rise to inflammation resulting from hypersensitivity either to a foreign protein or to one or more of the body's own proteins (auto-immunity).

A. *Foreign protein hypersensitivity* may be immediate, episodic (reaginic) or delayed.

(i) *Immediate hypersensitivity* follows the injection of antisera, foreign proteins, e.g. insulin (usually obtained from pigs), or substances, e.g. penicillin, that combine with body protein to produce what is in effect a foreign protein to which the patient has become sensitised.

(ii) *Episodic (reaginic) hypersensitivity* includes hay fever and asthma which usually occur after exposure to certain pollens, also various skin allergies and gastro-intestinal allergies (e.g. to shellfish) with vomiting and diarrhoea.

(iii) *Delayed hypersensitivity* occurs after infection with certain viruses, bacteria or fungi. The patient's lymphocytes become sensitised to the organism. It occurs in tuberculous infection or after immunisation with BCG (Bacille Calmette Guérin, a modified tubercle bacillus) and accounts for a positive Mantoux test. In this test a small quantity of the extract from tubercle bacilli is injected into the skin. A positive reaction is a red, slightly raised area at the site of injection reaching its maximum 48 hours after injection.

B. *Auto-immunity* is an immune reaction produced by the body against its own tissues. Examples are thyroiditis, atrophic gastritis, rheumatoid arthritis and chronic active hepatitis. They may be considered as examples of a misdirected protective mechanism which actually produces inflammation.

ACUTE INFLAMMATION

A mild form of acute inflammatory reaction is produced by making a firm stroke across the skin with a metal spatula. This produces a transient pallor followed by a dull red line (the *flush*), with an irregular surrounding zone of redness (the *flare*); if the stroke is sufficiently firm a linear swelling (the *wheal*) is produced. The sequence of flush, flare and wheal formation was described in 1927 by Sir Thomas Lewis as the *triple response*. These changes gradually subside.

With more severe inflammation, as with an acutely infected finger, the four cardinal signs of inflammation develop. They are redness (rubor), swelling (tumor), heat (calor) and pain (dolor). These changes do not subside until the infection is controlled, and can cause loss of function (*functio laesa*) of the affected part.

The inflammatory reactions described above are related to a sequence of changes in which the small blood vessels supplying the area play a crucial part. They have been studied in living tissues which are sufficiently transparent for the blood vessels and cells to be seen, as in the web of a frog's foot.

Initially there is a momentary arteriolar constriction producing the transient pallor. This is followed by arteriolar dilatation, with increased blood flow, dilatation of capillaries and venules and resultant redness (rubor) and heat (calor). The walls of the vessels become more permeable, allowing the escape of protein-rich fluid. This causes the swelling (tumor) and the resulting pressure on the nerves is the main cause of the pain (dolor). With the loss of fluid the blood cells become more densely packed together (haemoconcentration) and the blood flow slows. The leucocytes, mainly polymorphs, leave the centre of the capillaries and move to the margins of the vessels. They then pass through the walls of the capillaries by squeezing between the endothelial cells. Having left the vessels the leucocytes actively move towards the site of infection. At this stage virtually all the leucocytes are polymorphs. They have the ability to engulf bacteria and dead tissue cells, a process known as phagocytosis (Greek, *phago*, I eat).

To summarise, the acute inflammatory process has four major components which will be described in detail:

Blood flow changes
Exudation of protein-rich fluid
Leucocyte emigration
Lymphatic drainage.

BLOOD FLOW CHANGES

The blood supply to a part is controlled very largely by the muscle tone in its arterioles. Increasing the muscle tone constricts the arterioles so that less blood can flow through, producing the transient pallor which precedes the triple response. This is followed by a relaxation of the muscle tone in the arterioles which is a major factor in the inflammatory process. The lumen of the vessels becomes wider. This reduces the resistance to blood flow and allows a larger volume of blood to flow more rapidly through the arterioles (hyperaemia). This increased blood flow reaches the capillaries under a higher pressure than previously. As a result many capillaries which were partially or completely shut down are opened up and so the affected part becomes engorged with blood (Fig. 2/2(1)). There is a phase of rapid blood flow which may persist for an hour or so. It is followed by a gradual slowing of the rate of flow.

There are a number of factors which cause this slowing. The loss of fluid causes the cells to become concentrated (haemoconcentration); water and other small molecules are lost more rapidly than larger ones, leading to increased protein in the plasma which makes it more viscous. The increased protein causes the red cells to come together in rouleaux, like heaps of pennies (Fig. 2/2(2)).

The leucocytes attached to the walls of the vessels, sometimes in several layers, reduce the effective size of the lumen.

EXUDATION OF PROTEIN RICH FLUID

In normal tissue there is some fluid in the spaces between the cells (tissue fluid) which contains little protein. The blood pressure at the arterial end of capillaries is sufficient to filter this fluid out through the vessel walls. By the time blood has reached the venous end of the capillaries the blood pressure has fallen sufficiently for the tissue fluid to be absorbed back into the vessels by the osmotic effect of the plasma proteins.

In inflammation the dilatation of the arterioles causes a rise in the capillary blood pressure so that more fluid is exuded from the capillaries and little is reabsorbed. In addition the vessel walls become more leaky so that plasma proteins can pass out through small holes between the endothelial cells (Fig. 2/2(3)). These holes are visible with the electron microscope. They open very occasionally in the absence

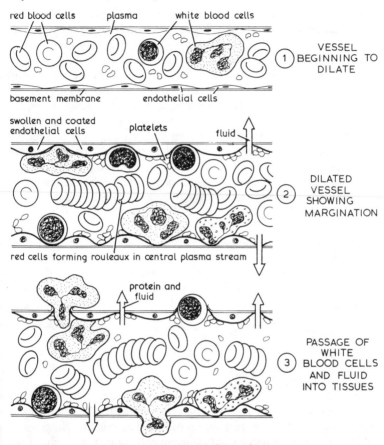

Fig. 2/2   The vascular changes which occur in inflammation

of inflammation to release a molecule of protein into the tissue spaces. In the early stage of inflammation, lasting about 30 minutes, protein exudation occurs from the venules but not from the capillaries.

There is evidence that histamine is the substance which produces this effect. In mild inflammation the changes may then gradually subside. In more severe inflammation protein exudation then occurs from the capillaries as well. It is not certain which substance produces this effect. It may be at least partly due to direct damage to the capillaries by whatever is causing the inflammation.

LEUCOCYTE EMIGRATION

During the early stage of rapid blood flow the leucocytes are mainly in the centre of the bloodstream (axial flow) (Fig. 2/2(1)). As the blood flow slows the leucocytes move towards the margin of the vessels (margination) (Fig. 2/2(2)). This occurs mainly in the venules and nearly all the leucocytes are polymorphs. They extend pseudopodia into the junctions between endothelial cells, actively forcing a gap through which they squeeze (Fig. 2/2(3)). The gap then closes behind them and they are guided chemically towards the site of tissue damage (chemotaxis). In pyogenic infections, such as pneumonia, there is a strong chemical stimulus to polymorphs, not only causing them to move to the infected site but also stimulating the body to produce large numbers of polymorphs from the bone marrow. In other types of infection, such as typhoid, there is little stimulus to polymorphs and instead the main cell to respond is the monocyte, which emigrates into the tissue to become a macrophage (Greek, large eater).

LYMPHATIC DRAINAGE

The lymphatics are thin-walled vessels which assist in the drainage of tissue fluid. In resting tissue many of these channels are collapsed and inactive. During inflammation these collapsed lymphatics open up and assist in the removal of excess fluid, protein and breakdown products of inflammation. The promotion of lymphatic drainage, e.g. by raising the affected limb to allow gravity to assist, will often relieve excess swelling and so reduce pain and discomfort.

Outcome of inflammation

The interaction between the infection and the body's defence now enters a critical phase. The outcome is determined by the number and virulence of the infecting organisms balanced against the effectiveness of the body's resistance. The balance may be tipped in favour of the patient by appropriate treatment such as the administration of an antibiotic to which the organism is sensitive. The most favourable outcome is complete resolution. Other possibilities are incomplete resolution, suppuration, chronic inflammation, spread of inflammation and death.

Suppuration

If there is much tissue destruction a hole or cavity is produced, an abscess. The cavity is filled with semi-liquid material called pus which is composed of dying or dead polymorphs, known as pus cells, dead tissue cells and bacteria, both living and dead. The process of pus formation is known as suppuration. When it occurs in the skin it is called a boil or a carbuncle. Although this may appear very unsightly it has the effect of walling off the infection instead of allowing it to spread through the body. Before the days of antibiotics abscesses were frequent and it was often necessary to drain them surgically. Even today it is occasionally necessary.

CHRONIC INFLAMMATION (Greek, *chronos*, time)

A chronic inflammation is one which persists for a long time, e.g. a year or more. An example is tuberculosis. As the infection continues the cells at the site of infection change. The short-lived polymorphs disappear and are replaced by macrophages. These larger cells live longer than polymorphs and are able to phagocytose larger particles, including tubercle bacilli which can remain alive inside them.

The macrophages come from the blood where they initially circulate for a day or two as monocytes and then leave the vessels to become histiocytes (Greek, *histos*, tissue and *cytos*, cell). They form the epithelioid cells and giant cells which are characteristic of tuberculous infection. They also give rise to the fibroblasts, cells which form collagen and produce fibrous tissue, a feature of chronic inflammation.

Lymphocytes, too, migrate to the site of chronic inflammation, often in large numbers. Some lymphocytes of the type called T cells are sensitised to kill specific organisms such as the tubercle bacillus. Lymphocytes of T-cell type can even become sensitised against tissue cells as in a heart transplant rejection or kidney rejection and also in auto-immune inflammations such as thyroiditis, causing myxoedema, or atrophic gastritis, sometimes causing pernicious anaemia.

In many inflammations which persist for more than about a week a number of lymphocytes of the type called B cells turn into plasma cells and produce specific antibodies against an organism or its toxin. They are produced in viral infections, subacute bacterial infections, syphilis and also in rheumatoid disease and other auto-immune inflammations.

IMMUNITY

Lymphocytes provide immunity in two different ways, known as 'cellular' and 'humoral' (by antibodies). The T-cell type are involved in cellular immunity. They cause the death of organisms or cells against which they are sensitised either by direct cellular contact as 'killer cells' but more often indirectly by stimulating the macrophages to do the killing. The T-cell lymphocyte is dependent upon the presence of the thymus gland, hence T cell.

The B cells are lymphocytes which have not passed through the thymus. They produce antibody either as small lymphocytes or after conversion into plasma cells. The antibody may be against organisms, e.g. agglutinins which cause the organisms to clump together, or against toxin, e.g. tetanus antitoxin, or against cells or cell components, e.g. anti-mitochondrial antibodies in auto-immune disease. They are called B cells because in birds they were found to be produced in the bursa of Fabricius, although in humans they are produced in the bone marrow or lymph nodes, like the other lymphocytes.

PERSISTENCE AND PROGRESSION OF INFLAMMATION

Subacute inflammation occurs with an intermediate type of infection, halfway between acute and chronic inflammation. It is characterised by infiltration of the affected tissue by plasma cells. Thus an acute inflammation of the Fallopian tubes may persist and become subacute salpingitis.

Further stages in the progression of infection are the entry of bacteria or viruses into the bloodstream (bacteraemia or viraemia), multiplication of organisms in the bloodstream (septicaemia) and the production of further abscesses as a result of organisms spreading in bloodstream (pyaemia). Some degree of bacteraemia or viraemia occurs in a number of infections and contributes to the fever and malaise.

The more severe conditions of septicaemia and pyaemia give rise to rigors. These are attacks of uncontrollable shivering in which the patient feels cold while at the same time the body temperature is rising rapidly. He may then suddenly feel very hot and sweat profusely with resultant fall in temperature. With uncontrolled infection, e.g. of the urinary tract a patient may suffer bout after bout of rigors and become extremely debilitated.

Sometimes rigors may persist until the temperature reaches a dangerously high level called hyperpyrexia (over 41°C) which may damage the temperature control centre so that the temperature continues to rise. Unless steps are taken to bring down the temperature artificially, e.g. by tepid sponging, the patient will die.

Types of chronic inflammation

Inflammation persisting for a year or more may be due either to recurrent attacks of acute inflammation or to inflammation which is essentially chronic from its onset.

Recurrent acute inflammation can affect the bronchus, gall bladder, kidney, bladder, cervix and large intestine. Each attack of acute inflammation produces local and general symptoms similar in nature to those already described, modified by the anatomical site involved. In the bronchus for example, it causes cough and expectoration of purulent sputum.

Essentially chronic inflammation includes many major diseases. Tuberculosis, leprosy and syphilis are examples in which the bacterial cause is known. The dust diseases such as silicosis characterised by fibrosis of the lung also have a clearly recognised cause. Rheumatoid disease, Crohn's disease and sarcoidosis are chronic inflammatory conditions whose cause is unknown and whose nature is only partially understood. Each of these conditions tends to cause progressive damage to the affected organs. As a result there is scarring and impairment of function which if untreated may become progressively worse, as with the grossly deformed joints which can occur in rheumatoid arthritis. Physiotherapy can play an important part in the prevention of such deformities and in encouraging the maximum mobility in affected joints.

HEALING

Tissue repair may take place by *resolution, organisation* or *regeneration.* When tissue damage is slight, healing takes place by *first intention.* When damage is more extensive or the healing process is complicated by infection, it takes place by *second intention.*

Resolution

The inflammatory process resolves and the tissue returns to its original state. This may occur in lobar pneumonia: the pneumococci are phagocytosed by the polymorphs, the polymorphs are liquefied by their own enzymes, the fibrin undergoes lysis and the liquefied exudate is reabsorbed to leave an intact lung which can function normally again. Not all cases of pneumonia will resolve so completely. Where there is tissue damage and abscess formation, healing occurs at the affected sites by organisation, resulting in a scarred lung.

Organisation

If resolution is incomplete, organisation of residual fibrin occurs. Fibroblasts and capillary loops grow into the fibrin from the margin. New capillaries grow out from existing capillaries, initially in the form of solid buds. They link up with adjacent new capillaries to form loops and arcades. Within hours of their appearance blood starts to flow through them. Red cells, leucocytes and proteinaceous fluid escapes from these new capillaries. Excess fluid is removed from the site by newly formed lymphatics which bud out from adjacent pre-existing lymphatics, linking up with each other to form a lymphatic drainage system (and apparently never linking up with a blood capillary by mistake). This vascularised tissue is called granulation tissue. While this blood supply and lymph drainage is developing, the fibroblasts multiply and start to lay down collagen, at first of primitive and later of more mature type. The blood supply is remodelled and eventually greatly reduced to form relatively bloodless scar tissue. This restores the continuity of the organ but never replaces the function of the tissue it replaces, e.g. lung or skeletal muscle.

Regeneration

In some organs damaged tissue can be replaced by functioning normal tissue. In addition to fractured bone and torn fibrous ligaments, thyroid, liver, pancreas and salivary glands are all capable of regeneration, provided the general alignment of the supporting tissues is retained. Peripheral nerves are able to regenerate provided the severed proximal end of the nerve is in continuity with the distal end which dies, leaving a neural tube up which the regenerating nerve grows at the rate of one millimetre a day. It has always been considered that there is no possibility of regeneration if the brain or spinal cord is

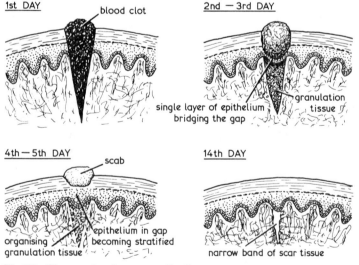

Fig. 2/3   The stages in primary wound healing

damaged. Recent work, however, suggests that some regeneration is possible by reproducing the conditions present in the fetus, but this is still at the experimental stage.

Healing by first intention (Fig. 2/3)

The healing of a clean operation wound is a typical example of healing by first intention. Slight haemorrhage occurs into the narrow space between the wound margins and so the gap becomes filled with blood clot (first day). The clot is composed mainly of fibrin which undergoes organisation as already described. At the same time epithelial cells spread over the surface from the adjacent epidermis (second to third days).

After covering the surface with a single layer they multiply to form the stratified squamous epithelium of which epidermis is composed (fourth to fifth days). This is the first tissue to restore continuity (14th day). Meanwhile fibroblasts lay down collagen in the granulation tissue which eventually becomes converted into a narrow band of scar tissue.

Healing by second intention

When the gap between the wound margins is wide or when the occurrence of infection interferes with the healing process a large amount of granulation tissue is formed. If the surface of the wound is large the spread of epithelial cells over the surface and eventual formation of stratified squamous epithelium may take a long time. The delicate epithelium may even be ripped off if care is not taken when changing dressings. The large amount of granulation tissue results in the formation of a large amount of scar tissue. The scar tissue may later contract and produce distortion, interfering with function, as in an infected wound of the hand.

Factors influencing tissue repair

The factors affecting the repair of tissue damage are its site, size, supply and support, also sepsis, sinuses, sutures and other foreign bodies ('odds and swabs'), to which may be added age and temperature.

SITE

The site of tissue damage determines whether it can regenerate as occurs in bone, fibrous tissue, mesothelium (peritoneum, pleura, synovium), liver, pancreas and peripheral nerves, or be replaced by scar tissue, as occurs in skeletal muscle, heart muscle and lung. Joint cartilage is a halfway tissue, being replaced by fibrous tissue when it is damaged which may then convert into fibrocartilage. Skin and the mucosa of the alimentary tract have variable regenerative ability.

SIZE

Where the size of tissue damage is small repair can take place with the minimum of scarring. Extensive tissue damage may lead to extensive scarring. In the case of skin this may be overcome by skin grafting. Extensively damaged kidneys may require to be replaced by a kidney transplant from a donor of the right tissue type.

SUPPLY

Blood supply to the site of tissue damage is a crucial factor in its repair. A good blood supply promotes rapid healing. The scalp is well supplied and sutures in scalp wounds may be removed after only five to six days. A part which has been irradiated may have a poor blood supply so that tissue repair is slow.

Poor venous and lymphatic drainage may also lead to slow healing as in the case of varicose ulcers in the region of the ankle where gravity and incompetent valves in the leg veins produce venous stasis. Physiotherapy may improve the circulation by means of ultraviolet light, ultrasound, moderate exercise and appropriate posture (raising leg).

Nerve supply to the damaged part apparently needs to be intact for healing to occur. If the nerve supply is impaired, as in syringomyelia or tabes dorsalis, trophic ulcers occur. The exact mechanism is not fully understood, but loss of pain sense allows tissue to be damaged more readily.

Food supply to the part by the bloodstream is dependent on adequate nutrition of the body. Adequate proteins and vitamins in the diet, particularly vitamin C, are essential.

Hormone supply is again provided by the bloodstream, particularly thyroxin. Deficiency of thyroxin, as in myxoedema and cretinism, impairs healing.

SUPPORT

Fractures require firm support and alignment if bone union is to take place. The support may be by internal fixation or external splintage usually plaster of Paris. It has been found that union is more rapid if support is not too rigid. Internal fixation by carbon fibre plates, which allows a very slight flexing, induces firmer and more rapid union than metal plates which allow no movement at the fracture site.

Protection from injury and infection by the use of petroleum jelly gauze, sterile dressing and bandages promotes wound healing. Good management requires sufficient immobilisation for repair to proceed, yet allowing sufficient movement to assist circulation and reduce muscular wasting to a minimum.

SEPSIS

Sepsis delays healing. *Asepsis* is the avoidance of infection by using sterile instruments, sheets, gowns, gloves and swabs and a non-touch technique in the changing of dressings. *Antisepsis* is the removal of infection by appropriate chemical agents. Because of their effects on living tissue some of these agents may impair healing, e.g. carbolic (phenol).

SINUSES AND FISTULAE

A sinus is a blind tract leading to an epithelial surface, e.g. to the skin from a foreign body embedded in a wound. A fistula is a tract leading from one epithelial surface to another, e.g. a rectovaginal fistula (from rectum to vagina) which occasionally complicates Crohn's disease. Surgical removal of the lesion and its cause (if removable) is indicated.

SUTURES AND OTHER FOREIGN BODIES

Initially sutures promote healing by bringing tissue surfaces together. Sutures which are left in too long (unless they are absorbable (catgut)) act as foreign bodies. Surgical swabs, pieces of clothing, dead tissue or any other foreign material left in a wound prevent healing and may give rise to sinus formation.

AGE

Healing tends to be more rapid in childhood than old age.

TEMPERATURE

Healing is impaired by excessive heat or cold.

Summary

From the above it can be seen that healing is promoted by:

1. Control of infection.
2. Removal of any foreign material, dead tissues, sinuses or fistulae.

3. Facilitation of repair with the minimum of scar tissue (first intention) by suturing together clean cut un-infected wound tissues and where appropriate by skin grafting.

4. Rest and protection of the affected part and if necessary immobilisation, e.g. for a fracture.

5. The maintenance of good general health with adequate protein and vitamins (especially C) in the diet.

6. Encouraging a good circulation and ensuring venous and lymphatic drainage by appropriate posture.

7. Where appropriate, physiotherapy to hasten the healing process, e.g. by the use of ultraviolet irradiation, infra-red irradiation, short wave diathermy, local massage in the case of varicose ulcers; and graded exercise(s) to maintain and/or restore muscle tone.

BIBLIOGRAPHY

See end of Chapter 5, page 65.

Chapter 3

Infection

by D. M. D. EVANS, MD, FRCP, FRCPath

The types of organism which cause infection are described on page 26. All such organisms are called pathogens (Greek, *pathos-gen*, disease producer). There are also many organisms present on the surface of skin, hair, nasal cavity, mouth, intestines and vagina of healthy people. They are called commensals (Latin, *con-mensa*, sharing the same table) and live in peaceful co-existence with their host.

Whether or not infection is produced depends partly on the organism (the 'seed') and partly on the relevant tissue (the 'soil'). The nature of the 'soil' often determines whether the 'seed' multiplies and produces an infection. *Staphylococcus aureus* is an organism which is quite often present on the skin or in the nose of healthy people without producing any ill effect. But if it gains access to an open wound it will probably cause sepsis. Preventing such access by using aseptic techniques is a major factor in the control of cross-infection.

MODES OF INFECTION

Transmission by direct contact, droplets, water, food and fomites are the main ways in which infection is spread.

Direct contact

There is a danger that infection may be spread by direct contact from the skin of the hand to an open wound in hospital. It is prevented by scrubbing the hands adequately, putting on sterile gloves and using sterile instruments to avoid direct contact. A physiotherapist with a boil (*Staphylococcus aureus* folliculitis) or other skin infection, particularly if it is on the hand, should avoid handling patients. Long hair which may infect a wound should be controlled by a cap. The sexually transmitted diseases are spread by direct contact.

Droplets

It is well known that coughs and sneezes spread diseases. It is not so generally appreciated that talking also spreads fine droplets for a distance of eight feet or so. The use of an adequate face mask cuts down the risk of such spread. A plain gauze mask which does not include a cellophane barrier is inadequate to prevent the spread of fine droplets. A patient with a dangerous respiratory infection, such as open tuberculosis, should be isolated.

Water

In civilised communities tap water is generally considered safe, particularly if it has been chlorinated. Cholera and typhoid have been transmitted by water in the past and have not yet been eliminated. Recently there have been occasional cases of Legionnaire's disease, even in hospitals, from infection of the water in air-conditioning systems or from showers, by fine droplets (aerosols). Taps and water filters may themselves become infected. When dressing wounds, infection is avoided by the use of sterile saline, etc.

Food

Contaminated food can spread food poisoning, dysentery, typhoid and other diseases. A boil on the hand can infect food or milk with *Staph aureus*. If this is then given a chance to multiply, particularly in warm conditions, it can cause severe gastro-enteritis. Selection of clean food, cleanliness in food handling and refrigerated storage help to prevent food-borne infection.

Fomites (Latin, *fomites*, tinder)

A fomite is the term used for any material which is infected and can then spread infection. Dirty dressings, swabs and utensils may all transmit infection. Care in the disposal of used dressings and the cleansing of utensils prevents such transmission. Clothing can act as a fomite. Where appropriate this is prevented by the use of sterile gowns.

PREVENTION OF CROSS-INFECTION

Once the modes of infection are understood, the prevention of cross-infection is essentially applied common sense, as outlined above. The strictness with which precautions need to be applied depends very much on the circumstances. In dealing with open wounds strict asepsis is indicated. When deciding whether a patient with a given infection should be isolated the guiding factors are its *infectivity* and the *virulence* of the infecting organism.

Infectivity

The infectious diseases, many of which are due to viruses, such as chickenpox, measles, mumps and rubella ('baby blight'), have a high degree of infectivity. Leprosy is often thought to be highly infectious but in fact has a low degree of infectivity. When assessing the infectivity of an individual case it is helpful to consider the mode(s) of spread of the infection concerned, the stage of the disease and whether the infection is still active.

Virulence

Virulence is the term used of an organism to indicate the severity of infection which it produces. The smallpox virus is an example of a highly virulent organism which produced a high mortality rate. By giving it to a cow its virulence was greatly reduced and the modified virus so produced was used for vaccination which gave its recipients immunity against smallpox. Rubella is an infection which can prove highly virulent for the unborn human fetus but causes only a mild infection during postnatal life. The virulence of an organism is related to its *invasiveness* and *toxin production*.

INVASIVENESS

An example of a highly invasive organism is the *Streptococcus pyogenes* which is a common cause of tonsillitis. If it infects an open wound it spreads readily through the tissue, digesting away barriers which might obstruct its progress by enzymes. It spreads along the lymphatics to produce a lymphangitis, reaching lymph nodes to cause a lymphadenitis, and penetrates the bloodstream (bacteraemia) where it multiplies (septicaemia), and can then settle in various tissues producing multiple abscesses (pyaemia). Invasion of tissues by an organism is assisted by its having a protective capsule or sheath. The tubercle bacillus has a lipid sheath which resists digestion by macrophages. So the macrophage transports living tubercle bacilli and actually assists the spread of infection.

TOXIN PRODUCTION

A toxin is a poisonous substance. A toxin present within an organism which does not escape into the host's tissues until the organism dies is called an endotoxin (Greek, *endon-toxin*, internal poison). The tubercle bacillus produces such an endotoxin. A number of organisms produce exotoxins (Greek, *exo-toxin*, external poison). These spread through the body while the organisms themselves remain more or less localised at the initial site of infection. An example of an exotoxin is tetanus toxin. This produces an effect on the nervous system, making it unduly sensitive to any stimulus such as a noise which causes uncontrollable and painful muscle spasm, often including spasm of the masseter muscles (lockjaw). Other examples of exotoxins are diphtheria toxin and the enterotoxin produced by *Staph aureus* which causes the gastro-enteritis mentioned earlier.

DEFENCE MECHANISMS AGAINST INFECTION

The natural defence mechanisms against the infection are: (1) intact skin and mucous membranes; (2) the acute and chronic inflammatory reactions; and (3) the immune responses. To this may be added (4) the artificial defences provided by immunisation, antiseptics, antibiotics and the preventive measures of aseptic techniques and isolation.

Skin and mucous membranes

The skin provides mechanical protection against many infections. A small cut is sufficient to allow organisms to enter and *Staph aureus* is able to infect an intact hair follicle to produce a boil. The eyes are protected by secretion from the tear glands which contain lysozyme, capable of killing many bacteria and fungi. The respiratory tract is protected by the secretion of mucus which forms a protective blanket, continually moved along by cilia. The stomach secretes hydrochloric acid which is strong enough to kill many organisms. The urethral sphincter is normally sufficient to prevent organisms from entering the urinary tract. The shorter urethra in the female urinary tract makes it more susceptible to infection than the male tract.

Inflammatory reactions

The acute and chronic inflammatory reactions described in Chapter 2 are important defence mechanisms. Phagocytosis of organisms by polymorphs and macrophages is often successful in killing them although some organisms, such as the tubercle bacillus, are resistant. Further protection is provided by the immune responses which are closely linked with the inflammatory reactions (see p. 33).

Types of immunity

Immunity may be *passive* or *active*. Each type of immunity may occur *naturally* or be induced *artificially*. In addition there is a *species* immunity. Thus man as a species has a high degree of immunity against foot and mouth disease, whereas animals with cloven feet such as cattle are very susceptible. There is also some degree of *racial* immunity. Jews tend to have a higher degree of immunity to tuberculosis than the Irish. Eskimos tend to have a lower degree of immunity to infectious diseases than most town dwellers.

PASSIVE IMMUNITY

Natural: A baby receives passive immunity in the form of antibodies from its mother. These are immunoglobulins whose molecules are small enough to cross the placenta or be transmitted in breast milk. This gives temporary immunity to the baby, lasting three to six months, against infections to which the mother had herself developed immunity.

Artificial: If a pregnant woman is exposed to rubella and does not have immunity against this infection it is advisable to give her (and her baby) passive immunity by injecting her with antibody. This is particularly important in the early months of pregnancy when the fetus is most susceptible to damage. The giving of antitoxin against diphtheria or tetanus toxin are also examples of passive immunisation. They have also been used successfully in the treatment of these infections. The antisera were often made by immunisation of horses. Unfortunately a number of patients became sensitive to the horse serum and suffered anaphylactic shock or serum sickness, so purer forms of antibody are now being produced.

ACTIVE IMMUNITY

Natural: The recovery phase of many infections is associated with the formation of antibodies against the relevant organism and its toxins. This provides an immunity which in the case of infections like measles and diphtheria is normally long lasting, although it may wane in later life. The cells which produce the antibodies are lymphocytes and plasma cells of the type called B cells. In other types of infection such as tuberculosis immunity is mainly of the cellular type provided by lymphocytes called T cells (see p. 33). Sometimes both types of immunity are involved, as in syphilitic infections: the detection of the syphilitic antibody produced provides the basis of diagnosis in all but very early cases.

Artificial: The body's defences against an infection such as tetanus are greatly enhanced by previous artificial immunisation through the injection of tetanus toxoid. It results in production of antitoxin by B cells at a very early stage of the infection so that tetanus toxin is immediately neutralised, thus preventing the painful muscle spasms and lockjaw. Artificial active immunisation against poliomyelitis, measles and whooping cough either protects against these infections completely or greatly reduces their severity.

ARTIFICIAL ANTIBACTERIAL DEFENCES

Antiseptics: The chances of a wound becoming infected may be greatly reduced by debridement. This involves cleaning the wound surface and the surrounding skin. Any foreign material is removed and an appropriate antiseptic such as hydrogen peroxide is used to kill organisms which may have entered the wound. In general, antiseptics are applied to the site of possible infection. Their effect is purely local and they have no effect on organisms which have penetrated more deeply into the body. Many antiseptics are poisonous if swallowed. Suitable antiseptics may, however, be used for sterilising instruments which have been previously cleaned.

Antibiotics: Antibiotics, like antiseptics, can kill susceptible organisms. Unlike antiseptics they can reach organisms that have penetrated deeply into the body tissues. They are given either by mouth or by injection, reaching the tissues via the bloodstream. They can also be applied locally when appropriate. Some antibiotics have a narrow range of organisms against which they act: thus penicillin is effective against *S. pyogenes* but useless against Gram negative bacilli.

Some antibiotics (broad spectrum) have a wide range of organisms against which they act. This apparent advantage has the drawback that it causes diarrhoea by removing the bacteria normally present in the gut and allowing the proliferation of fungi. Before any antibiotic is given to a patient, a swab or specimen should be sent to the bacteriology laboratory to culture the organism concerned and test its sensitivity against an appropriate range of antibiotics.

Asepsis: Prevention is better than cure. It is better to avoid the introduction of organisms than to treat the resultant infection by antiseptics which may damage the tissues or antibiotics which may have harmful side-effects. Modern surgery has only been made possible by the use of rigid aseptic techniques. These include scrubbing up to remove excess organisms from the hands, the wearing of sterile gowns, caps, masks and gloves, the use of sterilised instruments, swabs, dressings and towels and the practice of a non-touch technique. The latter is the use of sterile instruments, rather than hands, for holding swabs, dressings and tissues, and carefully discarding any potentially contaminated materials or instruments. A similar technique is used in the dressing of wounds or changing dressings postoperatively.

An important adjunct to aseptic techniques is the cleansing of skin adjacent to a wound or pre-operatively by skin antiseptics.

An extension of the aseptic technique is the early skin grafting of extensive burns which would otherwise become infected, producing scarring and deformity. This is a great advance, both cosmetically and functionally. It is particularly important for the physiotherapist who has to ensure that as much mobility as possible is retained, especially following burns of the hand.

BIBLIOGRAPHY

See end of Chapter 5, page 65.

Chapter 4

Circulatory Disturbances

by D. M. D. EVANS, MD, FRCP, FRCPath

Circulatory disturbances may be divided into general and local.

The most important *general* disturbance of the circulation is cardiac failure. Its main causes are excessive load, damaged heart muscle and conduction system, and inefficient heart valves. Excessive load is most commonly due to high blood pressure, the immediate cause being increased tone in the muscular arteries and arterioles. Damaged heart muscle and conduction system is most commonly due to obstruction of the coronary arteries which supply the heart, by atheroma and thrombosis. Inefficient valves may be due to congenital effects or to damage resulting from infection. Rheumatic fever was a common cause but has now become rare as a result of treating streptococcal infections by antibiotics. Whatever the cause, one effect of cardiac failure is slowing of the circulation. This in turn can contribute to local circulatory disturbance such as thrombosis. Another common effect of cardiac failure is oedema due to the increased venous pressure.

The most important *local* disturbance of circulation is obstruction of the blood supply. This is usually due to thrombosis or embolism but may be due also to disease of the vessel wall, compression, invasion by a growth or vascular spasm.

THROMBOSIS

Thrombosis is the formation of a thrombus (Greek, *thrombos*, a clot). Normally blood does not clot when it flows through healthy blood vessels. Factors which promote thrombosis are stasis (slowing of the bloodstream) and injury or disease of the vessel wall. Stasis may be part of general slowing of the bloodstream, as from cardiac failure or from prolonged recumbency without the benefit of physiotherapy.

Local factors include the compression of veins by tight clothing, the bar of a deckchair, a pregnant uterus or a tumour, and the narrowing of the lumen of coronary arteries by atheroma. Damage to a vessel wall, usually a vein, may be due to a fracture or an operation in its close vicinity. Following an operation there may be a period of recumbency with a consequent slowing of the circulation, although nowadays this is kept as short as possible, with early mobilisation. Following childbirth and surgical procedures, particularly splenectomy, there is a rise in platelet count which increases the patient's susceptibility to thrombosis temporarily.

The formation of a blood clot results from conversion of the soluble blood protein fibrinogen into insoluble fibrin which forms a web of fine threads in which the blood cells become enmeshed. This conversion is brought about by thrombin. Normally circulating blood contains no thrombin, otherwise it would clot. Instead it contains an inactive substance called prothrombin which, in the presence of calcium, is converted into thrombin by thromboplastin (also called thrombokinase). Normally circulating blood contains no thromboplastin, otherwise it would clot. Instead it contains a number of factors, platelets being one of these factors. If there is any damage to the blood vessel wall platelets tend to stick to the damaged vessel wall and the clotting process may be triggered off by the production of thromboplastin. This clotting tendency is increased if the circulation is slowed. It is diminished by regular physiotherapy with exercise. It is also diminished by carefully controlled anticoagulants which interfere with the clotting process outlined above.

Once a thrombus has formed in a vein the stasis resulting from the blockage of the lumen causes further clotting (propagated thrombus) which usually extends to the point at which the next tributary joins the vein. Initially such thrombus may be only loosely attached to the vessel wall and there is a danger that part of it may become detached. Later an inflammatory reaction develops. Capillary buds and fibroblasts grow into the clot so that it becomes organised and firmly attached to the vessel wall. Eventually the thrombus may become re-canalised, with one or more channels extending through the length of the clot so that circulation is re-established. Alternatively the vein may end up as a fibrous cord.

EMBOLISM

When a clot occurs in a leg vein there is a danger that part of the clot may break away and form an embolus (Greek, *embolos*, a wedge or stopper). This is carried off in the bloodstream until it becomes wedged, usually in the pulmonary artery or one of its branches. The process is then referred to as pulmonary embolism. A large pulmonary embolus is often fatal.

INFARCTION

Infarction is tissue death due to a blocked vessel. The extent of the tissue death reflects the distribution of the vessel. In the case of a blocked artery in an organ such as the kidney it is often cone-shaped, as is the tissue supplied by the artery. It is called an infarct (Latin, *infarctum*, stuffed) because in the early stages it is stuffed with blood, at least in soft tissues such as the lung. Infarcts in firmer tissues are only haemorrhagic at the edges due to seepage of blood in to the dead tissue from vessels at the margin of the infarct. The blood gradually becomes absorbed and it changes from a red into a white infarct. It also becomes fibrotic and shrinks in size.

Infarction only occurs in tissues which do not have an adequate collateral (secondary) blood supply. Thus, in addition to pulmonary vessels, the lung has a secondary supply from bronchial vessels. So a small pulmonary embolism may not produce an infarct unless there is also cardiac failure, making the bronchial supply inadequate. It is patients who have poor circulation, as in cardiac failure, who are more likely to get leg vein thrombosis with the possibility of pulmonary embolism and resultant pulmonary infarction.

Infarction may occur from a blocked vein such as a mesenteric vein undergoing thrombosis or from blockage of both artery and vein, as from torsion of an ovarian cyst when the whole cyst becomes infarcted. A common cause of death is infarction of heart muscle due to blockage of a coronary artery by atheroma and thrombosis. The brain may undergo infarction either from embolism due to a clot released from a damaged heart or from thrombosis of a cerebral artery. Gangrene of an extremity due to arteriosclerosis is another example of infarction.

Signs: symptoms: management

Thrombosis, embolism and infarction are closely related conditions, any one of which may give rise to signs and symptoms. Leg vein thrombosis may give rise to pain and tenderness at the site of thrombosis with swelling of the affected limb. Management is a compromise between resting the limb to avoid dislodging an embolus and sufficient movement of the rest of the body to discourage further thrombosis, assisted by anticoagulant administration. Prevention is by adequate movement and physiotherapy for recumbent patients, particularly postoperatively and especially if they are obese.

Not uncommonly leg vein thrombosis may be symptomless and the first indication of its existence may be the effects of pulmonary embolism. A large embolus causes extreme distress, shock and breathlessness and may be fatal within minutes.

A smaller embolus may give rise to transient pleuritic pain which may be associated with signs and symptoms resembling pneumonia. Sometimes there is little clinical evidence that pulmonary embolism has occurred and a puzzling shadow on the chest radiograph may be the first clue to what has happened. Pulmonary infarction may be complicated by chest infection which will then require treatment as for pneumonia. Otherwise management is mainly directed to the prevention of further pulmonary embolism by anticoagulants and physiotherapy.

Thrombosis of a coronary artery may give rise to a typical heart attack, with chest pain and shock, often with breathlessness and cyanosis. Quite often the pain is described as indigestion or back pain; it may radiate down the arm or into the neck. Management depends on severity and available facilities. It varies from intensive care with cardiac monitoring in a coronary care unit, possibly with dramatic resuscitation procedures, to bed rest at home. Once the acute phase is over, graduated exercise plays an important part in the recovery phase.

Embolism from the heart to the brain or thrombosis of a cerebral artery can cause cerebral infarction, i.e. a stroke. A small infarct may cause slight weakness on one side (hemiparesis), sometimes involving only one limb. A larger infarct may cause complete paralysis of one side (hemiplegia). Physiotherapy and occupational therapy play an important part in regaining maximum movement and control. This may include training the left hand to undertake functions previously performed by the right hand.

Embolism from the heart to a leg artery causes pain and discolouration of the leg. Immediate operation to remove the embolus (embolectomy) is sometimes successful. If this cannot be done, keeping the limb cool with minimal movement (to reduce metabolism) may keep gangrene at bay and allow a collateral circulation to develop. If gangrene develops, amputation may be necessary; the rehabilitation and training in the use of the prosthesis is described in Chapter 18.

OEDEMA

There is normally a small amount of tissue fluid in the intercellular spaces. Oedema occurs when tissue fluid is formed more rapidly than it is reabsorbed. This commonly presents clinically as swelling of the feet and ankles. A finger pressed on the swollen tissues produces an indentation which persists for a while after the finger is removed (pitting oedema).

Tissue fluid is formed by filtration from the blood as it flows through the capillaries. The capillary lining acts as a semi-permeable membrane. It allows water and electrolytes to pass through but holds back the cells and virtually all the proteins. At the arterial end of the

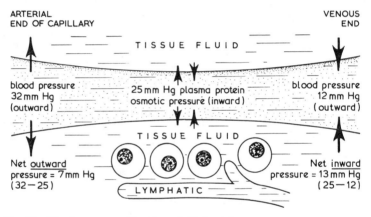

Fig. 4/1   The factors controlling tissue fluid circulation

capillaries the blood pressure is higher than the osmotic pressure of the plasma proteins and so fluid passes through the capillary wall into the tissue spaces. By the time blood reaches the venous end of the capillary the blood pressure has normally fallen sufficiently for the osmotic pressure of the plasma proteins to draw the tissue fluid back into the vessels (Fig. 4/1). Tissue fluid drainage is also provided by reabsorption into the lymphatics. This tissue fluid circulation enables the cells to be provided with food and oxygen and also removes waste products. Oedema occurs when the reabsorption of tissue fluid cannot keep pace with its formation. There are four main causes: (1) increased venous blood pressure; (2) reduced plasma protein osmotic pressure; (3) increased permeability of the capillary wall, allowing more protein to pass through; and (4) obstruction of lymphatic drainage.

Increased venous pressure

GENERAL

The venous pressure is increased in cardiac failure. The causes for this have already been outlined at the beginning of this chapter. The raised pressure at the venous end of the capillary counteracts the osmotic pressure of the plasma proteins, thus impeding the reabsorption of tissue fluid. Oedema results. Its treatment involves the appropriate management of cardiac failure, including the use of drugs such as digoxin and diuretics.

LOCAL

Gravity: An important factor in determining the site of oedema. Even in healthy people oedema of the feet and legs can occur if the limbs remain dependent for too long, as on a long flight. Change of posture can be of great importance in controlling oedema. An example is the prevention of oedema of the lungs in a patient with left ventricular failure by sleeping propped-up in bed against pillows.

Inactivity: The venous return, especially from the legs depends on compression of the veins by muscular activity in conjunction with competent valves in the veins which prevent reverse flow. If the muscles are inactive the venous return is poor, the venous capillary pressure is raised and so oedema occurs. An extreme example is paralytic oedema. A less extreme example is the oedema due to poor muscle tone. In the latter instance the physiotherapist can help to restore the strength and tone of the muscles by teaching graded exercises. If there is also laxity of the fascia the limb is elevated and a firm (but not tight) elastic bandage may be used. In the case of paralytic oedema passive measures to promote venous return will be required. These include: (1) elevation of the affected limb; (2) passive movement of joints; (3) artificial exercise of the paralysed muscles by interrupted direct current (now rare); or (4) light massage which is sometimes effective in dispersing the fluid into regions not affected by the paralysis. Care must be taken neither to increase the paralytic vasodilation nor to bruise or stretch the atonic muscle fibres.

Varicose veins: These greatly impair venous return from the legs. The dilatation of the veins causes valves to become incompetent so that even with muscular activity the venous return is poor. Venous return can be improved by raising the legs or by providing support, e.g. with an elastic stocking. Surgical treatment of varicose veins is often effective.

Pressure: Tight clothing, e.g. garters and elasticated hosiery, may obstruct both veins and lymphatics. Pressure may also be produced by the pregnant uterus, tumours or by inflammation. Treatment is to educate the patient about clothing, and investigate the medical causes of pressure.

VENOUS THROMBOSIS

Factors involved in venous thrombosis have been described already. When thrombosis occurs in the deep veins of the leg it obstructs the venous capillary pressure behind the obstruction so that tissue fluid cannot be reabsorbed and oedema results. The leg becomes swollen and painful (white leg or phlegmasia alba dolens).

In the initial stages the leg has to be rested to avoid provoking embolism and anticoagulant therapy given to prevent extension of the thrombosis. By elevating the leg the severity of the oedema can be reduced. Not until the danger of embolism is past is it possible to introduce more active measures to promote reabsorption of oedema, e.g. alternating muscle contraction and relaxation.

TRAUMATIC OEDEMA

The swelling which occurs after minor trauma is usually mainly due to oedema. The discomfort may be alleviated by simple measures such as cold compresses. Reabsorption of the oedema fluid is often quite rapid. With more severe trauma including fractures much of the swelling is due to haemorrhage (a bruise or haematoma) which takes considerably longer to reabsorb. The swelling associated with extensive burns is usually mainly oedema; it will be considered further under increased capillary permeability.

Reduced plasma proteins

The plasma proteins may be reduced by inadequate intake as in starvation, or excessive loss as in protein-losing nephritis. Management includes raising the level of plasma proteins, particularly albumin, by intravenous infusion, and treatment of the cause.

Increased capillary permeability

The sluggish circulation associated with raised venous pressure tends to cause anoxia of the endothelial cells. The resulting increased capillary permeability is thus a factor in circulatory oedema. Damage to the capillary endothelium is also a factor in the oedema occurring in nephritis, e.g. peri-orbital oedema. Allergy, e.g. wasp sting may also damage the endothelium of capillarics and produce local oedema which can be a hazard to life if the sting involves the tongue. The oedema of nettle-rash is similar and may be controlled by antihistamine drugs, histamine being one of the main substances causing damage to the capillary endothelium in allergic states.

Burns are an important cause of increased capillary permeability. The resulting oedema fluid has a high protein content so that it clots and organises readily. This may result in permanent disfiguration if appropriate steps are not taken to promote its reabsorption. The underlying principles and practical measures have already been described but unfortunately their application may be impeded by the extent of injury caused by the burns. An over-riding consideration is the maintenance of blood pressure by the infusion of plasma or plasma substitute to replace the fluid and protein lost from the circulation into the tissue spaces as oedema fluid.

Obstruction to lymphatic drainage

In addition to the factors already mentioned under raised venous pressure, which obstruct both veins and lymphatics, there may also be selective lymphatic obstruction. This occurs after repeated attacks of lymphadenitis and lymphangitis; following radical surgery, e.g. for carcinoma of the breast; and as a long-term effect of filarial infection (elephantiasis). The oedema produced by lymphatic obstruction is usually of the non-pitting variety due to fibrosis. Unless treated early it rarely responds significantly to physiotherapy.

Important precaution

In all forms of oedema the vessels in the oedematous region should not be encouraged to dilate since this exacerbates the oedema. The application of heat to the affected part is therefore to be avoided.

BIBLIOGRAPHY

See end of Chapter 5, page 65.

Chapter 5

Cellular Pathology

by D. M. D. EVANS, MD, FRCP, FRCPath

The human body is a complex organisation of cells. If cellular function in any part of the body is impaired the whole body may suffer. Cell death is called necrosis. Lesser degrees of cell damage from which recovery is possible are called degenerations.

NECROSIS (Greek, *nekrosis*, a killing)

Necrosis means death of cells while they still form part of a living body. It implies permanent cessation of function of the affected cells. Anything which damages cells can cause necrosis. This includes all the factors described in Chapter 2 as causes of inflammation, especially infection, infarction and injury. One example of necrosis is the pressure sore which may occur over a bony point in a bedridden patient.

Gangrene

When necrosis affects a mass of tissue such as a digit or limb it is called gangrene. An example is the gangrene of a toe resulting from an obstructed blood supply. The toe becomes purplish and may eventually go black. The main cause of the necrosis is lack of oxygen (tissue anoxia). Two types of gangrene are recognised, dry and moist.

DRY GANGRENE

This occurs when there is no oedema or infection. The affected digit or limb mummifies and there is a clear line of demarcation due to an inflammatory reaction in the living tissue next to the dead tissue.

MOIST GANGRENE

This occurs when oedema and infection are present. The affected part undergoes swelling and putrefaction. It is seen in infarction of a loop of bowel as in a strangulated hernia. Moist gangrene may also complicate dry gangrene of a digit or limb if it becomes infected. This is particularly likely to happen if the patient has diabetes mellitus.

ATROPHY (Greek, *a-trophē*, without nourishment)

Atrophy is a wasting away of part of the body. It may simply be a reduction in the size of the affected cells but if severe may also involve a reduction in the number of cells. Atrophy may be generalised or local.

Generalised

This occurs in starvation and in protein deprivation (kwashiorkor). In starvation, body fat and protein are mobilised to provide the essential energy requirements for life. Practically all the soft tissues and organs of the body become reduced in size. In kwashiorkor there is insufficient protein for the growth and replacement of tissues which normally take place. It is characterised by wasting and weakness of the muscles which is in marked contrast to the associated swelling of the abdomen.

Generalised muscular wasting also occurs in patients who are confined to bed for any length of time. Muscular inactivity is the main cause and the legs, being relatively more immobile than the arms, tend to be more severely affected. Appropriate physiotherapy can prevent or greatly reduce such muscular wasting.

Other causes of generalised atrophy include toxaemia due to prolonged infection such as tuberculosis; systemic conditions such as rheumatoid disease; endocrine deficiency such as myxoedema; ulcer or carcinoma of the oesophagus or stomach; and cardiac failure. The latter has been known to cause cachexia (severe wasting) leading to a diagnosis of a carcinoma when in fact there was no evidence of one.

Senile atrophy is of importance to physiotherapists because not only is there atrophy of the soft tissues but also the skeleton undergoes atrophic change known as osteoporosis. Elderly women are particularly susceptible. Their bones may become so fragile that they fracture spontaneously; the neck of the femur is a common site. Vertebrae are also affected; vertebral bodies can collapse causing compression of nerve roots with considerable pain. It is important to recognise this condition. Handling frail elderly women requires special care. The progression of the bone fragility may be controlled by appropriate hormone therapy.

Local

Local atrophy results from a number of conditions which interfere with the nourishment or health of the affected part. They include impaired blood supply, disuse, pressure, impaired nerve supply and primary muscle disease.

IMPAIRED BLOOD SUPPLY

Partial loss of blood supply to a group of muscles causes them to waste and, if severe, results in replacement fibrosis. Its most serious form is seen in the heart as myocardial ischaemia. It can cause progressive cardiac failure or a heart attack which may be mild, severe or fatal. Carefully controlled exercise under medical supervision may improve the blood supply to the affected part by encouraging the development of an alternative blood supply by collateral vessels. This applies to the heart as well as to skeletal muscles.

DISUSE

Disuse atrophy of muscles is one of the most important conditions that a physiotherapist may be called upon to treat or, infinitely better, to prevent. Untreated it can progress with remarkable speed. Active exercises provide the most effective treatment; but in the case of paralysis, passive measures, including electrical stimulation of muscles, may have to be used. This is particularly important where the paralysis is temporary and eventual recovery is anticipated.

PRESSURE

Pressure atrophy is produced when there is prolonged pressure on a group of cells. The more serious condition of pressure sores has already been mentioned under necrosis. Lesser degrees of pressure cause atrophy of the compressed tissues. Constant awareness of the danger, particularly in elderly bedridden patients, is the key to its prevention.

IMPAIRED NERVE SUPPLY

In addition to the disuse atrophy already described, the absence of a nerve supply can, in itself, lead to tissue atrophy. It is minimised by taking steps to restore the nerve supply as quickly as possible. This may require surgical intervention to suture a severed nerve together, so that nerve axons may grow down the tube provided by the dead distal part of the nerve at the rate of about one millimetre a day.

PRIMARY MUSCLE DISEASE

Myopathies (primary muscular dystrophies) are a group of diseases of skeletal muscle, many of which are due to an inherited enzyme deficiency. They are often present in early childhood with progressive muscular weakness. The affected muscles may not appear wasted but instead may appear enlarged, particularly the calf muscles, due to the presence of fat. It is important to recognise myopathies because misapplied physiotherapy may be harmful.

DEGENERATIONS

Cell degeneration results from damage which is insufficient to cause cellular necrosis and from which recovery is possible. Two of the commoner forms of degeneration are cloudy swelling and fatty degeneration.

Cloudy swelling

This occurs in many febrile conditions, e.g. acute specific fevers such as measles and whooping cough. It also occurs in anaemia, anoxia, malnutrition and minor grades of poisoning by chemical substances. If the kidney is examined the cut surface is seen to pout. Under the microscope the kidney cells appear swollen with a hazy, granular cytoplasm; the granules are protein from damaged cell organelles. Normally it is a transient condition and complete recovery is the rule.

Fatty degeneration

This form is evidence of more severe cellular damage. It is a change commonly seen in the liver of alcoholics. The liver is large and pale and the cut surface is greasy. Under the microscope the liver cells are seen to contain fatty droplets. In the early stages the cytoplasm of the cells contains a number of small droplets. These coalesce to form one large droplet which may push the nucleus to one side resembling the appearance of a fat cell in adipose tissue. If the alcoholic gives up drinking the fatty liver cells return to normal. Often, however, the condition is complicated by cirrhosis of the liver, a condition with nodules of liver surrounded by fibrosis, which does not revert to normal. The heart and kidneys may also be affected by fatty degeneration. In Western society alcohol is probably the most important cause of fatty degeneration, the liver being the main target. Other causes include infections, anaemia, anoxia and kwashiorkor. In the latter the liver is greatly enlarged, in marked contrast to the wasting of the limbs.

NEOPLASIA (Greek, *neos plasis*, new moulding)

Neoplasia means tumour formation. It includes both benign and malignant forms of tumour. When a benign tumour grows it may compress surrounding tissue but does not invade it. Malignant tumours (cancers) not only invade surrounding tissues but may also spread to more distant tissues either along lymphatic channels to produce lymph node deposits; or through the bloodstream to produce deposits in liver, lungs, brain or bone; or else across spaces such as the peritoneal cavity to implant at other sites and on other organs in the cavity.

The term intra-epithelial neoplasia has recently been introduced to describe the changes that occur in the lining of the uterine cervix before an invasive growth or cancer develops. There has been some objection to this terminology since many examples of cervical intra-epithelial neoplasia (CIN) do not develop into cancer. However, the term neoplasia includes both benign and malignant tumours and so it is not entirely inappropriate. The recognition that such changes may be detected and treated before the neoplasia becomes invasive is an important step in the control of malignant growth.

Tumours may be divided broadly into two groups, those which arise from epithelial cells and those arising from connective tissue.

Epithelial tumours

BENIGN

The benign epithelial tumours are papillomata and adenomata. A *papilloma* is a protuberant tumour arising from an epithelium such as skin. A *pedunculated* papilloma is one with a stalk. A *sessile* papilloma is one without a stalk which appears to sit on the epithelium from which it is arising.

An *adenoma* is a benign tumour arising from glandular tissue such as salivary gland or gastro-intestinal tract. An adenoma arising in the gut usually protrudes into the lumen as a polyp. Although an adenoma is a benign tumour it is likely to recur if it is not completely removed, particularly one arising from the salivary gland.

MALIGNANT

Malignant epithelial tumours are all called carcinomas (Greek, *karkinos*, a crab). If the epithelium from which they arise is glandular and the tumour is of glandular type the term adenocarcinoma is appropriate, being the malignant version of an adenoma; this more clearly defines the type of carcinoma. Other types of carcinoma are defined by their component cells such as squamous cell carcinoma or oat cell carcinoma. They are also defined by their site of origin, e.g. squamous cell carcinoma of lung. From experience it is known that a squamous cell carcinoma grows more slowly and is more likely to be cured by surgery than an oat cell carcinoma of lung.

Connective tissue tumours

Benign connective tissue tumours are designated by the ending *-oma* following a prefix indicating the tissue involved. Thus fibroma arises from fibrous tissue, lipoma from fatty tissue, myoma from muscle and osteoma from bone. *Malignant* connective tissue tumours are all called sarcomas. One arising from fibrous tissues is a fibrosarcoma, one from bone is an osteosarcoma and from skeletal muscle a rhabdomyosarcoma. Like carcinomas, sarcomas infiltrate surrounding tissues; they have a much greater tendency to spread by the bloodstream, particularly to lungs, than carcinomas which more frequently spread by lymphatics to the related lymph nodes.

Patterns of tumour growth

There is a group of malignant connective tissue tumours arising in the central nervous system called gliomas. They infiltrate the surrounding nervous tissue of brain or spinal cord but do not spread outside the nervous system.

Another important group of tumours arise from the pigment-forming cells (melanocytes) of the skin or eye. The benign form is called a pigmented naevus. The malignant form is a malignant melanoma. Any pigmented tumour which starts to grow, itch or bleed should be looked upon with suspicion and excised with a wide margin of clearance. These tumours can spread both by lymphatics, like carcinomas, and by the bloodstream, like sarcomas. They have an unpleasant reputation for malignancy. Sometimes there is an interval of several years between the initial tumour, thought to have been removed completely, and the appearance of secondary deposits (metastases). Breast cancer can behave similarly.

The tissues of which benign tumours are composed are similar to the normal tissue from which they are formed. Malignant tumours are variable. If they are well differentiated they closely resemble their tissue of origin but if they are poorly differentiated their tissue type may be difficult to recognise. In general, poorly-differentiated cancers invade and spread more rapidly than well-differentiated cancers.

The term benign suggests that such tumours are not harmful. This is not always true. A meningioma is a benign tumour arising from the meninges, the membranes enclosing the brain and spinal cord. As a meningioma grows it compresses the adjacent nervous tissue, causing progressive damage to the brain or spinal cord. If diagnosed early it can be removed before irreparable harm is caused. A benign thyroid adenoma may suddenly enlarge due to haemorrhage into its substance and compress the trachea, causing asphyxia unless prompt action is taken.

Conversely the diagnosis of malignancy does not imply a sentence of death if it is diagnosed at an early stage. Cancer of the cervix can cause death by infiltrating the ureters which run nearby, producing uraemia. Yet many cases of cervical cancer are now being prevented or cured by early recognition and treatment. Other malignant tumours such as Hodgkin's disease of lymph nodes and even the highly malignant Ewing's sarcoma of bone have been successfully treated by surgery, radiotherapy and chemotherapy.

Cancer causation

In recent years there has been considerable advance in the understanding of the nature of cancer. It is now known that there is no single cause, but many causes. A number of cancers are due to factors in the environment – these factors are known as carcinogens and in certain cases are controllable, the most notable factor being tobacco smoke.

There are also intrinsic and extrinsic factors concerned with the development of tumours.

INTRINSIC FACTORS

Genetic factors are involved in the development of certain rare tumours such as retinoblastoma. Polyposis coli and xeroderma pigmentosum are inherited conditions which predispose to the development of cancer. It appears that there is a high incidence of a particular cancer in a family, but at present there is little evidence of a hereditary factor in most of the common tumours. High risk families should be screened regularly.

Malignant disease occurs in all races but the types of cancers vary. Carcinoma of the liver is rare in Europeans but common in Bantus. People whose skins are pale and who do not tan easily are more likely to develop skin cancer if they live in a hot climate where their skin is exposed to the sun.

There is also a different incidence of certain cancers according to the sex of the person. Carcinoma of the bronchus has been more common in the male than the female. At present, the numbers occurring in the female population are increasing which suggests that it was relative to smoking habits rather than the sex of the individual. Age is significant in relation to the development of tumours. The majority develop or become apparent over the age of 50 although some types can occur at any age. Sarcomas tend to develop in younger people and likewise some types of leukaemia develop in children.

EXTRINSIC FACTORS

Substances which are known to contribute to the formation of malignant tumours are known as carcinogens. There are an enormous variety of ways in which these carcinogens work and the production of a tumour depends on their concentration and the length of exposure or the interaction of various substances which are not carcinogenic on their own but are when combined. The following are examples of carcinogens:

1. *Chemical*: Hydrocarbons such as benzpyrene (active compound of soot and tar).
2. *Physical*: Radiant energy – x-rays, alpha, beta and gamma rays.

Alterations in the level of hormone secretions which cause hyperplasia of tissue may lead to the formation of a malignant growth. There is certainly a connection between oestrogen levels and the development of endometrial and breast cancer, and in the male a connection between hormones and prostatic carcinoma.

Chronic inflammation such as ulcerative colitis can increase the risk of a cancer developing.

Over many years researchers have hoped that a virus would be found to be responsible for cancer as it might then be possible to protect people by vaccination. A number of virally-produced tumours have been found in animals although the evidence for similar cases in man is not well proven.

Development and control of early cancer

There is growing evidence that the development of cancer is preceded by cellular changes occurring in a series of steps, usually extending over a long period of time. Some of these steps are reversible. Smoking produces squamous metaplasia in the bronchial epithelium. Giving up smoking before irreversible change has occurred allows the bronchial epithelium to revert towards normality, with a corresponding reduction in the risk of developing cancer.

It appears probable that the uterine cervix undergoes progressively severe dysplasia before it reaches the stage of carcinoma in situ and eventually invasive cancer. As the degree of dysplasia becomes more severe so the chances of invasive cancer developing are found to increase; but even at the stage of carcinoma in situ spontaneous regression can occur. However, since it is not possible to distinguish between cases which will regress and those that will progress the usual procedure is to remove such lesions, e.g. by cone biopsy. Less severe cases are now being treated more conservatively, e.g. evaporation of the abnormal epithelium by laser beam.

Just as the early stages of cervical cancer can be detected by cervical cytology so the early stages of urinary tract cancer can be detected by urine cytology. This is of particular value in detecting early cancer in industrial or laboratory workers who have been exposed to carcinogens such as aromatic amines, perhaps many years previously. Multiple biopsies have shown that atypia, hyperplasia, dysplasia and early cancer may be present simultaneously in the same bladder. Their detection has become even more important now that the early changes can be reversed, e.g. by giving intravesical doxorubicin.

Treatment

Some cancers may be prevented by the removal of the relevant carcinogen from the environment. There is considerable evidence about the effect of carcinogens as seen by the dramatic rise of deaths from lung cancer which relates to the smoking habits of man. Great efforts are being made to reduce smoking by advertising the health risks. Similarly, preventive measures are being taken where carcinogens are involved in work situations. Protective clothing and masks are compulsory for workers in asbestos industries, and similar rules apply in furniture-making factories where wood dust has been found to be a cause of cancers of the nasal sinuses. These known industrial carcinogens are now listed and Acts of Parliament embody preventive measures as well as procedures for compensation should it be proved that a cancer has been caused through working with a specific substance.

It is of note that if two carcinogens are present in the environment their effect may be multiplicative. Thus if smoking increases the lung cancer risk by 10 times and asbestos by five times, the two together increase it by 50 times (Selikoff et al, 1968).

The main forms of treatment are surgical excision, radiotherapy and chemotherapy. Successful treatment depends on early diagnosis so that the malignant tumour may be removed before it spreads. This is not easy as many tumours do not have significant effects on health until they have spread. Early diagnosis is itself dependent on tests such as regular chest radiographs (in situations where there is a known hazard) or through early diagnostic units to which 'well persons' may be referred for preventive check-ups and instruction in, for example, breast self-examination.

PHYSIOTHERAPY

This is largely related to patients undergoing surgery and the treatment will depend on the particular surgical procedure. The physiotherapist may also be concerned with helping a patient who is terminally ill with cancer (see p. 441). This may involve help and advice on maintaining independence for as long as possible – provision of walking aids or helping to remove secretions from the chest to improve respiration.

REFERENCE

Selikoff, I. J., Hammond, E. C. and Churg, J. (1968). Asbestos exposure, smoking and neoplasia. *Journal of the American Medical Association*, **204**, 106.

BIBLIOGRAPHY

Anderson, J. R. (ed) (1980). *Muir's Textbook of Pathology*, 11th edition. Edward Arnold (Publishers) Limited, London.

Robbins, S. L., Angell, M. and Kurmer, V. (1981). *Basic Pathology*, 3rd edition. Holt-Saunders, Eastbourne.

Spector, W. G. (1980). *An Introduction to General Pathology*, 2nd edition. Churchill Livingstone, Edinburgh.

Thomson, A. D. and Cotton, R. E. (1982). *Lecture Notes on Pathology*, 3rd edition. Blackwell Scientific Publications Limited, Oxford.

Tiffany, Robert (ed) (1978). *Oncology for Nurses and Health Care Professionals*. Volume 1, *Pathology, Diagnosis and Treatment*. George Allen and Unwin, London.

Walters, J. B. and Israel, M. S. (1979). *General Pathology*, 5th edition. Churchill Livingstone, Edinburgh.

Chapter 6

Drugs

by D. B. McHUTCHISON, BPharm, MPS

A drug may be broadly defined as a substance which modifies the activity of living tissues. The study of this activity in relation to the diagnosis, treatment or prevention of disease is termed *pharmacology*, while the application of the principles of pharmacology in clinical practice is known as *therapeutics*. A very large number of substances known to exert a pharmacological action have been studied, but only a small number of these are suitable for therapeutic use.

ADMINISTRATION AND ABSORPTION

In order to exert its therapeutic action a drug must first be absorbed by the body and transported to the tissues where its activity is required. Administration of drugs may be by one or more of the following routes.

Gastro-intestinal tract

The majority of drugs are absorbed into the bloodstream from the gastro-intestinal tract, and may be given as a solution, suspension or solid dose form, i.e. tablet or capsule. The rate at which a drug is absorbed after oral administration is dependent on a complex set of factors such as the chemical nature of the drug, the rate at which it dissolves, the pharmaceutical form used, and the contents of the gut at the time the dose is given. When more than one drug is given at the same time their rates of absorption may be further modified. Some preparations are designed specifically to delay absorption, to prevent gastric disturbance, or to prevent chemical change during passage through the gut. Enteric-coated tablets pass through the stomach unchanged and release their active ingredients in the small intestine. Slow-acting, or sustained-release, tablets or capsules prolong absorption by delaying the release of the drug from an insoluble matrix during passage through the gut. This allows a single dose to exert action for much longer, perhaps all day or all night.

A small number of drugs are absorbed from the buccal cavity, and in these cases absorption is often very rapid. This effect is exploited by the use of sub-lingual tablets which dissolve quickly under the tongue, for example glyceryl trinitrate used for the rapid relief of anginal pain.

Some drugs are also absorbed from the rectum when given as suppositories or as a retention enema. Aspirin, indomethacin and aminophylline are examples of drugs which may be given successfully by this route. (Suppositories are also widely used where purely local action on the rectum is required.)

The lungs

Administration via the lungs is a long-established practice. Traditionally inhalations were used, but modern pharmaceutical techniques have refined this and aerosol therapy is now common, particularly in the treatment of asthma. Solutions may be given by nebuliser, or dry powders by metered pressurised aerosols which can deliver exact doses of highly active drugs such as salbutamol.

By injection

The use of drugs by injection is widespread in hospital practice and, though generally a more expensive therapy, has many advantages over the oral route. The possibility of erratic absorption or chemical breakdown in the gut is avoided; this is particularly important in the use of antibiotics to treat severe infections. The intravenous (IV) route ensures total absorption and achieves desired tissue levels rapidly, and can be used even with drugs which would cause necrosis if concentrated in muscle tissue, e.g. some cytotoxic agents. Intramuscular (IM) and subcutaneous (SC) routes also ensure total absorption, but distribution to the tissues is slower than the IV route. Depot injections can be given by the IM route, with the drug in an oily solution or as a suspension, allowing slow absorption from the injection site over a period of days or even weeks. Special techniques of injection such as intrathecal (IT) into the cerebrospinal fluid, and intra-articular (IA) into joints allow adequate doses to be delivered directly to the tissues where the action is required.

Topically

In a suitable formulation many drugs will be absorbed through the skin and the mucous membranes. This method of administration is normally used where drug action is desired at the site of application, for example creams and ointments to treat skin conditions, or treatment of the eye with drops or ointment.

DISTRIBUTION

As a general principle, drugs, once they are absorbed into the bloodstream, will be distributed to all tissues in the body; the object of therapeutics is to give a dose such that a sufficient concentration of the drug is present in the particular tissue where action is required. Several factors control the rate at which this distribution takes place, and thus the time needed to achieve adequate tissue levels. Blood flow varies in different parts of the body, and in disease may change significantly in specific tissues, for example the liver or kidneys. When in the bloodstream a drug may exist freely in solution or be chemically bound to plasma proteins, and the stronger the protein binding the slower the rate of distribution. Different drugs may bind to different proteins, but complications can occur when two drugs given together bind to the same protein. One will usually be bound preferentially and thus the other will be distributed more rapidly, achieve higher than expected tissue levels and hence exert a greater therapeutic effect than anticipated. For example, the anticoagulant warfarin is more active in the presence of aspirin because the latter displaces the warfarin from its binding sites. Transfer through membranes occurs in the capillaries, when the drug passes into the interstitial fluid, and at the cell wall where the drug diffuses from the interstitial fluid into the cell itself. The rate at which this transfer takes place may depend on the chemical nature of the drug, physical properties such as the size of the molecule (its molecular weight) and its degree of protein binding.

METABOLISM AND EXCRETION

During the course of their distribution many drugs will undergo biochemical changes, i.e. will be metabolised. These changes may reduce or even eliminate the pharmacological activity of the drug by producing inactive metabolites, or may convert the administered drug into pharmacologically active compounds which exert the actual therapeutic effect. A few of these changes may occur in the gut during absorption and in some cases in particular organs such as the kidney, but the vast majority of metabolic changes take place in the liver.

Breakdown of the drug may be by reduction, oxidation or hydrolysis in the first phase of metabolism. In the second phase the drug, or the phase one breakdown product, may combine (be conjugated) with other molecules such as glucuronic acid or amino acids such as glycine.

Reference will often be seen to *hepatic first-pass metabolism*, a factor of importance in deciding the best route of administration. When absorbed from the gut drugs enter the hepatic portal system and thus all the dose goes through the liver. If the drug is rapidly metabolised by the liver the amount reaching the systemic circulation may be significantly reduced. This is known as the first-pass effect. In such cases it is often desirable to give the drug by injection, which allows passage around the systemic circulation before entering the liver.

When two or more drugs are given at the same time interactions may result from their effect on liver enzymes. Some drugs are known to enhance the activity of liver enzymes, either by stimulating their production or delaying their breakdown. If the affected enzyme is involved in the metabolism of a second drug being used at the same time the rate of metabolism of the latter drug may be increased and its therapeutic effect therefore reduced. For example, barbiturates inhibit the action of the anticoagulant warfarin and phenytoin reduces the efficacy of oral contraceptives by this mechanism.

After metabolism, and having exerted their pharmacological action, drugs and their metabolites will be eliminated from the body. The most important route of excretion is via the kidney. As with their absorption, the mechanism and the rate at which drugs and their metabolites are excreted by the kidneys is dependent on their chemical composition, molecular weight, and degree of protein binding. Some drugs are excreted by this pathway unchanged and this may be of considerable importance if the desired site of action is in fact the kidney itself, for example, antibiotics used to treat urinary tract infections. Some drugs are excreted by the liver, usually as metabolites which are passed into the bile and thus to the small intestine. Excretion is then via the faeces, though in some cases the drug or metabolites may be reabsorbed and return to the liver again. This may have the effect of prolonging the activity of the drug since some will continue to pass around the entero-hepatic circulation until all has been metabolised. Examples of drugs which undergo entero-hepatic re-cycling are phenytoin and rifampicin.

In a few cases some drugs may be excreted by other routes such as in the sweat, via the lungs if the drug is a gas, e.g. anaesthetics, or in breast milk. The latter is particularly important in breast-feeding mothers when the baby could receive doses of unwanted drugs.

BIO-AVAILABILITY AND PHARMACOKINETICS

These terms will often be seen in information on drug activity. They are concerned with the mathematical considerations of a drug's absorption; the rate at which it becomes available, the length of time the action is maintained, the rate at which the action falls off, and finally how rapidly the excretion occurs. These studies can therefore lay down broad guidelines on how patients are likely to respond to a particular drug. It must always be remembered however that no two human bodies are the same and that the response to a particular drug in a particular dose will always vary slightly from one patient to another. Where factors are known to exist which will affect the rate of metabolism or excretion, e.g. liver or kidney disease, pharmacokinetic studies will provide the information to adjust dose regimes suitably for particular patients.

MECHANISM OF ACTION AND DRUG RECEPTORS

In the body the functions of the tissues and organs are controlled by a variety of substances produced in the body itself and usually known as messengers or endogenous regulators. Some examples are acetylcholine, histamine, insulin and the catecholamines, e.g. noradrenaline. Many drugs act in a similar way to these endogenous substances. The basic concept is that once the drug or messenger has reached its site of action it will react in some way with a group of molecules forming a receptor site in the tissue. Drugs or messengers which by their action at the receptor sites stimulate the activity of the tissues are referred to as agonists, while those which inhibit activity are known as antagonists or blockers.

Many types of receptor are now recognised and an important consideration is that the same type of receptor may influence different tissues in different ways; receptors are also now divided into sub-types. Histamine receptors are divided into types H_1 and H_2. At H_1 receptors histamine causes constriction of smooth muscle, e.g. in the bronchioles, tissue oedema, inflammation, and pain. These effects are antagonised by H_1-receptor blocker drugs, usually known as antihistamines. At H_2 receptors histamine causes an increase in gastric acid secretion, and this effect is not controlled at all by antihistamines, but is antagonised by the recently introduced H_2-receptor antagonists such as cimetidine or ranitidine.

Adrenergic receptors (those at which the catecholamines act) are divided into α and β sub-types. α-receptor stimulation causes, for example, inhibition of intestinal or bladder movements, vasoconstriction of the arterioles and dilation of the pupils. Stimulation of β_1 receptors increases the rate and force of heart movements, while β_2-receptor stimulation leads to decreased bronchial secretions, relaxation of bronchial muscle and dilation of the coronary and peripheral arterioles.

Much drug research is now aimed at producing substances in which parts of the molecule are structurally similar to parts of the molecule of known endogenous regulators. The hope is that such substances will be pharmacologically active in either mimicking or inhibiting the action of the natural regulator. The term *structure activity relationship* is often used in this context.

If a drug acts at receptors that are common to many tissues, or on more than one sub-type of receptor, it may produce undesirable side-effects as well as effects of therapeutic benefit. The ideal therefore is to use a drug which is selective and will act only at receptors of a specific sub-type or in a specific tissue. Selectivity can sometimes be improved by chemical modification of an existing drug or by pharmaceutical formulation.

While most drugs are thought to act at tissue receptor sites a few are known which act by comparatively simple chemical or physical means. For example, chelating agents used to treat heavy metal poisoning, such as by lead, combine chemically with the poison allowing it to be excreted. Mannitol, a carbohydrate used to reduce intracranial pressure or to promote diuresis, acts physically by changing the osmolarity of body fluids.

ADVERSE REACTIONS AND INTERACTIONS

Any substance used to interfere with a biological process in a desirable way is also likely to produce unwanted effects as well, usually referred to as side-effects or adverse reactions. In drug treatment it is usually necessary to consider a balance of advantage. In treating life-threatening conditions a quite high incidence of side-effects may be accepted. These effects may be many and varied, some minor and a nuisance, such as skin rash or gastric disturbance, others more serious and even potentially fatal, such as liver damage or suppression of the bone marrow. New drugs in particular are closely monitored to attempt to detect all adverse effects, though where the incidence is low it may be many years before the effect is recognised. A recent example was the β-blocker practolol, found after some years' use to cause eye and intestinal damage in a very small number of patients.

DRUG GROUPS

Drugs are usually considered in groups relating to their effect on a particular organ or body system. It is not possible here to more than outline some groups which will be of particular relevance to the physiotherapist's practice.

DRUGS ACTING ON THE RESPIRATORY SYSTEM

Mucolytics

These are agents which reduce the viscosity of sputum and therefore make expectoration easier. Traditionally, inhalations were used, such as menthol and eucalyptus or compound benzoin tincture in hot water. The volatile ingredients help to clear the nasal passages, while the inhaled steam reduces the viscosity of the sputum, and expectoration can be facilitated by postural drainage. Drugs have been developed which attempt to achieve a similar effect when administered by nebuliser, and are thought to act by breaking down sputum proteins. The two commonly used are acetylcysteine (Airbron) and tyloxapol (Alevaire).

Carbocisteine (Mucodyne) and bromhexine (Bisolvon) are examples of mucolytics which act systemically and are thought to alter the composition and increase the flow of bronchial secretions. They may be administered as tablets or syrup, and bromhexine may also be given by IM or IV injection.

Antitussives

Many cough medicines are prescribed and sold, some of which may increase bronchial secretions but there is no good evidence that any will stimulate the cough centre to increase expectoration. Cough suppressants are drugs used for the opposite effect, that is to depress the cough centre in the brain and relieve dry unproductive coughs which may be painful and distressing. Examples are codeine, diamorphine and pholcodine, all administered as linctus. Such preparations are not recommended in patients where expectoration is necessary, as retention of sputum and inhibition of ventilation may result.

Respiratory stimulants

Where inhibition of respiration occurs in patients with chronic obstructive airway disease, respiratory stimulants may be used as an adjunct to physiotherapy. Such drugs are usually given by IV injection or infusion and their use requires careful medical supervision. They are often used for short-term treatment in association with oxygen therapy. Examples are nikethamide and doxapram (Dopram) both of which act on the respiratory centre in the brain to increase the rate and depth of respiration.

Drugs in asthma

In an asthma attack the bronchi contain thickened mucus, their walls are oedematous and the bronchial muscle is constricted. Asthma may be inherent or intrinsic and treatable with corticosteroids; or triggered by some outside stimulus (antigen) and known as extrinsic asthma, and treatable, for example, with β_2 stimulants.

CORTICOSTEROIDS

The anti-inflammatory glucocorticosteroids are used in asthma for their action of reduction of capillary permeability, bronchial congestion and oedema. In severe cases they may be given by injection, for example as hydrocortisone, or as short courses of oral treatment, for example as prednisone tablets. When given orally steroids may exert other effects, some undesirable; as an alternative, inhalation therapy has been developed. Beclomethasone (Becotide) and betamethasone (Bextasol) are examples of potent steroids administered either from pressure-metered aerosols or powder inhalers. By this technique a small controlled dose is given, sufficient only to act in the lung and avoid undesirable systemic effects. In many cases sufficient control can be achieved to avoid the use of oral steroids entirely.

BRONCHODILATORS

The bronchodilator drugs play the major role in the treatment of asthma, bronchitis and other diseases causing bronchospasm. Drugs once widely used, and still in limited use today, such as adrenaline, isoprenaline or ephedrine are non-specific, having both α- and β-agonist properties. Thus while they do produce bronchodilation they also give rise to unwanted side-effects by their action on the heart, gastro-intestinal tract and bladder. The drugs now most widely used are the more selective β_2 stimulants; fenoterol (Berotec), isoetharine (Numotac), reproterol (Bronchodil), rimiterol

(Pulmadil), salbutamol (Ventolin), and terbutaline (Bricanyl). These are available in a variety of formulations for administration orally as tablets or syrup, by injection, by metered aerosol, powder inhaler or by nebuliser.

Salbutamol is probably the most widely used. Given by aerosol or powder inhaler it produces prompt bronchodilation, relieves bronchospasm and reduces bronchial secretions. It may also be given orally or by injection, but the inhaled route is considered to have the advantage of rarely producing side-effects, and the bronchodilation is more prolonged. The side-effects of oral or injected doses result from the limited β_1-agonist activity that salbutamol also exhibits. Tachycardia and tremor are the most noted, though night cramps and increased insulin and free fatty acid levels have been observed also. The other drugs listed above have broadly similar effects to salbutamol, though with some variation in their rates of absorption and duration of action. Though some would hold that to have several different drugs of similar type available is unnecessary it can often help the prescribing physician, as if one becomes ineffective another in the group may enable the patient's treatment to continue.

An alternative treatment in some forms of asthma is a prophylactic one using sodium cromoglycate (Intal). This acts by preventing the release of histamine, and other substances which cause bronchospasm, from sensitised cell membranes. Treatment, which is by aerosol, needs to be regular since the drug is of no value in treating an attack. A newer drug ketotifen (Zaditen) has similar effects and is active orally, given as tablets or capsules.

Respirator solutions: In hospital, and occasionally in the home, respirator solutions of salbutamol or terbutaline are often used in the treatment of status asthmaticus, severe bronchospasm resulting from acute episodes of bronchial asthma and bronchitis, or in bronchial infections. The undiluted solutions, 2ml of salbutamol 5mg/ml, or 1ml of terbutaline 10mg/ml, may be given up to four times daily in oxygen-enriched air over a period of about three minutes. A suitable intermittent positive pressure ventilator such as the Bird respirator is used. Alternatively these solutions may be administered continuously with equipment such as the De Vilbiss or Wright's nebuliser and the Ventimask. In these cases the solutions are diluted with sterile water or saline to a concentration of 100 micrograms per ml and are given at the rate of 1 to 2mg per hour. To avoid contamination and infection such solutions in nebulisers should be replaced with fresh material at least every 24 hours. It is important to remember that these drugs are Prescription Only Medicines (see p. 79) and may therefore *only* be administered by the physiotherapist *when prescribed by a physician*. On completion of the treatment the details, such as dose and time given, must be recorded by the physiotherapist in the appropriate section of the patient's treatment card or case notes.

DRUGS IN RHEUMATIC DISEASE

Patients suffering from the rheumatic diseases will form a significant portion of the physiotherapist's workload. Drugs are used extensively, but none have to date effected a cure. They may be considered in two groups; those affecting the course of the disease, and those relieving the symptoms of pain and inflammation.

The actions of those drugs affecting the course of the rheumatic diseases are not well understood. Those used are penicillamine, sodium aurothiomalate (a gold salt), chloroquine, hydroxychloroquine and the immunosuppressant azathioprine. They are effective only when the disease is active and their benefits may take many months to appear. Side-effects are common and may be severe, requiring withdrawal of the treatment. All are given orally, as tablets, except the gold salt which can only be given by IM injection. Close medical supervision, blood and urine tests are all necessary when therapy is undertaken with any of these agents.

Non-steroidal anti-inflammatory agents are widely used to relieve the symptoms of pain and inflammation, but these drugs have no effect on the course of the disease.

The relief of pain is probably the most widely used therapy. In theory it can be achieved in one of several ways, for example by suppressing the perception of pain in the brain or by overcoming the stimulus at the actual site of pain. An important modifying factor is the significant emotional content and individual variation in the perception of pain. Possibly for this latter reason the choice of analgesic/anti-inflammatory drug for a particular patient can often be a matter of trial and error. It is therefore fortunate that a wide range of such drugs are at the physician's disposal. Most of these drugs are administered by mouth as tablets, capsules or syrup and a few are also available as suppositories which can be a useful adjuvant to treatment in that they help to reduce morning stiffness by their long action.

Non-steroidal anti-inflammatory agents are all considered to exert their action at the site of pain production. To a greater or lesser degree they all inhibit the production in the tissues of prostaglandins, the endogenous regulators responsible for the production of fever, pain and oedema in inflammatory disease. In addition to relieving pain and inflammation some of these drugs, notably aspirin and its derivatives, also exert a significant antipyretic action. This is also thought to result from suppression of prostaglandin release, in this case in the temperature regulating centre in the brain. Table 1 lists those drugs currently in use in the United Kingdom.

TABLE I: NON-STEROIDAL ANTI-INFLAMMATORY AGENTS

Approved name	Daily oral dose range in adults	Proprietary name
aspirin	up to 8g	
azapropazone	1.2g	Rheumox
benorylate	4 to 8g	Benoral
choline magnesium trisilicate	1 to 1.5g	Trilisate
diclofenac	50 to 150mg	Voltarol
diflunisal	500mg to 1g	Dolobid
fenbufen	600 to 900mg	Lederfen
fenclofenac	600mg to 1.2g	Flenac
fenoprofen	900mg to 3g	Fenopron
feprazone	200 to 600mg	Methrazone
flufenamic acid	400 to 600mg	Meralen
flurbiprofen	150 to 300mg	Froben
ibuprofen	800mg to 2.4g	Brufen : Ebufac
indomethacin	50 to 200mg	Indocid : Imbrilon
ketoprofen	100 to 200mg	Alrheumat : Orudis
mefenamic acid	1.5g	Ponstan
naproxen	500mg to 1g	Naprosyn
oxyphenbutazone	200 to 600mg	Tandacote : Tanderil
phenylbutazone	200 to 600mg	Butacote : Butazolidin
piroxicam	20 to 40mg	Feldene
salsalate	1.5 to 4g	Disalcid
sodium salicylate	up to 10g	Entrosalyl
sulindac	200 to 400mg	Clinoril
tolmetin	600mg to 1.8g	Tolectin

NOTE: The daily dose is normally divided into two or four doses, and is often best taken with or after food to avoid gastric upset

Corticosteroids have a significant part to play in the treatment of rheumatic disease. They have a powerful anti-inflammatory action, but are only used systemically where the non-steroidal agents have been unsuccessful. Prednisolone in tablet form is usually used, at the lowest dose which will control the symptoms. If treatment is prolonged, tolerance may lead to the need to increase the dose with the consequent danger of side-effects. Steroids exert their anti-inflammatory action locally if given by intra-articular injection, when relief of pain and improved joint movement can be quite spectacular. They act by reducing fluid production and cellular exudates in the joint. To maintain the effect repeated injections are necessary every few weeks, but this is approached with caution as joint damage can ultimately result. Aseptic technique is essential with intra-articular injections, since infection introduced into a joint will increase the inflammatory process and may prove very difficult to treat. Table 2 lists those steroids available as intra-articular injections in the United Kingdom.

TABLE II: CORTICOSTEROIDS FOR INTRA-ARTICULAR INJECTION

Approved name	Dose range	Proprietary name
dexamethasone sodium phosphate	0.8 to 4mg	Decadron
hydrocortisone acetate	5 to 50mg	Hydrocortistab
methylprednisolone acetate	4 to 80mg	Depo Medrone
prednisolone acetate	5 to 25mg	Deltastab
prednisolone sodium phosphate	1.6 to 24mg	Codelsol
prednisolone pivalate	10 to 50 mg	Ultracortenol
triamcinolone acetonide	2.5 to 40mg	Kenalog
triamcinolone hexacetonide	2 to 30mg	Lederspan

NOTE: The dose required depends primarily on the size of the joint involved

Although not often used in rheumatic disease the rubifacients or counter-irritants are popular for symptomatic relief of musculo-skeletal pain, for example in sports injuries. They act by producing irritation of the skin itself and this has the effect of relieving pain deeper in the tissues. Poultices such as kaolin, and liniments or ointments containing methyl salicylate are widely used.

CANCER CHEMOTHERAPY

The drug treatment of cancers involves the use of substances which will interfere with cell multiplication or will stop the synthesis of DNA or RNA. Unfortunately these agents, usually known as cytotoxic drugs, cannot be confined in their actions to the malignant tissues and will therefore adversely affect the normal cells of the body as well. This is particularly a problem in tissues where the cells are normally dividing rapidly, such as the ovaries, testes, gut or bone marrow.

Different groups of these drugs act at different points in the dividing cell cycle and it is common therapeutic practice to use several agents in a regime designed to attack the malignant cells at several points at the same time. The cytotoxic agents currently in use may be divided into the following groups.

Antimetabolites. These act by interfering with the synthesis of essential cell constituents such as folic acid and pyrimidine. Examples of such drugs include methotrexate and cytarabine.

Alkylating agents. These interfere with the synthesis of DNA and include such drugs as busulphan, cyclophosphamide and melphalan.

Cytotoxic antibiotics. Antibiotics are substances produced by micro-organisms which interfere in some way with the growth of other cells. The majority in therapeutic use act against bacterial cells and are therefore used to treat infections. A small number however act against human tissue cells by inhibiting formation of nucleic acids and proteins, for example actinomycin, bleomycin and doxorubicin.

Vinca alkaloids. These alkaloids are extracted from the periwinkle plant and are thought to act by interfering with the synthesis of micro-tubular protein, thus preventing cell division. Three drugs have been isolated, vincristine, vinblastine and vindesine. They are widely used and exhibit a particular side-effect which is of significance to the physiotherapist, in that they give rise to peripheral neuropathy. This probably arises from their mode of action in that they also interfere with micro-tubular protein in nerve tissue. The incidence of neuropathy is usually dose related, and patients treated for lymphoma are generally much more susceptible than others. The symptoms may present in various forms including autonomic, e.g. constipation; motor, e.g. muscle weakness and loss of tendon reflexes; or sensory, e.g. jaw pain and paraesthesia. The symptoms normally disappear on withdrawal of the drug, and of the three agents vincristine is the most often implicated.

In addition to the main groups there are several other agents with varying uses and modes of action. A few examples are procarbazine used in Hodgkin's disease; tamoxifen, an anti-oestrogen used in breast cancer; and cis-platin used in testicular and ovarian cancers. The latter drug is notable as the first platinum salt used therapeutically, and like the vinca alkaloids may also give rise to peripheral neuropathy.

PHOTOSENSITISERS

Some drugs have the effect of increasing the sensitivity of the skin to ultraviolet light. This reaction may be an unwanted side-effect but in some cases can be of therapeutic use.

Methoxypsoralen is an example of a drug used for its photosensitiser effect. It may be given orally as tablets or capsules or applied topically as a lotion, and subsequent exposure to ultraviolet light or sunlight results in increased melanin formation in the skin. It has therefore been used to treat idiopathic vitiligo. In addition exposure to long-wavelength ultraviolet light following topical or oral methoxypsoralen results in an inflammatory phototoxic reaction in the skin and this effect is utilised in the treatment of resistant psoriasis.

LEGAL ASPECTS

In the United Kingdom all drugs for human use are controlled at all stages of their development, import, manufacture or use by the Medicines Act 1968. Drugs may only be licensed for use after they have satisfied stringent safety requirements; they must be manufactured in approved premises by approved procedures; and they may only be promoted for treatment of conditions for which successful clinical trials have been completed.

For supply to the patient the Act divides medicines into three categories:

General Sales List. A very small group of materials which may be sold by any retailer, e.g. small packs of analgesics such as aspirin or paracetamol.

Pharmacy Only Medicines. These are drugs which may be sold without prescription, but only from a registered pharmacy.

Prescription Only Medicines. These are drugs which may be sold or supplied only against a prescription from a medical or dental practitioner. The majority of drugs fall into this category. In hospital practice this differentiation does not normally apply, as all drugs are administered only in accordance with a prescription.

In addition more stringent controls are applied to the small group of drugs which are liable to cause addiction, for example the amphetamines and narcotic analgesics such as morphine and diamorphine (heroin). These controls are contained in the Misuse of Drugs Act 1972.

FURTHER INFORMATION

Succinct information on the majority of drugs in current use in the United Kingdom will be found in the British National Formulary (BNF) which is now published every six months.

The pharmacies in most large hospitals have a drug information section capable of answering the majority of queries for information on drugs which may arise in day to day practice. Links are also established with regional and national centres where more detailed information is needed.

BIBLIOGRAPHY

Hopkins, S. J. (1983). *Drugs and Pharmacology for Nurses*, 8th edition. Churchill Livingstone, Edinburgh.

Hopkins, S. J. (1983). *Principal Drugs: An Alphabetical Guide to Modern Therapeutic Agents*, 7th edition. Faber and Faber, London.

Martindale: The Extra Pharmacopoeia, 28th edition. (1982). The Pharmaceutical Press, London.

Wilkes, E. (ed) (1982). *Long-Term Prescribing: Drug Management of Chronic Disease and Other Problems*. Faber and Faber, London.

British National Formulary is published six-monthly by the British Medical Association and the Pharmaceutical Society of Great Britain. Available through book shops. All pharmacy departments receive a supply to be distributed free to specific personnel in the hospital.

MIMS (Monthly Index of Medical Specialities). Only lists proprietary products, and is distributed free to GPs, pharmacy departments and selected medical personnel. It may be supplied on subscription to others who write. Published monthly by MIMS, Haymarket Publishing, 38/42 Hampton Road, Teddington TW11 0JE.

Chapter 7

Cardiac Arrest and Resuscitation

by J. R. PEPPER, MChir, FRCS

CARDIAC ARREST

This may be defined as a sudden cessation of a functional circulation. It is an emergency which demands prompt recognition. The absence of carotid or femoral pulses is sufficient. There is no need to listen for the heart beat or look for dilated pupils.

Aetiology

The heart arrests either in asystole or in ventricular fibrillation. Asystole is due usually to hypoxia, for whatever reason, or complete heart block. Ventricular fibrillation is commonly the result of an electrolyte imbalance, e.g. hypokalaemia.

The common causes of cardiac arrest are:

1. Massive pulmonary embolus which obstructs the circulation and produces myocardial hypoxia.
2. Myocardial infarction which can lead to sudden death probably due to ventricular tachycardia and fibrillation.
3. Pericardial tamponade which restricts filling of the heart.
4. Tension pneumothorax which produces an acute shift of the mediastinum compressing the opposite lung and the heart.
5. Increased vagal tone which can occur during induction of general anaesthesia and may lead to a cardiac arrest when associated with hypoxia and acidosis.

Less common causes include anaphylactic reactions to drugs and air embolism.

RESUSCITATION

Unless the circulation can be rapidly restored, irreversible brain damage will occur within three (3) minutes. The priority therefore is to restore the circulation and ventilate the lungs.

If there is no board under the mattress the patient is transferred to the floor so that effective cardiac massage can be given. External cardiac massage in adults is applied by placing one hand over the other at the lower end of the sternum. The arms should be held straight as this is less tiring for the operator who may have to continue massage for several minutes before further help is available. A rate of massage of 60 per minute is the aim in adults; 80 to 90 per minute in children. In infants and small children the heart lies higher in the thorax so that the massaging hands should be placed over the mid-sternum. Care should be taken to avoid sudden compression of the abdomen as this may cause the liver to rupture.

Initially ventilation is achieved by mouth-to-mouth breathing or a face mask and Ambubag, taking care to maintain an airway. The patient should be intubated with an endotracheal tube swiftly and skilfully; until such skill is available it is safer to continue ventilation by face mask, keeping a close watch on the airway.

While this is going on, medical help will have arrived and an intravenous line and ECG monitor will be set up. If the heart rhythm is ventricular fibrillation, DC counter-shock is given starting at 100 Joules (in adults) to restore sinus rhythm. If asystole is present, 1 in 10 000 adrenaline is injected either directly into the right ventricle through the chest wall or into a central venous line to induce ventricular fibrillation which can then be treated by DC shock. Sodium bicarbonate is given to correct the acidosis which invariably develops following a cardiac arrest.

The patient who has recently undergone open heart surgery is in a special situation. If after giving adrenaline and continuous external massage for one minute there is no improvement the chest is re-opened via the recent wound. There are many recorded instances of patients surviving this procedure and leaving hospital in good health.

Once a cardiac output has been restored as shown by the return of the carotid or femoral pulses a search is made for the cause of the arrest and appropriate action taken. An anti-inflammatory steroid, dexamethasone, is generally given as prophylaxis against the development of cerebral oedema. However, the patient may slide into a state of low cardiac output which is insufficient to meet the needs of the vital organs; brain, kidneys and heart.

Low cardiac output

When such a state exists a vicious cycle develops (Fig. 7/1).

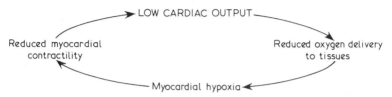

Fig. 7/1   The vicious cycle resulting from a low cardiac output

If this cycle is allowed to continue, cardiac arrest will inevitably recur. On an intensive care unit such a state should be recognised early from the following features:

1. Poor urine output; less than 30ml per hour in an adult.
2. Cool peripheries and if the core and toe temperatures are being measured there will be an increase in the core:toe gradient.
3. Mental confusion deteriorating eventually to unconsciousness.
4. An increasing tendency to acidosis.

Although the causes of low cardiac output are many, the basis of treatment is the same. Initially the filling pressure of the heart is examined by measuring the central venous pressure (right atrial pressure). In some cases it is useful to measure the left atrial pressure as well. Due to the relationship between cardiac output and the filling pressure of the heart as described in Starling's law of the heart, there is a critical range for optimal function of the heart. If the right atrial pressure is below this range which is $+5$ to $+15$mmHg, blood, plasma or plasma expanders are given to raise the pressure. By raising the right atrial pressure to the upper limit of this range the heart is placed in the optimal physiological situation. In many instances this simple measure will suffice to restore a normal circulation.

If this is not enough, attention is directed to the state of myocardial contractility. This can be altered by the administration of synthetic catecholamines of which the commonest are isoprenaline and adrenaline. Recently dopamine has come into regular use because of its special beneficial effect on the kidneys. Other drugs in use include salbutamol and noradrenaline. A further drug has appeared recently called dobutamine. All these drugs increase the rate and force of contraction of the myocardium but in practice it is their effect on heart rate which is the limiting factor.

If after applying these measures the patient has not improved an attempt may be made to reduce the peripheral resistance. The aim of this treatment is to reduce the minimum pressure which the left ventricle has to generate in order to open the aortic valve; and thus to reduce the work done by the left ventricle. This is achieved by the administration of peripheral vasodilator drugs which reduce the sympathetic vasoconstrictor drive to arterioles. Hence, whole new vascular beds which were closed are opened up and the capacity of the circulation increases. For this reason the central venous pressure will fall and in order to maintain the heart at its optimal filling pressure, several units of blood or plasma will need to be given. This type of treatment is potentially lethal unless the central venous pressure is maintained. Examples of the drugs which are used include chlorpromazine (Largactil), phentolamine (Rogitine), nitroprusside (Nipride).

In addition the patient may be placed on intermittent positive pressure ventilation (IPPV), to reduce oxygen requirements by taking over the work of the respiratory muscles and to gain better control of the arterial oxygen tension. The acid base balance is also closely maintained and corrected when necessary.

Chapter 8

An Introduction to General Surgical Care

by P. A. DOWNIE, FCSP

THE TEAM CONCEPT

The total care necessary for patients who undergo any form of surgery involves many people – nowadays called the team. Not everyone will be required for each patient but all are available as and when necessary. The physiotherapist is included in this team and she should be aware of the skills of the others and how they may be utilised to the best advantage of the patient and his family. She must realise that she herself may only have a minor part to play and in many instances no part at all. Some types of surgery will require that the physiotherapist is a very important team member, e.g. cardiothoracic and orthopaedic surgery, while other types of surgery, e.g. ear, nose and throat will only require limited physiotherapy. However much she is involved or not in the care of the patient the physiotherapist must always be prepared to co-operate with other members – for example she will need to discuss with the speech therapist what particular breathing exercises are most helpful for a patient who undergoes laryngectomy and subsequently requires to be taught oesophageal speech. Equally she will combine with the occupational therapist to ensure that patients can return home and that the necessary equipment and aids are provided.

In hospital the team will include the following:

1. The medical staff, e.g. the anaesthetist, the surgeon and his registrar and houseman, and in cases of malignant disease the radiotherapist and medical oncologist.
2. The nursing staff including nurse specialists such as stoma therapist, mastectomy liaison nurse and others.
3. The occupational therapist, speech therapist, remedial gymnast, physiotherapist, and radiographer.
4. The social worker; the disablement resettlement officer (DRO).

5. The prosthetist will be a vital member of the team where mutilating surgery has been necessary, e.g. amputation of a limb or extensive head and face surgery.
6. The dietician.
7. Other ancillary staff including porters and cleaners.

There should also be links with the community team which will include:

1. The district nurse (community sister).
2. The health visitor.
3. The community physiotherapist.
4. The social services, who usually have an occupational therapist in their team.

At all times the patient, relatives and general practitioner are to be considered as the most important members of the team; the GP can often act as the co-ordinator of services and the patient and relatives really determine the extent to which the team is required. The hospital chaplains and parish clergy and ministers should not be overlooked and they should be involved as and when required.

It is not proposed to discuss the individual roles of these team members but it is hoped that each physiotherapist will make it her responsibility to find out what everyone in the team is able to offer and how they can best be used. Participation in ward rounds, in clinics and in case conferences is to be encouraged. Whenever a patient is transferred either to a different hospital or back to the community full details of all treatment as well as an assessment of the patient should be sent to the relevant services.

There has been considerable discussion as to the value of physiotherapy for patients undergoing surgery. Nichols and Howell (1970) undertook controlled trials and the result showed that upper abdominal surgery in particular is likely to inhibit the function of the diaphragm. They concluded that physiotherapy has an accepted part to play in the treatment of established bronchitis by physically aiding the drainage and expulsion of bronchial secretions. They also felt that the problem of postoperative complications was more that of selecting those patients 'at risk', and treating them vigorously *before* surgery, rather than providing unnecessary postoperative treatment in a routine fashion to all surgical patients.

An Editorial (1982) in the *British Medical Journal* discusses postoperative pneumonias and comes to the conclusion that prophylactic treatment of any kind seems scarcely justifiable for all patients since more than 80 per cent will suffer no complications.

PHYSIOTHERAPY IN GENERAL SURGERY

Bearing in mind the previous comments, patients who undergo surgical procedures may or may not be referred for physiotherapy. Those patients who are referred for pre- and postoperative physiotherapy need to be adequately assessed so that unnecessary treatments are neither carried out nor continued indefinitely. Unless the surgical procedure is an emergency, it is to be hoped that when patients are referred for pre-operative training the physiotherapist will have sufficient time to prepare the patient adequately before the proposed surgery. Patients undergoing extensive abdominal surgery will certainly benefit subjectively and any patient who is known to be either a heavy smoker or who suffers from a chronic chest disorder should receive adequate pre-operative training. In many cases this preparation may be carried out as an outpatient, to save the patient occupying a hospital bed for a week prior to operation.

It is unlikely that patients undergoing minor surgery, endoscopic examination, haemorrhoidectomy, etc will be ordered physiotherapy *unless* they are known to have a chronic chest condition.

Principles of physiotherapy for patients undergoing surgery

The general principles involved are:

1. To prevent chest complications by maintaining lung function and aiding the clearance of secretions.
2. To prevent thrombosis of the legs by encouraging active leg movements, or, if necessary, by performing passive exercises.
3. To maintain muscle power by encouraging simple bed exercises.
4. To help maintain good posture by ensuring that pillows are arranged in a good supportive position.

The approach of the physiotherapist to the patient must be positive and firm, though sympathetic. Patients are very quick to sense when someone does not really know what she/he is doing.

COUGHING

One of the invariable questions will be 'Will I burst my stitches when I cough?' All patients must be reassured about this and shown how they may themselves support their wound when coughing. A sensitive yet firm hand to support the patient's own hands as he holds his wound, will give confidence as well as reassurance. The author has always found that sitting on the bed behind the patient, with the patient able to lean on her shoulder, enables her to use both her hands to support

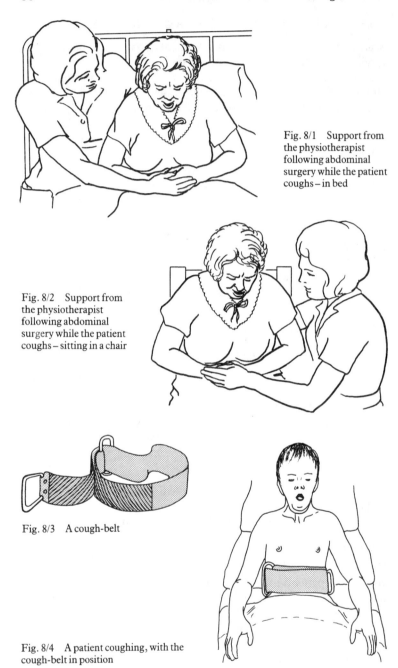

Fig. 8/1   Support from the physiotherapist following abdominal surgery while the patient coughs – in bed

Fig. 8/2   Support from the physiotherapist following abdominal surgery while the patient coughs – sitting in a chair

Fig. 8/3   A cough-belt

Fig. 8/4   A patient coughing, with the cough-belt in position the wound (Fig. 8/1). Sometimes patients are told to bend their knees up as they cough, but this is not always very easy. The head should be flexed as the patient coughs. Patients who undergo surgery are seldom in bed for very long and coughing is very much more easily performed when sitting (Fig. 8/2). Indeed, some patients will find sitting over the side of the bed with their feet supported on the locker a helpful position in which to cough. Sometimes it helps to give them a 'cough-belt' (Figs. 8/3 and 8/4). These belts are very useful when the patient is a chronic bronchitic with a productive cough as well as being stout. They can be worn loosely and then pulled up tight when they want to cough (Barlow, 1964).

It may be helpful to teach 'huffing' as a prelude to actually coughing. A 'huff' may be termed a type of forced expiration and is useful to loosen secretions and initiate coughing. To 'huff' correctly the patient should be taught to take a full inspiration using the diaphragm, and then to breathe out sharply contracting the abdominal muscles as he does so. Following two or three good 'huffs' the patient should then breathe in deeply and attempt two strong coughs with the mouth slightly open.

In all teaching of coughing it is important for the patient to appreciate the difference between an effective cough and a 'genteel' clearing of the throat.

It is not the act of coughing which causes a wound to burst occasionally, although it invariably seems to happen as the patient coughs and he naturally assumes that the coughing was the cause. A wound breaks down, i.e. the sutures give way, almost always because there is an infection or an increased serous fluid collection. Just occasionally the suture material may be faulty. If the patient is stout or is known to have a chronic chest disorder, the surgeon may insert some tension sutures as well. These are in addition to the normal suturing of the wound, and are usually threaded through thin rubber tubing so that they can remain in situ without cutting through the skin.

GENERAL POINTS TO BE NOTED BY THE PHYSIOTHERAPIST

Pre-operative

1. Before the patient is seen by the physiotherapist, the notes should be carefully read and any relevant facts noted. For example he may be a heavy smoker, he may have a past history of a leg thrombosis, he may have some disability which could influence his mobility, he may live

alone and this could influence how independent he would need to be before being discharged.

2. Introduce yourself to the patient and explain in language which he can understand, exactly what you are going to do and what he will have to do and why all this is necessary.

3. Assess the respiratory expansion of the patient and teach diaphragmatic and lateral costal breathing. It is wise to warn the patient that postoperatively it may be necessary to treat him in side lying and/or with the end of the bed tipped, and he should be shown how to reach this position. If this method has to be used, it is sensible to combine the physiotherapy at a time when the nurses are carrying out nursing procedures so that the patient is not moved unnecessarily.

4. As previously mentioned he should be shown how to hold himself when coughing.

5. Simple foot and leg exercises should be taught and the patient told why they are important. It is not necessary to talk about thrombosis; it is quite simple to explain that the legs will ache if they are kept still after the operation, and that if they are regularly moved this will not happen and they will feel less wobbly when he gets up. The patient should also be told not to sit in bed with his legs crossed at the ankles.

Postoperative

1. The notes must be read and the extent of the operation noted, together with the nursing record of the patient's condition since his return from the operating theatre.

2. The position of drainage tubes, intravenous lines, catheter and type of dressing should be noted.

3. If analgesic drugs have been prescribed, the physiotherapist should arrange that they are given *before* the physiotherapy. Occasionally Entonox (50% nitrous oxide and 50% oxygen) may be used – this has the advantage that the patient can control it, and its use can be very effective in pain relief where coughing is essential.

Chapter 9 discusses the application of treatments which the physiotherapist can use pre- and postoperatively. This chapter will now concentrate on some aspects of general surgical procedures and how the physiotherapist may find herself involved. Specialised care following gynaecological, head and neck, plastic and cranial surgery in addition to amputations will be discussed in separate chapters.

SURGICAL PROCEDURES

The actual surgical procedures for different operations will not be described as these can be studied in surgical textbooks. There are, however, certain aspects about which it is useful for the physiotherapist to have some knowledge.

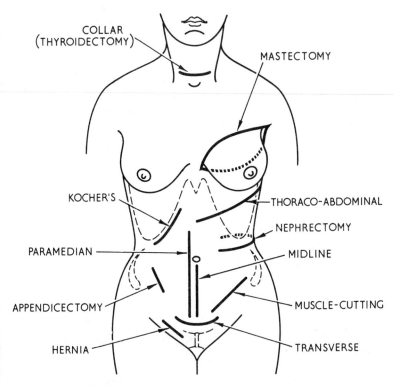

Fig. 8/5   Surgical incisions

Incisions

Figure 8/5 shows some of the basic incisions which are used in surgical procedures. The decision to use which depends on the surgeon as well as the prime requirement of giving adequate access to the diseased area.

CLOSURE OF THE INCISION

The incision may be closed in various ways:

1. Clips are used where an unsightly scar could be distressing to the

patient, e.g. following thyroidectomy. They are removed 48–72 hours postoperatively.

2. Sutures can be absorbable, e.g. catgut; non-absorbable, e.g. silk or nylon; invisible intradermal absorbable sutures; or tension sutures (p. 89).

3. The sutures can be tied as single stitches, as a continuous suture or as mattress sutures. The advantage of single sutures is that alternate sutures can be removed and if there is any danger of the incision gaping, stitches in the area at risk can remain longer.

4. The size of the suture material will depend on the site at which it is used. Plastic surgery will require very fine material and more numerous stitches, whereas abdominal muscles will require a strong material. Steel wire is used to suture the sternum after the sternum is split in heart surgery, and in some jaw surgery when the mandible is divided and then resutured. If steel wire is used, it is necessary to drill a hole in the bone ends which are to be wired together, through which the wire is threaded.

Drains

Almost all wounds will have some form of drainage left in situ, thus reducing the risk of haematoma formation and subsequent break-down of wounds.

Drainage tubes can take several forms:

1. A Redivac drain, which is a closed system of drainage using a vacuum principle.

2. Corrugated drains which are either rubber or polythene and drain into the dressing and can be shortened by pulling out gradually before final removal.

3. Intercostal drains which are inserted into the pleural cavity to drain blood and/or air following surgery involving the opening of the chest. They are attached to an underwater bottle(s) and this is a form of closed drainage. Where an empyema is being drained the wide-bore tubing is sometimes allowed to drain into a dressing (Innocenti, 1983).

4. Internal drains such as a T-tube which is inserted into the common bile duct following an exploration of the common bile duct. These are usually attached to a bottle or bag thus allowing the collection of bile or other fluid(s). They are usually in situ for 10–12 days.

A caecostomy is sometimes left following colon surgery – this is a drain inserted into the caecum which allows faecal fluid to escape instead of building up and possibly causing an obstruction. It is usually attached to a bag. It is withdrawn about 10–12 days postoperatively. It must *not* be confused with a colostomy. A caecostomy is essentially a safety valve.

Other tubes

Following surgery, the patient may also have an intravenous infusion – this is to maintain electrolyte balance as well as ensuring both nutrition and hydration. In surgery not affecting the alimentary tract such an infusion will be taken down the morning following surgery.

A nasogastric tube is almost always passed following surgery involving the alimentary tract. This has a dual purpose in that the stomach may be aspirated regularly and, at the appropriate time, feeding may be begun. The physiotherapist should acquaint herself with these essential nursing matters either by discussing them with her nurse colleagues or by reading about them in a nursing textbook.

A catheter may be passed while the patient is in the operating theatre, and particularly where renal, bladder, rectal or very extensive abdominal surgery has been carried out. It will drain into a bag which hangs from the bed frame. Sometimes the catheter tube may be strapped lightly to the upper thigh and the physiotherapist must ensure that there is sufficient play in the tubing before she starts on too active leg exercises!

SPECIAL POINTS TO BE REMEMBERED BY THE PHYSIOTHERAPIST

Abdominal surgery

Unless the surgery is specifically for gall bladder disease, inguinal or femoral hernia, or nephrectomy, the incision will be a paramedian or mid-line with extension as necessary to allow for adequate exposure.

After gastrectomy, the patient may develop left pulmonary atelectasis (p. 103) and the physiotherapist needs to emphasise localised breathing to both lower lobes but particularly to the left. The diaphragm will have been handled in the operative procedure and the patient will be reluctant to breathe deeply.

Following cholecystectomy in which a Kocher incision is used, the danger of atelectasis is to the right lower lobe, and so the emphasis must be to the right lower lobe. In addition, if the common bile duct has been explored, there will be a T-tube in situ. This can cause pain and discomfort when the patient breathes deeply. Adequate analgesia must be given *before* the main treatment is given by the physio-therapist and the patient *must* be continually reminded by both nurses and the physiotherapist to breathe deeply.

Adrenalectomy

A bilateral adrenalectomy is most often performed for patients suffering from disseminated cancer and particularly for those with metastatic bone disease. It is also performed for primary tumours of the adrenal glands. The surgical approach is either through the abdomen when the physiotherapy will be as for any abdominal operation, or through bilateral loin incisions, i.e. through the bed of the twelfth rib. If the latter approach is used there is always the danger of nicking the pleura with a consequent pneumothorax which may require an intercostal drain to be inserted. Breathing exercises are most important when the loin incision is used.

In addition, if the patient has metastatic bone disease care must be exercised if the deposits affect the ribs. Clapping, shakings and vigorous vibrations must NOT be used; gentle vibrations and resisted bilateral costal breathing should be given. Bed exercises are important, but again these must be active and care must be observed if there are deposits in the weight-bearing bones, particularly the femora. Downie (1978a) has described the treatment for these patients.

Breast surgery

Perhaps no other surgery causes so many reactions. Mastectomy is performed most often for malignant conditions but it should always be remembered that it is also performed for benign lesions, e.g. multiple fibromata. The type of surgery varies nowadays from the removal of a lump – 'lumpectomy' – to the full radical mastectomy (Halsted's operation). Probably the most commonly performed operation is the simple or extended simple mastectomy (Patey operation). This latter allows for the removal of the axillary glands with the breast tissue but without the excision of the pectoral muscles.

Whatever surgery is carried out, the physiotherapy allowed will be at the discretion of the surgeon and the physiotherapist MUST ascertain what each particular surgeon will allow by way of movement. If she is unfortunate enough to have little or no contact with the surgeon or if he tells her to 'do what you like', she will be well advised to steer a middle course with regard to arm movements.

Basic guidelines may be summarised as follows:

1. Following lumpectomy, or wedge resection, no treatment should be required.

2. Following local or simple mastectomy without axillary clearance, no treatment should be necessary, but occasionally physiotherapy may be required to help the patient overcome her fear of movement and thus to encourage a full range of shoulder movements.

3. Following an extended simple mastectomy (Patey), the patient should be encouraged to use her arm for normal daily activities. If stiffness develops, pendular type shoulder exercises are the most useful. In no circumstances must a shoulder be forced.

4. Following radical mastectomy (Halsted), physiotherapy will be aimed at restoration of shoulder movement, particularly elevation and rotation. The pectoralis major and minor muscles will have been excised and pure abduction of the shoulder should not be allowed until all the drains are out and the skin flaps firmly adhered to the chest wall. If abduction is allowed too soon, fluid will collect between the skin flaps and the chest wall and will require repeated aspirations. Apart from causing unnecessary discomfort for the patient, repeated aspirations carry the risk of infection. Pendular type shoulder exercises are the most useful, and all exercises should be active and the shoulder must never be forced.

Some surgeons will bandage the arm to the side for the first week, to prevent abduction and undue movement of the skin flaps. In this case finger, hand and wrist movements should be encouraged, also shoulder shrugging and isometric contractions of the deltoid.

Instruction should also be given in posture correction and how to lift without placing too great strain on the shoulder of the mastectomy side.

In all cases where the physiotherapist is involved in treating mastectomy patients, she must be prepared to enter into the total care of these patients. She should have a knowledge of breast prostheses, of how to adapt brassières and where to purchase suitable swimwear (Downie, 1978b). She should be aware of the emotional problems which can arise following mastectomy (Downie, 1976; Maguire, 1975), and she should always be ready to listen and to help in any way possible. Co-operation with nurses, social workers, and patient volunteers as well as the doctors is very necessary in this field of care.

LYMPHOEDEMA

In some cases following mastectomy, and particularly following radical mastectomy or where the patient has undergone radiotherapy, lymphoedema will occur. Physiotherapy may well be ordered and various methods of treatment are available including massage in elevation, faradism under pressure and the newer compression techniques. There is, as yet, no evidence that any of these has a lasting effect though there is no doubt that all can help to relieve the condition. As well as such specific treatment, the patient should be taught exercises in elevation and how to posture the arm so that drainage may be helped; particularly useful to the patient is to be shown how to position the arm at night in bed, and while sitting watching the television.

Colonic and rectal surgery

As with all abdominal surgery physiotherapy will be directed towards the prevention of chest complications but with lower abdominal surgery special attention must also be paid to the prevention of thrombosis. Leg exercises must be taught and supervised thoroughly postoperatively.

Following surgical intervention on the bowel, a paralytic ileus can result leading to great discomfort for the patient with distension of the abdomen. It is important that breathing exercises are encouraged during this period as well as the patient being persuaded to move around in bed as much as possible.

COLOSTOMY

A colostomy is the formation of an artificial anus on the surface of the abdominal wall which can be temporary or permanent. It is sited over the transverse colon or in the lower left quadrant of the abdomen. The lower the siting of the colostomy, the more formed will be the stool. The physiotherapist does not treat the colostomy itself but she should certainly have an understanding of the consequences of such an operation.

When the patient has undergone a combined synchronous abdomino-perineal excision for a carcinoma of the rectum, the colostomy will be permanent.

If a patient is admitted with an acute intestinal obstruction the first stage of relieving the obstruction is often the fashioning of a temporary colostomy. This is followed in about two weeks by an excision and end-to-end anastomosis of the affected colon and about two further weeks later the colostomy will be closed. Sometimes when a resection of the colon is carried out for a carcinoma of the colon, diverticular disease or Crohn's disease, a temporary colostomy may be fashioned so that the anastomosis of the colon can firmly unite before the continuity of the gut is re-established.

When the colostomy is permanent, the aim of rehabilitation must be to ensure that the patient can not only cope with the appliance but does return to a normal life and takes his place fully in society. The Colostomy Welfare Association has done great work in this area; their volunteers (all of whom have had a colostomy) are all carefully selected and trained and are willing to visit any patient at the request of the surgeon or general practitioner. Unlike the Ileostomy Association they do *not* hold group meetings of colostomists. In recent years nurses, who have undergone a post-graduate course in stoma care, have begun to be appointed in the larger hospitals. These are clinical nurse specialists more commonly referred to as the stoma therapists. Their role is to advise patients, their families and the nurses in the understanding of the colostomy and to ensure that the most suitable appliance is provided for each patient.

The physiotherapist should certainly teach these patients how to lift correctly and should help to ensure that they get dressed and are able to walk about not only in the hospital and its grounds, but out in the street as well, before being discharged home.

ILEOSTOMY

Like the colostomy this is an artificial anus on the abdominal wall but is sited in the right lower quadrant of the abdomen. It is always permanent and is usually performed following a total colectomy or pan-procto total colectomy – the latter includes the excision of the rectum and anus as well as the colon. These very extensive excisions are performed for patients with ulcerative colitis or extensive Crohn's disease. These patients are often extremely ill before surgery and will require a great deal of physiotherapy to help them maintain a good respiratory function and leg mobility.

As they improve, and in many cases this improvement can be dramatic, the physiotherapist should teach lifting and generally help with total rehabilitation prior to discharge.

For these patients the Ileostomy Association organise volunteers to visit in hospital and after discharge and they have groups all over the country who meet regularly for social events, holidays, as well as to discuss new appliances etc.

Genito-urinary surgery

NEPHRECTOMY

The removal of a kidney may become necessary when it is diseased as the result of a malignant tumour; pyonephrosis (gross infection);

tuberculosis; hydronephrosis (dilatation of the renal pelvis due to obstruction, leading to atrophy of the kidney tissue and impaired renal function); and occasionally for calculi (renal stones).

The remaining kidney must be healthy before nephrectomy is undertaken. The incision is usually through the bed of the twelfth rib but may be higher, through the bed of the tenth rib. Care of the chest is very important and it is not unknown for the pleura to be nicked at operation and for a pneumothorax to occur. An intercostal drain will be inserted and physiotherapy will follow the pattern as for thoracic surgery (Innocenti, 1983).

Whenever a loin incision is used, the physiotherapist should check carefully the posture of the patient, both when lying in bed and when he gets up and starts walking.

PROSTATECTOMY

This operation is usually performed on elderly men, many of whom will have a chronic chest disorder. Chest physiotherapy is therefore very important, and this is an instance where the cough-belt could be used (p. 89). Prostatectomy is usually performed for benign enlargement of the gland and is carried out through a transverse supra-pubic incision. Carcinoma of the prostate is usually treated by hormonal manipulation but if the condition is causing difficulty of micturition through pressure on the bladder neck, a trans-urethral resection (TUR) of the gland may be undertaken. This is performed endoscopically, and under direct vision the surgeon is able to resect the obtruding tissue.

Early ambulation of these patients is not only desirable but essential; drainage tubes and catheter will need to be secured safely and the elderly gentleman persuaded to walk. Nowadays catheters drain into bags which can be easily carried.

CYSTECTOMY

Surgery for a carcinoma of the bladder will entail removal of the bladder (cystectomy) and the fashioning of an ileal conduit. Not all bladder cancers will need to be treated with radical surgery; radiotherapy is used quite extensively and it is often following such treatment that cystectomy and the formation of an ileal conduit is carried out. An ileal conduit is the formation of an artificial bladder on the abdominal wall, in a manner similar to that of forming a colostomy. In this case a small segment of the ileum is fashioned into a tube and brought out through the abdominal wall, thus forming a stoma. The two ureters are inserted into the ileal conduit and an appliance into which the urine will drain is attached to the stoma.

Physiotherapy for these patients will include care for the chest, and, more especially, teaching them to lift and generally helping them to become active, mobile and capable of being independent before discharge.

An ileal conduit may also be fashioned for patients suffering from chronic incontinence due to certain neurological conditions, e.g. children with spina bifida.

GOLD GRAINS INSERTION IN BLADDER

Very occasionally radioactive gold grains may be inserted for treatment of a circumscribed bladder tumour. If physiotherapy is required the physiotherapist must observe the precautions which are laid down and particularly the time allowed for close treatment of the patient. Radioactive gold has a very short half-life and this time allowance will rapidly increase over five days.

These patients may well be in a poor general state of health and chest physiotherapy is often required. Provided the precautions are observed, there is no danger to the physiotherapist; a portable lead shield may be used to protect the physiotherapist while she encourages the patient to carry out exercises.

Repair of herniae

A hernia is a weakness in the musculature through which contents of a cavity may prolapse.

HERNIAE OF THE ABDOMINAL WALL

1. A *femoral* hernia occurs at the femoral ring. It is most common in women.
2. An *inguinal* hernia occurs at the inguinal canal. It is more common in men. There are two types: *Direct*, which occurs in older people due to associated muscle weakness and increase in abdominal pressure; and *Indirect*, which is congenital and occurs in younger people.
3. An *umbilical* hernia or para-umbilical hernia occurs either in childhood or at the fifth decade. In adults they are more common in obese patients.
4. An *incisional* hernia occurs through a previous incision and can be found anywhere.

Repair for these herniae involves excision of the hernial sac where necessary and strengthening of the abdominal wall by means of sutures. Fascia lata may be used like a darn, to repair the groin herniae; this latter procedure is rarely performed now.

Apart from chest physiotherapy as required, hernia patients must be taught to lift correctly. They may also be given abdominal exercises – isometric or inner range exercises but not outer range exercises.

Two other types of hernia are:

1. A *hiatus* hernia which is the prolapsing of the stomach through the hiatus of the diaphragm. Repair is usually through a thoracotomy incision and physiotherapy will be as for patients undergoing thoracic surgery (Innocenti, 1983).
2. A *strangulated* hernia which is always a serious surgical emergency. The contents of the hernial sac can become trapped if the neck of the sac is very narrow; if the blood supply is impaired, the trapped bowel can become gangrenous. Intestinal obstruction is a not infrequent complication of a strangulated hernia. Physiotherapy is as for abdominal surgery.

REFERENCES

Barlow, D. (1964). A cough-belt to prevent and treat postoperative pulmonary complications. *Lancet*, **2**, 736.

Downie, P. A. (1976). Post-mastectomy survey. *Nursing Mirror*, **142**, 13.

Downie, P. A. (1978a). *Cancer Rehabilitation: an Introduction for Physiotherapists and the Allied Professions*. Faber and Faber, London.

Downie, P. A. (1978b). *Rehabilitation*. Chapter included in *Oncology for Nurses and Health Care Professionals*. Vol 2 (ed Tiffany, R.). George Allen and Unwin, London.

Editorial. (1982). Postoperative pneumonias. *British Medical Journal*, **284**, 6312, 292–3.

Innocenti, D. M. (1983). *Cardiothoracic Surgery – 2. Physiotherapy*. Chapter in *Cash's Textbook of Chest, Heart and Vascular Disorders for Physiotherapists*, 3rd edition (ed Downie, P. A.). Faber and Faber, London.

Maguire, P. (1975). The psychological and social consequences of breast cancer. *Nursing Mirror*, **140**, 74.

Nichols, P. J. R. and Howell, B. (1970). Routine pre-and postoperative physiotherapy: A preliminary trial. *Physiotherapy*, **56**, 8.

BIBLIOGRAPHY

Ellison Nash, D. F. (1980). *The Principles and Practice of Surgery for Nurses and Allied Professions*, 7th edition. Edward Arnold (Publishers) Limited, London.

Feeley, T. M., Peel, A. L. G. and Devlin, H. B. (1982). Mastectomy and its consequences. *British Medical Journal*, **284**, 1246.

McFarland, J. (ed) (1982). *Basic Clinical Surgery for Nurses and Medical Students*, 2nd edition. Butterworths, London.

Maguire, P., Pentol, A., Allen, D., Tait, A., Brooke, M. and Sellwood, R. (1982). Cost of counselling women who undergo mastectomy. *British Medical Journal*, **284**, 1933.

Rennie, H. and Wilson, J. A. C. (1983). A coughing belt. *Lancet*, **2**, 138–9.

Taylor, S. and Cotton, L. (1982). *A Short Textbook of Surgery*, 5th edition. Hodder and Stoughton, Sevenoaks.

Chapter 9

Complications Following Surgery

by K. M. KESSON, MCSP

No matter how simple and straightforward an operation, or how physically fit the patient is before he undergoes it, there are always certain risks which cannot be avoided, though preventive measures can lessen their incidence. Some of the complications which may follow surgery are given here in their order of importance to the physiotherapist.

Respiratory problems

Whenever a general anaesthetic is administered there is the possibility of respiratory problems. The anaesthetic may act as an irritant; the cough reflex may be depressed and therefore expectorating secretions is difficult. Thoracic and upper abdominal surgery are most likely to cause respiratory problems.

Thrombosis

Thrombosis of the deep veins of the leg, which may lead to a fatal pulmonary embolism, is always a postoperative danger. The physiotherapist may be the person who discovers this during an exercise period, so must be always watchful for the symptoms.

Wound infections

These are due to the prevalence of bacteria, particularly resistant types. Infections occur even in clean, cold surgery despite the existence in most hospitals of teams whose task it is to combat infection.

Pressure sores

Any patient confined to bed must be watched constantly by all who care for him to prevent pressure sores occurring. These may have been precipitated by pressure while on the operating table or they may occur later. Pressure can be caused also from within the tissues by oedema. Vigilance is especially needed when the patient is old, unconscious, immobile, incontinent, or diabetic.

Haemorrhage

Another complication is haemorrhage. This can be primary, occurring within the first 24 hours, or secondary, when it can take place up to three weeks postoperatively.

Muscle wasting and impairment of function

If incisions are very extensive and divide, or in extreme cases damage, muscle or nerve tissue, there may be resultant muscle wasting and impairment of function. This can lead to faulty posture, deformities and, occasionally, stiff joints.

Cardiac arrest

Cardiac arrest requires immediate action to prevent irreversible brain damage. It is vital that it should be recognised at once by everyone who comes in contact with the patient, and that the appropriate action is known and instantly followed (see Chapter 7).

RESPIRATORY PROBLEMS

Respiratory complications are liable to follow any operation in which general anaesthesia is used. They are most common in thoracic surgery since, in many cases, the lung function may be impaired already. After thoracic surgery the highest incidence is probably in abdominal operations, particularly those which require a supra-umbilical incision.

Postoperative respiratory complications are due to retained secretions and/or decreased thoracic expansion due to pain. Sometimes these secretions are stringy and viscid and therefore difficult to expectorate. Following operation the patient is drowsy, making deep breathing and coughing difficult, and if the incision is thoracic or abdominal, coughing is voluntarily inhibited through fear of pain.

Provided the patient is reassured that his stitches will not break through coughing (see p. 87), and his pain relieved by adequate analgesia, a good effective cough will clear these secretions. Postoperative analgesics make the patient lethargic and the presence of drains, intravenous lines or other tubes may make him relatively immobile and less likely to be able to clear his chest of secretions. Retained secretions may lead to the following problems:

Atelectasis or postoperative pulmonary collapse

This occurs when a plug of mucus becomes lodged in an airway and the air distal to it is absorbed, causing the area to collapse. Collapse of a whole lobe is rare. Segmental collapse is more common and is usually unilateral and basal. Postoperative atelectasis occurs within the first 24 to 48 hours. There is a rise in temperature and respiratory rate followed by a cough with purulent sputum. Patchy atelectasis may be seen on the chest radiograph.

Postoperative pneumonia

This occurs when the retained secretions become infected and an inflammatory process takes place. It usually presents two to three days postoperatively with a gradual rise in temperature, reduced expansion and radiographic changes. A productive cough follows and purulent sputum may be produced. Bronchopneumonia frequently occurs in elderly patients following surgery.

Aspiration pneumonia

This type of pneumonia occurs following the inhalation of vomitus or infected secretions from the respiratory tract. It may occur in comatose patients when it can be fatal, unless prompt action is taken. A particular form occurs in obstetric patients – Mendelson's syndrome (1946).

Inhalation can occur pre-operatively as in elderly patients awaiting surgery for intestinal obstruction. Reflux of gastric contents into the trachea via the oesophagus can also occur during operation when the cough reflex has been abolished by the anaesthetic, or early in the postoperative period. An aspiration pneumonia may be accompanied by severe airways obstruction and pulmonary oedema.

The reduction in depth of each breath, i.e. vital capacity (VC), which inevitably follows operations on the thorax or abdomen is a further factor in predisposing towards these complications. The diaphragm is responsible for as much as 60 per cent of the normal respiratory movements, but in the first 24 hours after the operation, its movement may be only 20 per cent of the normal. The result is that the lungs, particularly the bases, are not fully ventilated and, with a decrease in the action of the thoracic suction pump, the circulation is slowed with consequent congestion. Not only is the vitality of the lung lowered, but there may be increased filtration of tissue fluid and slight oedema of the lung bases.

Postoperative pulmonary complications delay the patient's recovery; whenever possible they must be prevented and should they occur they need to be treated immediately.

Physiotherapy

The aim of pre- and postoperative physiotherapy is to prevent complications, but should they occur then they must be treated effectively. Respiratory complications are due to:

Decreased thoracic excursion due to pain
Retained secretions
Inhibition of cough reflex
Disruption of the cough mechanism by abdominal incisions

The physiotherapist must encourage thoracic expansion and teach effective coughing.

DEEP BREATHING EXERCISES
Deep breathing exercises should be taught pre-operatively while the patient is alert, pain-free and fully co-operative. Emphasis is laid on diaphragmatic and lateral costal expansion with a good, deep inspiration, followed by a relaxed expiration. An understanding by the patient of the value of the correct breathing is essential so that he will co-operate as soon as he recovers from the anaesthetic.

EFFECTIVE COUGHING
The patient should be taught how to cough effectively and with as little pain as possible. This is again best taught pre-operatively. Two points need to be emphasised when teaching coughing. First, strain on the wound will be relieved if the patient supports the operation site with his hands, draws up his knees and leans his trunk slightly towards the area of incision. Second, following a good, deep inspiration, a short, sharp expiration produces the easiest and most effective cough. If the patient is still unable to cough effectively, 'huffing', i.e. several short forced expirations, may be sufficient to move the secretions.

Humidification may be necessary to moisten the secretions and facilitate their removal, especially if the patient is to have 'nil-by-mouth' for any length of time. Humidification may be achieved in several ways:

(a) The simplest method is by Tinct. Benz. Co. (Friars Balsam) inhalations given three times daily. Ideally these inhalations should be given immediately before chest physiotherapy is carried out.

(b) Humidifiers which add water, usually warmed, to the oxygen or air of the environment in which the patient is nursed.

(c) Where there is a tracheostomy, 1–2ml of normal saline may be injected into the trachea.

(d) By the use of a nebuliser (e.g. Wright's, Hudson, Inspiron, Turrett, Bird) in which a bronchodilator, e.g. salbutamol (Ventolin), or a mucolytic agent, can be nebulised for inhalation. Indications for their use are bronchospasm or to thin down thick, sticky sputum.

ADMINISTERING DRUGS

All drugs for use by nebuliser or intermittent positive pressure breathing machines (IPPB) have to be prescribed and written up by a medical practitioner. The routine for the administering of such drugs by the physiotherapist will be laid down by the hospital pharmacy and the medical committee. This is known to vary from unit to unit and each physiotherapist must learn what is required in her hospital or unit. As a standard rule the procedure will follow the rules laid down for nurses and may be summarised as follows:

1. The drug must be written up by the doctor.
2. The physiotherapist will draw up and prepare the drug as prescribed.
3. The physiotherapist should then have it checked by either a state registered nurse (SRN) or by a learner nurse who has passed her drug assessment. (It is this checking which will vary: many specialised units certainly do not adhere to this routine.)
4. The administration of the drug must be recorded on the patient's drug sheet: dose; time and the giver's signature.

Student physiotherapists *must* always be checked.

MECHANICAL ASSISTANCE FOR THE REMOVAL OF SECRETIONS

When in spite of adequate coughing and practise of breathing exercises, mucus does collect and there is danger of collapse, then mechanical assistance will be necessary to remove secretions.

The methods used are percussion, deep breathing exercises with vibrations and postural drainage. Usually there is no reason why a patient should not be posturally drained if it is necessary, but in certain conditions, such as hypertension, hiatus hernia and some aortic surgery, it is contra-indicated. The physiotherapist must be absolutely certain of the patient's condition and where necessary must confirm with the medical officer in charge of the patient whether or not postural drainage is permitted.

If the patient is nursed in the half-lying position, he should be positioned in crook lying or crook side lying for treatment. The foot of the bed may need to be elevated. The breathing exercises, and the movement generally, usually help to relieve the flatulence which so often causes abdominal distension and further hampers breathing.

It must be remembered that practising breathing exercises once a day is useless. To be effective in preventing chest complications, they should be practised for at least five minutes in every hour so that correct breathing becomes a habit. It rests with the physiotherapist to establish a good rapport with the patient and gain his interest, understanding and co-operation. Frequent short visits are essential until it is clear that the patient is sufficiently enthusiastic to work on his own.

Nasopharyngeal suction may be necessary in some circumstances where the patient is unable to cough up secretions, despite the assistance of physiotherapy, e.g. inability to co-operate, weakness which makes coughing ineffective or sticky sputum which, though the patient is able to cough, he cannot expectorate. In the case of drowsy or unco-operative patients, a catheter may need to be introduced into the trachea in order to stimulate a good cough. (Where there are particularly obstinate secretions bronchoscopy may have to be carried out.)

If major chest problems are anticipated, e.g. before extensive pulmonary, cardiac or upper abdominal operations or where there is pre-existing lung disease, it may be decided to intubate and even ventilate the patient postoperatively for a short while. In this case he will return from theatre with an endotracheal tube in situ. Chest physiotherapy is performed regularly on these patients and secretions removed by suction through the endotracheal tube using a sterile technique. Once the patient is awake and co-operative the endotracheal tube is removed, and since this is often within the first 24 hours, the physiotherapist must persist with frequent treatment to keep the chest clear.

Early mobilisation is an important factor, not only in preventing respiratory complications, but also in the general rehabilitation of the patient. As soon as they are able, patients should be encouraged to move about the bed as much as possible and in the absence of major complications, they usually sit out of bed within the first 24 hours. Infusion lines and drains need not prevent patients from moving from bed to chair, or from walking in the ward. As soon as these lines, drains and tubes are removed, the patient should be encouraged to be freely mobile.

DEEP VEIN THROMBOSIS

Thrombosis of the deep veins of the lower limbs may occur in any patient immobilised for any length of time but occurs more frequently in high risk groups, e.g. elderly patients, those with a history of previous deep vein thrombosis and those with malignant disease. It can have an insidious onset with no clinical signs or symptoms in the early stages when the main danger is of a fatal pulmonary embolus occurring. A deep vein thrombosis may present with local signs in the lower leg, the calf becoming swollen, tender and cyanosed. Passive ankle dorsiflexion causes pain in the calf muscles (Homan's sign). It may however only show itself when the thrombus becomes suddenly detached and is carried through the right side of the heart to occlude the pulmonary artery, causing a pulmonary embolism.

When a deep vein thrombosis is suspected the patient is treated with anticoagulants; once he is adequately anticoagulated and any calf pain has eased the surgeon usually allows the patient to resume exercising and mobilising wearing an elastic stocking. He should not stand about, and when sitting he should have the leg elevated with adequate support.

Other medical treatment will include the correction of dehydration (this increases the risk of thrombosis) or cardiac failure, if either is present.

The physiotherapist should be alert to any pain or tenderness in the calf while treating the patient and must report it to the nurse in charge of the ward immediately.

WOUND INFECTIONS

Normally, surgical incisions heal quickly with little formation of scar tissue and it is perfectly safe for the patient to cough and move around (see p. 87).

The presence of infection in a previously clean wound is indicated by pain, throbbing and tenderness; the area may become hot, red and oedematous. The sutures tend to cut through the tissues and the wound may gape either along its whole length or in between the sutures.

If the area is already infected, healing is likely to be less satisfactory. Sometimes the very presence of sepsis is an indication for surgery, e.g. a gangrenous appendix, or empyema. Such surgery will involve the use of drainage tubes to permit free drainage of the pus and ensure healing from the base upwards; if tubes remain in for any length of time they may cause irritation and consequent fibrous tissue formation. In such cases healing becomes difficult when the tube is eventually removed; for this reason tubes are usually shortened and removed as soon as possible, usually between three and seven days, except in the case of an empyema.

Where there is an incision of the abdominal wall, distension can cause bursting either of the whole wound or areas between the sutures; persistent distension is therefore to be avoided.

As a result of any of these factors, scarring may occur in the musculature of the walls of the abdominal or pelvic cavities and consequently there is always the possibility of the contents of the cavity protruding through the weakened area. This condition is known as an incisional hernia.

Physiotherapy

Active exercise is good, as some strain on the wound stimulates the healing process. Excess strain should be avoided. Outer range abdominal exercises or heavy work such as double hip and knee flexion should not be given immediately following abdominal surgery.

If a clean wound becomes infected, cleaning and healing may be stimulated by some form of dry heat. If the infection is superficial, infra-red or radiant heat are satisfactory; if the infection is deep-seated, short wave diathermy using a co-planar technique should be used. Treatment is best given after the sutures have been cut and the wound allowed to gape so that free drainage is established, and treatment should be given at least twice daily. Occasionally, ultraviolet irradiation may be requested.

The scar may be adherent to underlying tissue and will probably hamper movement, as well as causing discomfort as it pulls on other tissues. In time it may well contract and produce deformity. To prevent this occurring, massage with lanolin may be prescribed after the wound is well healed. Massage should be carried out over the surface of the scar in order to loosen it from the underlying tissue.

Ultrasound therapy is helpful in the treatment of particularly hard scars, such as can occur after surgery for the release of the flexor retinaculum in the carpal tunnel syndrome or after operation for Dupuytren's contracture. Paraffin wax treatment also helps to soften scars and the sooner the treatment can be started, the more successful it will be. Occasionally a scar may be painful, because a superficial nerve becomes entrapped in fibrous tissue. If other treatments fail the fibrous tissue is excised and the nerve freed.

PRESSURE SORES

Nowadays patients are mobilised quickly after surgery and pressure sores are unlikely to develop unless the patient is elderly, recovery is delayed or if the patient lies in one position on the operating table for a very long period.

Pressure sores can be divided into superficial and deep sores. Superficial sores begin in the skin and break down leaving a shallow, painful ulcer. Deep sores begin in the subcutaneous tissues, where muscle and fat have less resistance to pressure than skin; destruction may occur in these while the skin covering them shows only erythema. Eventually the skin breaks down and the deeper necrosed tissues are exposed. Both types of sore are due to pressure which occludes the blood vessels and deprives the tissues of nutrition. In a patient with normal sensation this pressure causes discomfort and he alters his position to relieve it, but if there is loss of sensation or he is unconscious or too ill to move, pressure will not be relieved. Other causes may be (a) ill-fitting splints; (b) friction from rucked sheets; (c) persistent soaking of the skin due to incontinence; and (d) poor skin. The most commonly affected sites are the heels, malleoli, greater trochanters, sacrum and elbows. If a patient is nursed in a propped-up position he tends to slide down and this causes a shearing force on the sacral area, rupturing deeper tissues and small blood vessels and consequently may lead to a deep sacral pressure sore.

Prevention

Pressure sores should be prevented and this can only be done by regular turning of unconscious or paralysed patients either by manual lifting or by nursing them on turning beds. If the patient is sitting in a chair, he should either be taught to relieve pressure by lifting himself on his arms, or be lifted by a nurse or attendant. Splints must be carefully made and well-finished so that there are no rough areas to cause an abrasion. Sheepskins are frequently used under paralysed or heavy patients to prevent friction and the oil content of a *real* sheepskin is also beneficial to poor skin. Ripple or water beds, in which the areas of pressure on the patient's body are constantly changed, are another aid to the prevention of sores. None of these supersede good nursing and regular turning. Physiotherapists can help in this prevention by teaching nurses how to lift and turn patients with minimum effort (Downie and Kennedy, 1981).

Physiotherapy

When treating a patient the physiotherapist should note any areas of redness or broken skin, and report these to the nurse in charge of the ward so that appropriate measures may be taken. If pressure sores occur the physiotherapist may be asked to treat them. If the pressure sore is only superficial, i.e. red and sore, then further erosion may be prevented and healing stimulated by infra-red rays. If the area has broken down, become infected or even necrotic, ultraviolet irradiation may be prescribed. Good team work is essential, and the task will be easier if the nurse prepares and cleans the area prior to the ultraviolet irradiation being applied and dresses it afterwards. If the pressure area is only reddened with no skin break, an ice cube may be used to massage the area (Marshall, 1971).

Traditional physiotherapeutic measures have been indicated, although it is appreciated that there is much discussion as to the most efficient way of treating and/or preventing pressure sores (Barton and Barton, 1981). See also page 192.

HAEMORRHAGE

Haemorrhage may complicate any operation, but is particularly liable when surgery has involved a vascular area, such as the thyroid gland or tonsils. If bleeding is excessive or prolonged, various signs and symptoms will arise; the pulse will be rapid and feeble, blood pressure low, and respirations fast and often of the sighing type. The skin will be cold, clammy and pale. The patient will be restless, feel thirsty and complain of faintness and giddiness. If haemorrhage occurs while the physiotherapist is treating the patient, further help should be summoned immediately and first aid treatment given. If possible the patient should be placed in the lying position and if bleeding is external, digital pressure may be applied above the site of haemorrhage, or directly over the bleeding part.

If sepsis is already suspected, active exercises should be avoided as this could precipitate a secondary haemorrhage particularly between the sixth and fourteenth day.

MUSCLE ATROPHY AND IMBALANCE

The musculature of patients undergoing surgery will vary according to their general health; some patients will be in poor condition such as the elderly patient and those who have been ill for some time, particularly if they are suffering from nutritional disturbances associated with ulcerative colitis or Crohn's disease; others will be in excellent condition but may be affected by the operation.

Muscles may be affected both generally and locally by surgery. Most operations lead to a lessening of general activity and this is as true for a meniscectomy as for a radical pelvic or brain operation. This inactivity can be increased by fear. Reduced muscular activity will lead to a lessened cardiac output, with consequent reduced metabolism.

Locally, muscles in the region of the operation may be affected either through division or through the local nerve supply being damaged. Provided that the muscles are adequately sutured, no lessening of power should result. If the nerve supply is only bruised, full muscle power will return; if however it is divided or excised then there may be residual weakness, e.g. a parotidectomy is quite likely to involve damage to the facial nerve and weakness of the facial muscles will result.

Occasionally during operation, stretching of, or pressure on a nerve may occur. If a relaxant drug such as tubocurarine (curare) is used during the operation there is complete absence of tone in the muscles, and consequently no protection for the nerves. If a position is necessary in which pressure on a nerve might occur, there will be a greater tendency for paresis to result and if an Esmarch's rubber bandage is used for a tourniquet in operations on the knee, a drop foot can occur due to ischaemia of the common peroneal nerve. Neurological damage will depend on the extent of the lesion.

In some operations certain positions may be necessary which prevent active use of the muscles, e.g. in operations for recurrent dislocation of the shoulder, where the arm may be fixed in adduction and medial rotation. Muscle power and movement can be inhibited by pain, fear, or as a result of reflex action. As the result of surgery on joints, distension or damage of the capsule can stimulate the nerve endings and reflex inhibition will result.

In the following chapters physiotherapy to prevent deformity occurring in certain conditions will be discussed.

Whatever the cause, atrophy and hypotonia of muscle will occur in varying degrees following any surgical procedure and the most outstanding effect of this is alteration in posture usually affecting the body as a whole. Atrophy and hypotonia of the spinal muscles will lead to a loss of the erect carriage of the trunk and if the gluteal muscles are also affected an increased pelvic tilt will be followed by spinal deformity. When the patient first gets up and walks, his general posture is likely to be poor; postural flat feet and round shoulders with poking head may be noticeable. If there is unilateral weakness of the trunk muscles then muscle imbalance is particularly noticeable, and may well lead to gross deformity. This is clearly seen following thoracic surgery or where there has been interference with the nerve supply of abdominal muscles. Scoliosis is a likely result and one which can be avoided.

Muscle atrophy can lead to diminished power, with possible serious results, since the muscles are the first line of defence of the joints. Inadequate musculature can result in continuous minor trauma to joint structures with chronic synovitis developing and this is particularly liable to happen following operations on the knee joint unless adequate isometric muscle work is taught.

If the abdominal muscles are affected then their function can be impaired also and not only will posture be disturbed but the intra-abdominal pressure will not be maintained. If intra-abdominal pressure falls, respiration, venous return, defaecation, and support of the abdominal viscera will all be affected. Scarring in abdominal muscles may lead to incisional hernia.

Finally muscle weakness may be a factor leading to stiffness of joints, for if the muscle has insufficient power to move the joint through its full range adaptive contractures can result.

Physiotherapy

Muscle atrophy can be avoided except in the case of nerve involvement. The principle is the practice of active movement, either in the form of active exercises or as static (isometric) work. This should be taught pre-operatively and encouraged for as long as necessary postoperatively. With early mobilisation following surgery, muscle atrophy is rarely seen today.

An important point to be observed is the wearing of shoes rather than slippers; this aids walking and correct posture once the patient is ambulant. The feet are frequently painful after bed rest or varicose vein surgery and exercises for the intrinsic muscles of the foot can be most helpful.

If crutches, sticks or a walking aid are needed, the physiotherapist should ensure that the item(s) selected fits the patient, and that he is taught how to use it.

REFERENCES

Barton, A. and Barton, M. (1981). *The Management and Prevention of Pressure Sores*. Faber and Faber, London.

Downie, P. A. and Kennedy, P. (1981). *Lifting, Handling and Helping Patients*. Faber and Faber, London.

Marshall, R. S. (1971). Cold therapy in the treatment of pressure sores. *Physiotherapy*, **57**, 8.

Mendelson, C. O. (1946). The aspiration of stomach contents into the lungs during obstetric anesthesia. *American Journal of Obstetrics and Gynecology*, **52**, 191.

BIBLIOGRAPHY

Godwin, R. J. (1978). Chest x-rays after abdominal surgery. *Physiotherapy*, **64**, 2, 34–9.

Schonell, M. (1974). *Respiratory Medicine*. Churchill Livingstone, Edinburgh.

Sykes, M. K., McNichol, H. W. and Campbell, E. J. M. (1976). *Respiratory Failure*, 2nd edition. Blackwell Scientific Publications Limited, Oxford.

Wallis, N. Z. (1978). Physiotherapy involvement in upper abdominal surgery. *Physiotherapy*, **64**, 2, 41–2.

Wiggs, S. M. (1978). IPPB with bronchodilators and Entonox. *Physiotherapy*, **64**, 2, 43–4.

See also Bibliography on page 100.

ACKNOWLEDGEMENT

The author thanks her physiotherapy colleagues at the Ashford and William Harvey Hospitals, Ashford, Kent, for their help and constructive advice in the revision of this chapter.

Chapter 10

Relaxation and Stress

by L. MITCHELL, MCSP, DipTP

What is stress? Why teach relaxation? Does relaxation help stress? What type of person becomes stressed? When does stress occur? What is the role of the physiotherapist – if any? This chapter offers a discussion on these questions and indicates how relaxation may be adapted to other conditions as well as being applicable for stressed individuals.

STRESS

This is the body condition in which the physiology is geared for activity. Stress is usually considered useful if the amount of stimulation is suitable for the work to be done, and that work is then done, for example driving a car, giving a lecture, giving birth, and so on. The term *psychosomatic* dates from 1818 and is used to describe bodily diseases of mental origin (Taylor, 1979).

Stress has been described as 'the non-specific (that is, common) result of *any* demand upon the body, be it mental or somatic demand for survival and the accomplishment of our aims' (Selye, 1980). Over the years research into stress and stressors has abounded, and many papers and books have been published. Physiotherapists have been involved in several symposia notably the Fourth Congress of the World Confederation for Physical Therapy in Copenhagen in 1963 and the Annual Congress of the Chartered Society of Physiotherapy in 1977 (Mills, 1978). It is inevitable that such an airing of the subject should produce a descriptive title – stressology.

Stress may be considered as a state of being threatened, either by a life shattering event or something absurdly small. It may be the death of a spouse with all the consequences of loneliness and poverty, or the dislike of the physiotherapist to whom the particular patient is referred. Indecision and the feeling of being trapped aggravate stress.

Holmes and Rahe (1967) drew up what has become a well-established scale of stress: it ranges from death of a spouse as 100 units to Christmas as 12 and minor violations of the law as 11. It demonstrates the point that stressors can arise through happy or unhappy circumstances (Benson, 1977). The menopausal woman may suffer stress not only through physical changes but also because of emotional changes such as children leaving home, death or disability of parents or spouse, or financial change.

Those who have become interested in stressology include doctors, sociologists, psychologists, physiologists, chemists, therapists (occupational, physical, music and art), as well as teachers of stress-relieving techniques.

Physiology

Stressors may be classed as:

1. Physical, e.g. heat or cold.
2. Non-physical, e.g. mental, emotional.
3. Social and psychological (Davison, 1978).

We depend upon our five senses, sight, hearing, smell, taste and touch to receive information from the environment, and relay it to the conscious brain. Information from within the body is conveyed to the mid- and hind-brain and spinal cord. Reflex actions determine the response to that information, e.g. an increase in the rate of breathing to remove the carbon dioxide due to increased muscle work. Joint position, skin pressure, pain and some temperature changes reach the conscious brain. As the result of all this information, plus the memory of past experiences (good and bad), mental and emotional states (grief, pain, happiness), so the state of stress, or lack of it, will be determined in a particular person at any particular moment.

Homeostasis

What then is the reaction of the body to stress? The most important function of the body is to remain in a state of homeostasis – the maintenance of constant conditions in the extracellular fluid derived from the blood that bathes all cells and upon which they depend for life (Guyton, 1974).

THE ALARM REACTION

When the body reacts to threat, the sympathetic nervous system goes into action for 'mass discharge', i.e. the 'fight or flight reflex', or stress reaction. This causes the anterior pituitary gland to secrete adrenocorticotrophic hormone (ACTH); the release of this into the bloodstream stimulates the thyroid gland to release thyroxine, and the medullae of the adrenal glands to release adrenalin and noradrenalin. These hormones will produce the following results:

1. Increase of heart action and blood pressure.
2. Increase in the metabolism of all cells particularly certain muscle groups.
3. Increased carbon dioxide (CO_2) in the blood.
4. Increase in rate of breathing.
5. Increased dilation of the bronchioles and the eye pupils.
6. Increase in blood glucose from the liver, and fatty acids from the fat reserves.
7. Increased sweating.
8. Increased blood supply to the voluntary muscles and the brain.
9. Decrease in the rate of peristalsis.
10. Decrease in gastro-intestinal glandular activity.
11. Decreased blood supply to the skin.
12. Decreased kidney and bladder function.

The sympathetic nervous system continues to act and enhances these results so that both hormone and nervous stimulation proceed simultaneously. Thus, in acute stress, homeostasis may be said to be endangered; in extreme cases actual pathology may result and death can occur.

General adaptation syndrome (GAS)

Selye (1975) showed that the body's resistance has a limit in its response to any stressor: he called it the General Adaptation Syndrome (GAS). This syndrome has three phases: (1) the alarm reaction (p. 116); (2) the stage of resistance; and (3) the stage of exhaustion. Selye says 'There are two roads to survival: fight and adaptation. And more often adaptation is the more successful'.

STAGE OF RESISTANCE

It is at this stage that adaptation can prevent the final stage of exhaustion leading to pathology. It must be remembered that stress is a normal part of life, without it we are barely alive. What is a threat to one person is a challenge to another. It is the *response* to the stressor that determines its results. Carruthers (1974) found during his research into stress in motor racing that 'noradrenaline levels were doubled immediately before the race, and were often more than quadrupled by the end', and yet 'it seems unlikely that they damage their hearts by subjecting them [the drivers] to these brief episodes of stress, as the emotional relief appears to last for several days. It is the overall emotional climate that counts'.

The stage of resistance has been likened to a tightrope walker balancing a suitcase in either hand, one labelled *work* and the other *leisure*, each filled with the necessary constituents. If these activities and satisfactions keep balanced or suitably adapted, he can safely walk across the tightrope. If a change occurs in either which is greater than the individual is able to adapt to, then he may go into the *stage of exhaustion* and finally actual pathology will result. If, however, he can cope by restructuring his lifestyle, possibly including relaxation, then he will be able to continue a balanced life. Wright (1975) has said 'executive health involves what is coming to be called "the whole man". A full medical diagnosis depends on enquiry into, and assessment of, the individual in relation to his environment, his work, home, leisure and social pursuits.'

The physiotherapist having seen the medical diagnosis will need to carry out her own assessment dealing with the following:

Lifestyle

Lifestyle will include the amount and type of work, relationship with associates, conditions of work, degree of job satisfaction or undue competition, monotonous or dangerous work, amount of daily travelling or travel abroad, and so on. Having assessed all these, the individual can then decide whether it is possible to change any of it, or what he would like to change. Quite small and simple changes can alter the stress level dramatically, for example, wearing ear plugs in a noisy work area, taking a walk in the park instead of lunching at one's desk, and so on.

There may have been a sudden alteration in the pattern of life – promotion may entail a different method of working, including a change of work place and associates. Sometimes the gain in prestige and money is not worth the stress engendered, and it may be wiser to refuse promotion. Redundancy presents its own problems.

Women who look after a home, children, and also have a job may be quite unaware of their pattern. The author has been asked frequently by such women for help in relaxing: their comment may be 'Can you help me relax? I am always tired and yet never seem to get through all I have to do'. When the woman is asked to explain further it becomes patently clear that she has gradually taken on the work of several people without realising it – home, children, husband, outside work, business entertaining, and so on. To learn to relax at will is valuable, but it should be part of a pattern of healthy planning of work and leisure.

All this should be discussed with the patient who seeks your help; he will then come to understand what is meant by 'the whole man' approach to stress.

Home and social life

Personal relationships are the foundation of any life. If there is disharmony there will be stress. While physiotherapists must not probe into a patient's personal life, they can *listen*: advice should not be offered except to suggest that it might be wise to seek skilled help.

Disability

Disabled persons, whether long term or recently affected by accident or illness, are often stressed. For these considerable tact is required: heartiness from the able-bodied is not helpful. Always remember that the disabled person has a personality as well as a disability. Personal independence needs to be encouraged at all times. It is no use trying to relieve stress by relaxation if you (the helper) are part of the cause through unthinking, over-robust or domineering behaviour.

The physiotherapist can be a vital link in helping the disabled person and his family to resume a happy association after traumatic changes in circumstances; she can indicate to the family when to give help and when to withhold it. By patience, knowledge and a sensitive understanding of the individual's needs, the physiotherapist can help greatly in this process of re-orientation. A sense of humour can lighten many occasions, and when teaching the disabled relaxation, try teaching it to the whole family as well.

Personal esteem

The sense of personal identity and being accepted by society are very important to the individual. The loss of either may well precipitate the onset of stress. Possible sources include pain, bereavement, disability, old age, lack of money or changed circumstances such as a mother having to cope with a handicapped child or an adult with elderly parents. The therapist has a great opportunity to help re-establish a sense of personal importance by encouraging a reassessment of the whole position and by teaching a method of relaxation to use when stressed. Other experts may be necessary to enable the patient to reach her own decision as to how best to improve conditions.

Diet: alcohol: smoking

There is much written about the value or otherwise of diet in stress, hypertension, and other metabolic disorders. There is conflicting evidence concerning cholesterol as a precipitating factor in coronary heart disease. Patients are best advised to be guided in all dietary matters by their general practitioner and/or dietician.

Alcoholic intake is difficult to assess, and is often a problem for those individuals who answer a stress situation with 'let's have a drink'. Although the physiotherapist does not deal with such matters she should know what treatment has been suggested for the individual alcoholic so that she may reinforce the advice. The same approach applies for those who smoke.

Exercise

Some form of physical activity is essential for a healthy body. A fit person tolerates stress better than an unfit person. Exercise leads to an increase in circulation and heart activity; increased carbon dioxide is given off by the working muscles, followed by increased breathing and general metabolic rate and a general sense of well-being. Exercise falls within the scope of the physiotherapist, though she must not be dogmatic. She should aim to help the patient understand why exercise, in some form, is necessary for everyone, and then help him choose whatever he prefers (Mitchell and Dale, 1980).

Probably the most important advice to give is to start any form of exercise gradually, and not rush from a lifetime of sedentary work to a marathon race overnight. Suggestions of walking one flight of stairs instead of taking the lift, of walking one fare stage instead of taking the bus from door to door, of standing up to dictate and so on; all these minor efforts may well prompt the businessman to take more exercise and enjoy it.

Sleep and rest patterns (Hartman, 1973)

There is much discussion about sleep: some opinions say that it is necessary for 'biological restoration', others that it has no function. All agree that the length and depth of sleep is essentially individual. Certainly one of the rules of nature is a cycle of activity alternating with rest, for example the heart beat.

Sleep may be classified as:

1. Orthodox or non-rapid eye movement for about one hour (NREM).
2. Paradoxical or rapid eye movement for about half an hour (REM).

It is thought that dreaming takes place during paradoxical sleep, because heart beat and breathing become faster and irregular, blood pressure rises and as more blood passes through the brain EEG waves show changes. It is not known whether the brain is sorting out past events or envisaging future ones. Dreaming is considered necessary for recuperation and emotional health. Some drugs interfere with sleep rhythms but the importance of this is not known. Other drugs are sometimes used to induce continual sleep for a limited period of enforced rest.

Regular sleep and rest periods interspersed with work and other activities appear to be normal, and a useful way of resisting stress. Both rest and sleep are essential for health. The substitution of physical effort for mental effort or vice versa, constitutes a rest; or rest may mean a period of calm from all kinds of activity during which relaxation techniques may be practised. For the busy person half an hour in the middle of the day or at the end of the day's work is the ideal routine. Stress is now almost a household word while relaxation is becoming more fashionable. No one will think less of anyone for practising relaxation during the day, indeed they may be envied.

Hobbies: holidays: pets

Some form of recreation is essential for general well-being so beware of those who say they have no time for 'silly indulgences' such as hobbies or holidays. It is quite likely that such people have been sent to the physiotherapist because they are hypertensive or suffering from stress. The physiotherapist, in her assessment, may well enquire about such matters from the patient, and if this is found to be the attitude she will certainly have difficulty in teaching relaxation.

However, she can explain in simple language how the body is affected by tension and relaxation, for example she can explain and demonstrate how merely clenching the fist causes the blood pressure to rise. Thus the patient may appreciate the importance of reviewing his lifestyle and agree to learn relaxation.

Drugs

In the United Kingdom the taking of tranquillisers and sedatives has reached appalling heights: in 1979 prescriptions for sedatives and tranquillisers numbered 24 million at a cost of over 24 million pounds; similarly prescriptions for hypnotics numbered 17 million at a cost of over 19 million pounds. Many patients are unhappy about taking drugs and prefer to stop them as soon as they begin to feel better; however, there are others who become addicted.

There is considerable interest in the discovery that the body itself is capable of manufacturing its own pain relievers and tranquillisers; endorphins are produced in the brain and considerable research is now being undertaken to ascertain how they function and how they can be stimulated to provide effective relief in patients.

The prescribing of any drug is the responsibility of the doctor but it is reasonable to assume that if tense and stressed patients could be encouraged to try 'relaxation' then the need to prescribe drugs could be reduced considerably.

RELAXATION

As this chapter is essentially for physiotherapists who may wish to apply the principles of relaxation to pathological as well as physiological circumstances, it is proposed to discuss fully the author's physiological method. This is suitable for all postoperative conditions involving stress, obstetrics, chest and heart conditions, arthritis where there is pain and tension, the terminally ill and patients with psychiatric conditions.

THE MITCHELL METHOD OF PHYSIOLOGICAL RELAXATION (Mitchell, 1977)

This method was devised by the author during the period 1957 to 1961, and is now widely used throughout the world. It is based on three premises:

1. That stress causes anyone to adopt a certain posture that is recognisable. Therefore not all muscles are tense – only those controlling the posture.
2. That by the application of physiological laws this posture can be changed at will to a position of ease. The muscles holding the tense positions relax by reciprocal innervation.
3. That the changes of stress physiology gradually subside.

POSTURE OF STRESS SITTING

The typical features of tension include:

Face is frowning; the jaw is clamped shut; the tongue is on the roof of the mouth, and there is possibly grinding of teeth.

The shoulder girdle is raised.
The upper and lower arms are adducted and flexed.
The hands are clenched.
The legs are adducted and flexed so that one crosses the other.
The upper foot is either held rigidly in the dorsiflexed position or is
moved up and down continuously.
The head and body are held flexed.
Breathing is of a rapid sighing nature, or gasping with diaphragmatic
spasm.
The person sits on the edge of the chair, often twisted on one buttock.
He may, when not sitting, walk up and down continuously.

TEACHING

When teaching the Mitchell method of physiological relaxation either
individually or in a class, it is helpful to ask people to build up a
picture of the tension position by asking them to remember what
happened in their own bodies or what they have seen in others who
were suffering from stress. In this way they are enabled to recognise
the stress posture and to be encouraged to observe others for signs of
stress. They are always able to remember the positions of shoulders,
arms and hands, often head, body and breathing changes, usually
facial changes but seldom leg and feet changes although when
demonstrated they are usually recognised.

PHYSIOLOGICAL LAWS APPLIED

1. The brain does not order muscle work; it only understands
   movement (Basmajian, 1982). Therefore, orders which are given
   to the body must be for positive activity in joints. They must not be
   for muscle action or relaxation, for example the command might be
   'stretch your fingers', but not 'relax your fingers'.
2. The body is accustomed to receive precise orders from the brain for
   specific performance, e.g. hop, skip, jump. These actions are
   brought about by different muscle work which has been learned by
   the body receiving exact orders carried out repetitively and
   enjoyably. The patterns are stored in the sensory areas of the brain
   as engrams (Guyton, 1972). After much repetition it is thought
   they may be transferred to the motor cortex or basal ganglia.
3. Sherrington's law of reciprocal innervation which states that if one
   group of muscles is voluntarily contracted, the opposite group
   relaxes.
4. Sensation from muscle contraction does not reach the conscious
   brain, only joint position and skin pressure are recognised by
   the cortex (Buchwald, 1967). The sensations become more

appreciated as they are repeated, and produce an engram of the ease position.
5. What the body has enjoyed it will remember and ask for repetition. What has been unpleasant it will forget, avoid or reject.

Treatment

The patient may be in bed, on the floor or sitting in a chair with a tall back and arms; he may be in lying, side lying or sitting leaning back or forward on to supporting pillows on a table.

The head should be supported by pillows, one only if lying on the floor. The arms rest on pillows if leaning forward, while if sitting leaning backwards or lying the hands rest on the thighs or abdomen and do not touch each other.

The principle of this treatment is to teach the patient body awareness following the physiological rules of the body. Therefore no added pillows for so-called comfort are used as this confuses the patient. The lighting should be normal and even bright. There should be no attempt at silence and the physiotherapist should use a normal voice, rather firm and exact, as no attempt is being made to soothe the patient. Music is never used.

The patient is learning to feel joint positions exactly and skin pressures. Probably he has never felt these before, so it is a completely new experience and always pleasurable as the tense muscles relax due to the in-built reciprocal relaxation. He must concentrate and realise he is in charge of his own body. The teacher is not giving him orders but simply saying them so that he may give the orders to his own body as he does every day when changing any position to another.

ORDERS

These orders are as follows:

1. Make an exact small movement in every joint in turn. These orders have been worked out so that they will induce relaxation in the tensed muscles. They will fit any position of the body and the words must *never* be changed. They are in lay language.
2. Stop the movement: the part remaining where it has arrived.
3. Feel the exact position of the joints in the new position and the skin pressures.

SEQUENCE

Shoulders: *Pull* your shoulders towards your feet. *Stop. Feel* your shoulders are further away from your ears.

Elbows:	Elbows *out* and *open*. *Stop*. *Feel* your upper arms touching the support and away from your sides. Feel the open angle at the elbows.
Fingers and thumbs:	*Long and supported*. The fingers and thumbs are stretched out 'long' with wrists extended. *Stop*. The fingers fall back on to the support. *Feel* the fingertips touching the support and the thumbs heavy.
Legs:	*Roll* your thighs outwards. *Stop*. *Feel* your turned out legs.
Knees:	*Move* your knees very gently if not comfortable. *Stop*. *Feel* your comfortable knees.
Feet:	*Push* your feet away from your face, bending at the ankle. *Stop*. *Feel* your dangling feet.
Body:	*Push* your body into the support. *Stop*. *Feel* your body lying on the support.
Head:	*Push* your head into the support. *Stop*. *Feel* your head lying in the support (pillow).
Breathing:	Breathe in gently lifting your lower ribs upwards and outwards towards your armpits, and a slight bulging above your waist in front. Breathe out easily and feel the ribs fall back. Repeat *once* only.
Face:	Keep your mouth closed and drag your jaw down. *Stop*. *Feel* your separated teeth. Place your tongue low in your mouth. *Close* the eyes by lowering the top eyelids only. *Stop*. *Enjoy* the darkness. *Smooth* the forehead up into the hair, continue over the top of the head and down backwards. *Stop*. *Feel* the hair move.

(A full description of these sequences may be found in *Simple Relaxation* (see Bibliography).)

The Mitchell method of relaxation can be adapted for any stressed patient – two groups of patients, obstetric and psychiatric, are discussed briefly.

Obstetric patients (see also Chapter 11)

ANTENATAL

Expectant mothers may be treated singly or in a group. It is wise to emphasise to them that fear of delivery is quite usual, and that this method will help the mother to cope with it. Relaxation is therefore given with the following objectives:

1. To obtain rest during pregnancy.

2. To help the mother during all stages of delivery.
3. To help the mother regain normal health afterwards by preventing unnecessary fatigue.

Pregnancy: The mother should practise the whole technique thoroughly in many positions, also timing.

Delivery: The mother begins relaxation as soon as the first contraction starts. She remains wherever she happens to be. As she has already learned many positions in which to perform the technique, she should adopt whichever is convenient. The mother maintains a slow sustained relaxation throughout the contraction. Immediately the contraction is over she moves and does whatever she wishes. At every contraction, no matter where she may be, she repeats the performance.

The final dilation of the cervix may be prolonged; she should try to obtain, and continue, total relaxation, checking each joint for '*move*', '*stop*', '*feel*' continuously, while breathing high in the chest 'pant, pant, sigh'.

During the second stage of labour, the mother may be in a variety of positions, and may or may not be pushing during the contractions. Immediately the contraction *begins* to pass off she seeks rest for her whole body and flashes the messages of relaxation in a wave down arms, legs, body and head all at once. She rests totally until the next contraction begins and is ready to resume relaxation for the birth of the baby's head. All this should be practised in the antenatal class.

Psychiatric patients

The physiotherapist in a psychiatric hospital or unit works as part of a team so that her part in treatments will dovetail with others.

She usually treats patients in a group for relaxation, and this consists of the usual techniques allied with varying suggestions, for example 'Think of the happiest moment of your life', 'Think of any unhappy experience you had last week', etc. Discussion is intermingled with bouts of relaxation, and each patient is encouraged to talk. Music is never used in these sessions as the patients are concentrating and thinking of body reactions, feelings and controls. If music therapy is used it would be at a different session.

Results of teaching relaxation

1. Tension and ease cannot exist at the same time in one section of the body. As the relaxation proceeds the physiological processes of

stress subside. Noticeable changes are the alteration in the rate of breathing, often preceded by a long sigh, and the eyes closing before the order for this is given. The blood pressure and heart beat are lower.

2. Patients enjoy the treatment, find it easy to learn, and practise willingly by themselves. They often willingly change their lifestyle for the better.

3. The technique can be used to ward off stress during work by using selected orders to relax some parts of the body, while continuing activity on others, or the full treatment can lead to sleep.

4. Often after practice, the patient can discontinue sedatives or tranquillisers under medical supervision.

Other treatments which physiotherapists may encounter are briefly discussed:

PROGRESSIVE RELAXATION (Jacobson Method)
(Jacobson, 1977)

The idea is to teach the patient to be aware of voluntary muscle contraction and relaxation of the same muscle group. 'Doing away with residual tension is the essential feature of the method' (Jacobson, 1977). The physician trained in this method teaches the patient for about an hour, and the patient is then asked to practise by himself for one or two hours a day between sessions. The sessions are continued for several months.

Practice consists of contracting a selected group of muscles, for example the wrist extensors by bending the hand back at the wrist and noting the sensation. Jacobson describes this as 'diffuse, indistinct and characterless'. He asks the patient to ignore the feeling of movement at the appropriate joint, in this case the wrist (Jacobson calls this 'strain') and says these and skin sensations are more noticeable than are the sensations from muscle. This is true because joint and skin sensations, but not muscle tension, are relayed directly to the cortex.

The patient then lets the hand fall back to its resting position on the couch and registers the lack of tenseness, i.e. relaxation in the same muscles. This is called 'going negative'. After repeating this several times, the patient rests for the remainder of the hour. This sequence is taught in subsequent sessions to all parts of the body.

An amended form of this system was taught in the United Kingdom in the 1930s and 1940s and often called 'tense and let-go'.

BIOFEEDBACK

This technique has been developed over the past 20 years and is now coming into the repertoire of the physiotherapist (see *Cash's Textbook of Neurology for Physiotherapists*). By the use of electrodes attached to the body and led into a machine (often portable) the patient is made aware of physiological effects. In the case of stressed patients these would include blood pressure, heart rate, muscle contraction and so on. The patient can be taught to control and change these by thought process. For stressed patients the electrodes register the amount of dampness on the fingers; a light or a buzzer indicates that sweat is present, and as the individual seeks to control his stress by thought, the light or buzzer becomes dimmer or more quiet indicating the measure of success.

There is considerable diversity of opinion as to the effectiveness of biofeedback in the treatment of stress.

MASSAGE AND HANDLING

In time past this was a frequent order in the treatment of patients suffering from stress – then called neurasthenia. It consisted of making the patient comfortable, using pillows and possibly some form of infra-red irradiation, then giving effleurage and stroking to each part of the body but concentrating upon the back. Such a treatment lasted about one hour; there appeared to be good immediate results, but long-term effects did not justify its continuance.

Today, massage is seldom prescribed, although it is still taught in the syllabus of training. There is little doubt that massage teaches the physiotherapist the skilful use of her hands, the awareness of touch and the ability to handle patients comfortably. Massage applied judiciously to a frightened and tense patient can work wonders. As physiotherapists we must remember that our methods of handling patients can cause distress or considerable relief. No machine can really be a substitute for a sensitive pair of hands.

Comfort of the patient extends to ensuring that he is properly supported when sitting up in bed and adequately covered. The head should be supported in the mid-position and not pushed forward or allowed to fall into extension. The physiotherapist should be able to spot the uncomfortable patient and help him, without asking the somewhat fatuous question 'Are you comfortable?' when it is clearly apparent that he is not. Skilled handling establishes the necessary trust and confidence between carer and patient which enables treatments, especially those to reduce stress, to be more effective.

HYDROTHERAPY

Hydrotherapy is exercise involving partial or complete submersion of the body in water, with active or passive movements of body parts, usually carried out by a physiotherapist. It is regarded as a useful method of developing movement and body awareness while supported. All physiotherapists are taught the principles and methods of hydrotherapy as part of their training.

While most patients enjoy relaxing in warm water and carrying out exercise, some do not: therefore be sure the patient will welcome the treatment before attempting it. For those patients who really enjoy water, hydrotherapy can provide an excellent form of exercise and stress relief.

Other techniques which are said to aid relaxation include hypnosis, breathing methods, autogenics, distraction and visualisation, meditation, yoga and so on, but all these fall outside the scope of this chapter.

REFERENCES

Basmajian, J. V. (1982). *Primary Anatomy,* 8th edition. Williams and Wilkins, Baltimore.

Benson, H. (1977). *The Relaxation Response*, pp. 39–41. Fount Paperbacks, London.

Buchwald, J. S. (1967). Proprioceptive reflexes and posture. *American Journal of Physical Medicine*, **46**, 104–13.

Carruthers, M. (1974). *The Western Way of Death*, pp. 44, 45. Davis-Poynter Ltd, London.

Davison, W. (1978). Stress in the elderly. *Physiotherapy*, **64**, 4, 113.

Guyton, A. C. (1972). *Structure and Function of the Nervous System*, pp. 211–12. W. B. Saunders Co, Philadelphia.

Guyton, A. C. (1974). *Function of the Human Body*, 4th edition, p. 4. W. B. Saunders Co, London.

Hartman, E. L. (1973). *The Function of Sleep*, pp. 23–5. Yale University Press, London.

Holmes, T. H. and Rahe, R. H. (1967). Social readjustment scale. *Journal of Psychosomatic Research*, **2**, 213.

Jacobson, E. (1977). *You Must Relax*. Souvenir Press, London.

Mills, I. H. (1978). Coping with the stress of modern society. *Physiotherapy*, **64**, 4, 109.

Mitchell, L. (1977). *Simple Relaxation*. John Murray (Publishers) Ltd, London.

Mitchell, L. and Dale, B. (1980). *Simple Movement*, chapter 7 and appendix. John Murray (Publishers) Ltd, London.

Selye, H. (1975). *Stress Without Distress*, p. 38. Hodder and Stoughton, London.

Selye, H. (ed) (1980). *Selye's Guide to Stress Research*. Von Nostrand Rheinhold Co, New York.

Taylor, G. R. (1979). *The Natural History of the Mind*, p. 135. Secker and Warburg, London.

Wright, H. B. (1975). *Executive Ease and Dis-ease*, p. 11. Gower Press, Epping, Essex.

BIBLIOGRAPHY

Bolton, E. and Goodwin, D. (1983). *Introduction to Pool Exercises*, 5th edition. Churchill Livingstone, Edinburgh.

Clare, A. (1980). *Psychiatry in Dissent*, 2nd edition. Tavistock Publications Limited, London.

Fenwick, P. B. C. et al (1977). Metabolic and EEG changes during transcendental meditation: An explanation. *Biological Psychology*, 5, 101–18.

Gowler, D. and Legge, K. (eds) (1975). *Managerial Stress*. Gower Press, Epping, Essex.

Illman, J. (1978). *Masks and Mirrors of Mental Illness*. National Westminster Bank on behalf of MIND, London.

Kearns, J. L. (1975). *Stress in Industry*. Priory Press, Hove, Sussex.

McLean, A. (1977). *Occupational Stress*. C. C. Smith, Springfield, Ill.

Mitchell, L. (1977). *Simple Relaxation*. John Murray (Publishers) Ltd, London.

Mitchell, L. (1984). *Health for the Over-Fifties*. John Murray (Publishers) Ltd, London.

Norfolk, D. (1979). *The Stress Factor*. Hamlyn Books, London.

Skinner, A. T. and Thomson, A. M. (eds) (1983). *Duffield's Exercise in Water*, 3rd edition. Baillière Tindall, London.

Cassettes and pamphlets on the Mitchell method of relaxation are available for purchase. All enquiries should be addressed to the author at 8 Gainsborough Gardens, Well Walk, Hampstead, London NW3 1BJ (a stamped addressed envelope will be appreciated).

ORGANISATIONS

REMEDIAL SWIMMING
Association of Swimming Therapy, 10 West Way, Wheelock, Sandbach, Cheshire

HYPNOSIS
The British Society of Medical and Dental Hypnosis, PO Box 6, Ashtead KT21 2HT

Chapter 11

Obstetrics

by J. McKENNA, MCSP

Obstetric physiotherapy is the oldest specialty in the profession. Originally it comprised only postnatal treatments but in the early 1900s a new development occurred; the then principal of the School of Physiotherapy, St Thomas' Hospital, London, Miss Minnie Randell, who was a nurse, midwife *and* a physiotherapist, had the foresight to realise that she could help new mothers to recover more effectively if she met them first in the antenatal period. Encouraged by the head of the obstetric unit, Dr J. S. Fairbairn, and helped by a physician, Dr Kathleen Vaughan, she established the first classes in antenatal education. Her book, *Training for Childbirth*, was first published in 1939 and remained for many years the standard textbook for those working in this field.

Since those early times there have been many different trends which, in varying degrees, have influenced today's teaching. In the 1930s the obstetrician Grantly Dick-Read achieved great popularity with his relaxation techniques by which he sought to break the cycle of fear, tension, pain, fear. In his foreword to the fifth edition of *Childbirth Without Fear*, Philip Rhodes describes it as 'A book that has changed the face of childbirth, immeasurably for the better, in the course of one generation' (Dick-Read, 1969). Indeed, to this day, throughout the many changes and modifications of antenatal education methods, relaxation has remained as an essential component.

In the late 1940s psychoprophylaxis came to London from Russia by way of Paris. The word means 'mind prevention', and its followers suggested that women felt pain in labour because they had been conditioned to expect it (Velvovsky et al, 1960). They sought to re-condition a woman to accept her contractions not as painful sensations but as stimuli to various activities, such as rather elaborate breathing patterns. No doubt many women benefited from the training, particularly those having a straightforward labour. But for many others it proved too rigid and dictatorial. Moreover, if the labour failed to conform to an expected pattern, a sense of personal let-down and failure could result.

At this point it is appropriate to quote from Lee Buxton, an American obstetrician, who studied various methods of education for childbirth and concluded: 'The involvement and enthusiasm of all who work with parents seems to characterise successful labour preparation and this is of greater importance than differences in methodology' (Buxton, 1962).

THE ROLE OF THE PHYSIOTHERAPIST

The work of the obstetric physiotherapist may be conveniently considered under the three headings: pregnancy, labour and the puerperium, but this demarcation should not be emphasised. The pregnant woman should be encouraged to look forward all the time to the pleasures of her new family relationship and her postnatal recovery, and this attitude will help her to face labour. In hospital the physiotherapist is often the one person who will see the mother throughout the whole period and is therefore in a position to encourage this positive attitude.

Pregnancy

As well as being a physical experience, childbirth is also a deeply emotional one. Brice Pitt (1978) in his book *Feelings About Childbirth*, cites *anxiety* as the prevailing emotion. He talks of the first trimester as being a time of anxiety for the woman about her own image and sexuality. The second trimester centres around the baby which has now become a reality. Fears of the birth itself and the outcome, feature in the third trimester. All these anxieties are exacerbated by the emotional instability so often associated with changes in hormone levels. Since a major part of preparation is aimed at encouragement and reassurance, the obstetric physiotherapist as well as the whole obstetric team must be aware of this aspect and sensitive to the very special needs of the expectant mother.

Antenatal education is best given in the form of classes of not more than 20 persons so that they can be conducted informally with time and opportunity for discussion. Small groups also ensure that those with particular problems, such as foreigners and single parents, can be given special attention. Wherever possible both expectant parents should be encouraged to attend. Usually six or eight two-hour classes are found adequate. These should be commenced not later than the

30th week of pregnancy and ideally be spread throughout the whole period. Besides advice on the maintenance or improvement of general health, the contents should include an account of the emotional and physical stresses of pregnancy and how they can be relieved. A description of normal labour should be followed by possible complications, a detailed account of the management of labour in the unit concerned and the pain relief available. Advice should be given on diet, breast and artificial feeding, and care of the new baby; often a newly-delivered mother can be introduced to tell the class of her experiences.

Sometimes it is possible to have evening classes: otherwise at least one evening session should be held for the benefit of those whose partners are unable to attend in the daytime. This should include a tour of the whole unit and a discussion of the father's role in labour. It is particularly important that both expectant parents should be aware of the different emotional stresses of pregnancy and the great benefits of a close supportive relationship. Such a wide span of information is ideally given by a team of specialists, the midwife, the obstetrician, the health visitor, the dietician and the physiotherapist. In this way not only do the couples have accurate teaching from those best qualified to give it, but also meet a variety of the staff who will be caring for them.

Since discussion forms an integral part of the programme, each member of the team must have a basic knowledge of the others' specialties. It is particularly important for the midwife and physiotherapist to work in close co-operation. They should plan the training for labour together, so that it integrates with the policies and practices of the unit concerned. It can then be reinforced by the midwife at all stages during labour. Ideally the physiotherapist should be continually in touch with labour procedures and have access to the labour ward to see the results of her work.

The specific role of the physiotherapist in pregnancy is to promote good health and a sense of well-being; to alleviate the physical stresses; and to instigate a training for labour. This should aim to raise pain tolerance, conserve energy and maintain control. The physiotherapist is uniquely trained to assess physical health and to advise on a correct balance between adequate exercise and rest. There are two views on exercise in pregnancy; one, advocated by Elizabeth Noble (1980) and also followed by many yoga teachers, is that special schemes should be practised throughout the period. The other considers that the woman should continue her normal sport or exercise with modifications as necessary, 'she should not alter her regime of exercise just because she is pregnant' (Llewellyn-Jones, 1982). The physiotherapist must be ready to give advice on these points and recommend that a woman should be sensitive to the changing demands of her body and respond to any symptoms of fatigue by resting.

The physical stresses of pregnancy are caused by the increased weight with an altered centre of gravity; an increased blood supply; hormonal changes; and mental anxiety.

The weight increase and the ligamentous laxity caused by hormonal changes can lead to postural problems if a woman is not helped to make the necessary bodily adjustments. The commonest of such problems is backache, for too long considered by the medical profession to be an inevitable consequence of pregnancy. The physiotherapist can bring a wealth of knowledge and skill to refute this view. Good posture must be encouraged throughout, and research has indicated that there is benefit to be gained in teaching prophylactic back care early in pregnancy (Mantle et al, 1981). A careful description of the abdominal muscles can be related to their role in maintaining good posture. Daily living activities must be carefully considered and related to the home and work. These include correct lifting, heights of working surfaces, comfortable positions in sitting and lying as well as in standing and walking. Particular attention must be paid to the sacro-iliac joint. Extra mobility caused by ligamentous laxity can cause torsion strains. These can result in one-sided pain which can extend from the posterior thoracic region down to the heel. In order to avoid this, the pregnant woman should be shown how to perform all *twisting* movements of the trunk (such as turning over in bed and pushing an electric floor cleaner) with the knees gripped together – not apart.

There are different methods of relieving backache, once serious pathology has been excluded, including mobilising exercises and manipulation. The latter is considered quite safe in the hands of experts and may be performed up until the last month of pregnancy. It can be particularly helpful in cases of sacro-iliac torsion. For this condition a medical practitioner in Ontario prescribes an exercise which he has found most successful. Treatment for the right side is as follows: 'In the supine position, the right ankle is grasped by the left hand and pulled into the left groin. The right hand is placed below the knee and the knee is drawn firmly to a point just outside the right shoulder, while maintaining the heel's position in the groin' (Fraser, 1976). Another form of treatment is by a pelvic support belt with or without manipulation according to the severity of the condition (Golightly, 1982). The belt is particularly helpful in cases of separation of the pubic symphysis. However, there seems no doubt that early *preventive* care is the best approach to these problems.

The physiotherapist should give a clear account of the anatomy and function of the pelvic floor (pp. 148–50). It is most important that a woman should be aware of these muscles both for the sake of her labour and the subsequent postnatal recovery. If she can adopt a habit of regular contractions in pregnancy there is a greater chance that she will continue afterwards in the busy postnatal days. Four contractions each time she uses the toilet is a suggested routine. This should be done both sitting and standing so that postnatally she will choose the most comfortable position. As a test of her awareness of the muscles she can sometimes try to stop and start midstream as she passes urine.

Labour training

A programme of training for labour forms an important part of the antenatal classes. Today's methods have evolved from various trends of the past and no doubt will continue to be changed and modified. Instruction must always be directly related to the labour ward routines of the unit concerned and ideally given in close co-operation with the midwife. The overall aim is to give a woman confidence in herself and confidence in those who will be caring for her. Some form of neuromuscular control has been part of the programme since the earliest days of antenatal preparation. The 'fight or flee' reaction of the body to pain must be overcome so that a woman 'goes with' rather than resists her contractions. Grantly Dick-Read (1969) taught that fear and tension lowered the pain threshold and it is sometimes suggested that it can actually prolong the first stage of labour. Those who work with animals have found that this is so and that contractions may even cease if the animal is frightened. It is sometimes helpful to encourage the pregnant woman to apply her relaxation to painful situations (when for instance she is in the dentist's chair) and see for herself if she is able to alter the pain sensation. There are various ways of achieving relaxation or neuromuscular control. The method most generally used and found to be successful in labour is that of Laura Mitchell (Chapter 10). However, *physical* relaxation can never be completely achieved in a state of anxiety; the ease of mind acquired with knowledge and understanding, reinforced by the support of the labour ward staff, is essential.

Formalised breathing patterns to be practised during first stage contractions have featured in many of the teaching programmes of the past. There seems to have been scant physiological basis for them and they have gradually been abandoned. In 1963 St John Buxton, then senior lecturer in physiology at the University of Bristol, undertook a research project in collaboration with the Obstetric Association of

Chartered Physiotherapists to investigate the effects of different types
of breathing being taught at that time. He found that the rigid pattern
of differing levels, such as featured in the psychoprophylaxis method,
caused hyperventilation and increased the stress and anxiety they
purported to relieve (Buxton, 1965). More recently the work of
Elizabeth Noble has supported these findings and resulted in a
completely different approach. As she says 'It is difficult to
understand the justification for altering something as fundamental as
normal breathing, especially during the increase in metabolic
demands that occur during labour' (Noble, 1981).

Rather than impose a regime of breathing patterns it is better to
encourage the woman to be sensitive to the demands of her body and
to concentrate on the *natural* breathing rate during her contractions.
Special breathing patterns should be confined to crises in labour, such
as the need to inhibit the pushing urge if it comes prematurely and for
control during delivery of the baby's head. Some form of gentle,
sighing-out breathing is usually recommended for these situations.
Position for delivery will be determined by the practice of the unit and
should be taught in collaboration with the midwife. Studies have
shown that forced pushing in the second stage with the glottis closed is
unproductive; it causes a marked fall in maternal blood pressure
which may be reflected in the fetal heart rate, and may increase the
need for episiotomy (Caldeyro-Barcia, 1978). As in the first stage it
seems a woman will do better to follow the directions of her own body
(guided by the midwife) rather than submit to a discipline of
behaviour imposed from without.

THE FATHER

For many years in the British Isles it has been recognised that the
father-to-be has an important function in the labour ward. In order to
play his part effectively, however, he must be trained to understand
the needs of a woman in labour. Emotional support is of primary
importance, but it can also be of help to remind her throughout of
what she has been taught in antenatal classes. Physical assistance,
such as supporting her in whatever position she may wish to adopt,
and rubbing her back, is likewise extremely valuable.

The puerperium

The best use of the physiotherapist's time in the postnatal period is in
taking group sessions. This enables her to give more time and
attention to the mothers who will also benefit from each other's
company. Formal exercise should be kept to a minimum: one

carefully chosen exercise for each group of the abdominal muscles is better than a long list. If the mother has had appropriate instruction antenatally, it is more likely that she will continue the habit of regular pelvic floor contractions. It is usually found that *very* gentle contractions done during the first six hours after delivery, while there is a certain amount of numbness, are easier to do than when these are started 24 hours later. The mother who has had stitches needs to be reassured that this exercising will not harm them but will do positive good by increasing the circulation. Occasionally, after a traumatic delivery, a woman may experience difficulty in passing urine. She should be taught to do gentle contractions in rhythm with breathing: 'breathe in, tighten and *hold*, sigh the air out and *relax*.' This method has been found very successful in re-establishing the reflex.

The physiotherapist must take a realistic view of the many pressures, physical and emotional, on the new mother, and where possible incorporate exercise into everyday situations. An example of this might be six abdominal contractions each time she feeds the baby. The main part of the session should be devoted to daily living situations with special reference to the new family commitments. This is similar to the instruction given antenatally: correct lifting, correct heights of working surfaces and protection of the sacro-iliac joint (remembering that the hormone imbalance causing ligamentous laxity can remain for many weeks after delivery). The new mothers should be reminded how periods of relaxation can relieve tiredness and a practice session during each class will be helpful. One aspect often causing tension, particularly in the mother who is most eager to succeed, is breast feeding. The physiotherapist can help her to find a comfortable relaxed position which is the first requisite for success.

Special cases will require individual treatment. The sore perineum following a tear or an episiotomy is usually relieved by salt baths or ice applications. Various physiotherapeutic methods are on trial such as interferential therapy and ultrasound; more work needs to be done before results can be considered conclusive. Ultrasound is often found to be very helpful in cases of dyspareunia following childbirth.

Back problems may need attention. Backache can cause fatigue and add to the considerable pressures on the new mother. Individual advice and treatment is similar to that given antenatally. A woman who has had a caesarean section may need routine postoperative chest and circulatory care although the increased use of epidural anaesthesia has largely obviated chest problems.

The physiotherapist must check each woman for divarication of the recti. If a gap of more than two fingers' width is felt when the woman raises her head in the crook-lying position, special precautions are needed. Exercise should be restricted to carefully controlled inner range contractions of the recti *only*, until the condition improves. In some cases faradic stimulation is to be recommended.

The success of postnatal rehabilitation depends largely on the enthusiasm of the physiotherapist who must supply the motivation to a woman who is often overwhelmed by the experience of motherhood. Sometimes it is many weeks before she feels sufficiently settled into her new life to think about herself. Postnatal support groups in the community are invaluable particularly if the physiotherapist can be involved.

The physiotherapist can make an important contribution to the field of preventive medicine. Two conditions in particular are often related by women to the childbearing period: chronic backache and pelvic floor laxity. It is the responsibility of the physiotherapist to apply her skills in the ante and postnatal periods knowing that good training can have far-reaching benefits. Women should be advised to report back or be referred back to the physiotherapist if either of these problems persist in the months following delivery. They must be told how to check the strength of the pelvic floor after three months in the following way: 'two or three hours after passing urine bounce up and down by bending and stretching at the knees and give two *deep* coughs at the same time'. If there is no leakage of urine one further month's routine exercise is advised. If there is leakage, a further three months' exercise is needed; if after then the test again fails the patient should be referred for further advice and treatment. (See Chapter 12, p. 157.)

POST-REGISTRATION TRAINING

The basic training for physiotherapists contains only the fundamental principles upon which obstetric physiotherapy is based. The need therefore arose for post-registration instruction in the subject. As early as 1948 a group of physiotherapists working in the specialty started meeting to exchange ideas and together formed the Obstetric Association of Chartered Physiotherapists. In 1978 the obviously allied subject of gynaecology was included and the title became the Association of Chartered Physiotherapists in Obstetrics and Gynaecology. The Association was the first specialty in physiotherapy to organise regular training courses, and by 1980 these were being held annually in six centres in the British Isles. Prospective members of the Association are now required to attend such a course and also undergo considerable in-service training.

Members of the Association are well aware of the importance of a close liaison with midwives. An agreement exists between them and the Royal College of Midwives defining the roles of the two professions in parenthood education. Unfortunately the demand for classes far exceeds the supply of obstetric physiotherapists especially in rural areas where classes are often held in remote centres. To meet this need the joint agreement further states that where no obstetric physiotherapist is available, a midwife may take the classes alone after having been taught the necessary physical skills by the physiotherapist. To this end, experienced members of the Association teach in the Education for Parenthood Courses held by the Royal College of Midwives.

REFERENCES

Buxton, L. (1962). *A Study of Psychophysical Methods for Relief of Childbirth.* W. B. Saunders Co, Philadelphia.

Buxton, R. St J. (1965). Breathing in labour: the influence of psychoprophylaxis. *Nursing Mirror,* **120,** 3128, 8–9.

Caldeyro-Barcia, R. (1978). *The Influence of Maternal Position on Labor, and the Influence of Maternal Bearing-down Efforts in the Second Stage of Labor on Fetal Wellbeing.* Included in *Kaleidoscope of Childbearing Preparation, Birth and Nurturing,* (Simpkin, P. and Reinke, C. (jt eds)). Pennypress, Seattle.

Dick-Read, G. (1969). *Childbirth Without Fear,* 5th edition. Pan Books, London.

Fraser, D. M. (1976). Postpartum backache: A preventable condition? *Canadian Family Physician,* **22,** 1434–6.

Golightly, R. (1982). Pelvic arthropathy in pregnancy and the puerperium. *Physiotherapy,* **68,** 7, 216–20.

Llewellyn-Jones, D. (1982). *Fundamentals of Obstetrics and Gynaecology,* 3rd edition, Vol 1 *Obstetrics.* Faber and Faber, London.

Mantle, M. J., Holmes, J. and Currey, H. L. F. (1981). Backache in pregnancy II: Prophylactic influence of back care classes. *Rheumatology and Rehabilitation,* **20,** 227–32.

Noble, E. (1980). *Essential Exercises for the Childbearing Year,* 2nd edition. John Murray, London.

Noble, E. (1981). Controversies in maternal effort during labour and delivery. *Journal of Nurse-Midwifery,* **26,** 2, 13–22.

Pitt, B. (1978). *Feelings About Childbirth.* Sheldon Press, London.

Velvovsky, I., Platanov, K., Ploticher, V. and Shugom, E. (1960). *Painless Childbirth Through Psychoprophylaxis.* Foreign Languages Publishing House, Moscow.

BIBLIOGRAPHY

Anderson, M. (rev) (1979). *The Anatomy and Physiology of Obstetrics: A Short Textbook for Students and Midwives,* 6th edition. Faber and Faber, London.

Bourne, G. (1972). *Pregnancy.* Pan Books, London.

Kitzinger, S. (1972). *The Experience of Childbirth*. Penguin Books, Harmondsworth.

Llewellyn-Jones, D. (1982). *Everywoman: A Gynaecological Guide for Life*, 3rd edition. Faber and Faber, London.

Llewellyn-Jones, D. (1983). *Breast Feeding: How to Succeed. Questions and answers for mothers*. Faber and Faber, London.

McKenna, J., Polden, M. and Williams, M. (1980). *You – After Childbirth: Exercises and Advice for the New Mother*. (Patient Handbook Series, No. 1) Churchill Livingstone, Edinburgh.

Williams, M. and Booth, D. (1980). *Antenatal Education*, 2nd edition. Churchill Livingstone, Edinburgh.

See also Bibliography on page 167.

SPECIFIC INTEREST GROUP

See page 167.

Chapter 12

Gynaecological Conditions

by S. M. HARRISON, MCSP

Gynaecology is the study of diseases peculiar to women especially those affecting the genital organs; obstetrics is the management of pregnancy, labour and the puerperium. It is important to bear in mind that the activity of the genital organs is controlled by the endocrine system, which itself is often influenced by the psyche (mind). While the symptoms of many diseases are psychosomatic, the mind plays a particularly important role in gynaecological conditions. There is a great deal of fear, anxiety and embarrassment associated with these conditions and their treatment. It is only when the patient is approached with sensitivity and understanding, and thought of as a complete person, that treatment may be expected to be effective.

The physiotherapist will meet gynaecological patients in the wards and as outpatients.

GYNAECOLOGICAL WARD

A wide range of conditions and operative procedures may be found on the ward. Vaginal termination of pregnancy and laparoscopic sterilisation are likely to be the most common operations requiring a short stay only; while hysterectomy and repairs are the major form of surgery. Threatened and inevitable abortion, ectopic pregnancy and conservation of pregnancy by insertion of a Shirodkar suture may also be encountered.

Investigations carried out in ward patients include cone biopsy of the cervix, dilatation and curettage (D and C), insufflation of the Fallopian tubes and laparoscopy.

SHIRODKAR SUTURE (Fig. 12/1)

A non-absorbable suture is placed around the internal os (cervix) during early pregnancy in women whose defective cervix has dilated

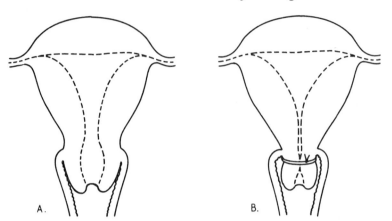

Fig. 12/1   Shirodkar suture. A. Uterus with an incompetent internal os.
B. Non-absorbable suture tied round the cervix at the level of the internal os

prematurely in previous pregnancies, leading to late abortion (18–20 weeks). The suture is removed about 14 days before term. Some authorities insert this suture before pregnancy.

LAPAROSCOPY

A means of visualising the abdominal contents after the induction of a pneumoperitoneum without making a large abdominal incision. Operative procedures can also be carried out by this method, e.g., ovarian biopsy or sterilisation when the Fallopian tubes may be cut by diathermy or occluded by plastic or metal ring clips (p. 162).

Pelvic inflammatory disease (PID)

This is an inflammatory condition of the Fallopian tubes, and often of the uterus, secondary to bacterial infection. The infection may be primary as in tuberculosis or secondary as in gonorrhoea. Infection may also follow abortion or parturition and occasionally follows such acute inflammatory diseases as appendicitis or diverticulitis.

The disease may present as an acute attack of abdominal peritonitis which is treated by chemotherapy and occasionally by the drainage of any abscesses by the vaginal or abdominal route.

As far as physiotherapists are concerned they are more likely to meet this condition in its chronic form, when they may be requested to give a course of short wave diathermy (p. 161). The symptoms of this chronic form of the disease are secondary dysmenorrhoea, dyspareunia and a disturbance of the menstrual pattern. Occasionally, under treatment, the condition may be exacerbated. This will be shown by the fact that the patient will be generally unwell and have an increase in her symptoms. Treatment must be stopped until the gynaecologist has been consulted. *Note*: This condition is often abbreviated as PID, and this may lead to confusion with the shortened form of the phrase prolapsed intervertebral disc.

Hysterectomy

This may be performed through an abdominal or vaginal incision. The latter route being most favoured when symptoms are menorrhagia, uterine prolapse or vaginal wall prolapse. More than one symptom may be present. The incision used for an abdominal hysterectomy can vary from median, paramedian to Pfannenstiel (bikini). Removal of the uterus *only* is a total hysterectomy; one or both Fallopian tubes and ovaries may be included and will be indicated in the title of the operation. When there is a proven carcinoma of cervix (and occasionally for carcinoma of the uterus) the whole uterus, tubes, ovaries, upper half of the vagina, broad ligaments and lymph nodes around the iliac vessels and lateral pelvic walls are removed; this is known as a Wertheim's hysterectomy.

Repairs

There are a wide range of corrective operations relating to the urethra, bladder and vagina.

ANTERIOR COLPORRHAPHY

This is a repair of the anterior vaginal wall for stress incontinence (p. 151) or prolapse of the bladder (cystocele, p. 153). It is sometimes accompanied by amputation of the cervix or vaginal hysterectomy.

COLPOPERINEORRAPHY

This is a repair of the posterior vaginal wall and deficient perineum. It may accompany vaginal hysterectomy or anterior repair and amputation of the cervix.

Operations for stress incontinence

VAGINAL

Anterior colporrhaphy.

ABDOMINAL

These are a series of abdominal or combined abdominal and vaginal operations, the principle of which is the construction of some form of sling to re-form the posterior vesico-urethral angle of the bladder (Fig. 12/2). Such operations are named after their originators, e.g. Aldridge, Millin, Marshall-Marchetti-Krantz, and others. These may be accomplished by the insertion of artificial substances, natural

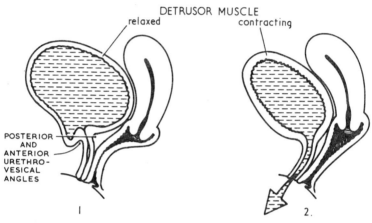

Fig. 12/2   The anterior and posterior urethrovesical angles showing (1) the normal and (2) their disappearance during micturition

transplanted tissues, or the use of contiguous tissues (vaginal). These materials are anchored either to the periosteum and ligaments of the bony pubis or the sheath of the rectus abdominis.

Vulvectomy

An excision of skin in the vulval area for skin disease such as leukoplakia. In the presence of malignancy the incision may be extensive to allow radical excision of the vulva with bilateral block disection of the inguinal nodes. As skin grafting is not often used to close the large raw area, infra-red irradiation is useful to prevent sloughing and speed granulation (p. 147), provided there is no contra-indication to its use.

PHYSIOTHERAPY

Physiotherapy cover on gynaecological wards varies throughout the country. In some hospitals the physiotherapist will only treat patients who develop a chest infection with an accumulation of secretions after a general anaesthetic; other hospitals will have a therapist in attendance for a short period every day.

Statistics indicate that 90 per cent of the major operations in a gynaecology unit are hysterectomies and vaginal repairs. Most of these women will have borne children; thus there are a large number of women, of all ages, whose pelvic floor and abdominal muscles and backs have been subjected to the strains of childbearing. It can be argued that these women will achieve a more complete recovery if they are shown how to strengthen their pelvic floor, abdominal and back muscles, and be given advice on self-care at home. The following points indicate differences in treatment regimes which may be used for other surgical patients.

Deep vein thrombosis

Patients who have had a pelvic operation appear to be particularly susceptible to deep vein thrombosis, therefore special precautions should be taken:

1. If Tubigrip or an elastic bandage has not been applied prior to operation or in the theatre, the physiotherapist may be asked to apply this when the patient returns to the ward.
2. The foot of the bed can be elevated and a bed cradle used to facilitate frequent foot and leg movements. These are most effective if practised slowly and strongly.
3. Extra emphasis should be placed on full chest breathing, practised frequently, to improve venous return and move secretions in readiness for coughing.

Coughing

Secretions are most effectively dealt with if a patient is in a curled-up position sitting up, or in side lying, with forearms 'cuddled' over the incision to prevent movement. They should be shown (preferably pre-operatively) how to move the secretions towards the bronchi with long, easy, slow breathing. Repeated 'huffs' (see p. 89) will project the mucus into the mouth with the minimum of discomfort. For vaginal operations, one hand should be placed on the sanitary towel with firm pressure upwards when coughing.

Pelvic rocking

This activity encourages the viscera to move away from the incision, prevents protective muscle spasm in the abdomen and back and decreases the pain from flatulence by speeding the dispersal of gases. Pelvic rocking should be commenced as soon as possible on recovery of consciousness. It is most easily taught as follows:

The patient is in crook lying with hands resting on hip bones; she is then told to 'Tilt your pubic bone towards your face – hold for four seconds and put it down slowly.'

Repeat in a rocking rhythm several times an hour. The patient will also feel the tilting of her pelvis under her hands and notice her lumbar spine flattening and hollowing. This is a simple, non-threatening and comfortable activity which can give patients confidence to make other movements even after extensive surgery, e.g. Wertheim's hysterectomy.

Correction of posture

As soon as drainage tubes allow ambulation the patient should be encouraged to adopt an upright posture using the phrase 'stand tall'. As the top of the head is pressed upwards, the vertebral column is stretched and opened, the pelvis tilts back and alignment of hips, knees and ankles is corrected automatically. This becomes the 'new posture' after a few days if it is practised whenever upright.

Further activity

The provision of an illustrated leaflet can be useful to promote further activity. If such a leaflet is available it should be given to patients in the pre-operative period so that they are able to understand that a programme of continuous care and activity in hospital and at home will reduce the effects of an anaesthetic and surgery and speed their restoration to normality.

SUGGESTED CONTENTS OF LEAFLET

1. Pre- and postoperative breathing and coughing.
2. Foot and leg movements.
3. Pelvic rocking.
4. Posture correction: 'stand tall'.
5. Pelvic floor information and exercises. Starting dates to be discussed with surgeon after vaginal repairs (see p. 143 for method).

6. Graduated exercises to strengthen abdominal and back muscles.
7. Advice for home care, see below.

ADVICE FOR HOME CARE

In addition to your exercises:

1. When you go home you will tire easily – lie on your bed for an extra rest during the day – for several weeks.
2. Do not return to full-time work until after your post-operation clinic visit (about six weeks after the operation).
3. It is common to have twinges of pain around the site of your wound for a few weeks.
4. Forceful pulling or pushing (vacuuming or opening swing doors) will seem difficult – start when you feel able.
5. Avoid straining to open your bowels – seek advice if necessary.
6. Your bladder will take a week or two to settle down – pelvic floor exercises will help.
7. No heavy lifting. Moderate lifting and carrying must be avoided for six to eight weeks. After this, if the pelvic floor is braced when lifting – especially after vaginal repairs – the effect of the downward thrust in the pelvis is reduced. Get help to lift whenever possible.
   Always remember:
   Bend your knees, hold heavy objects close to you, and twist from your feet and not your spine.
   Teach your family the 'safe' way as well!
8. All operations are different, so it is better not to compare your progress with friends.

Infra-red irradiation and short wave diathermy

Heat can be very effective in speeding the healing of infected and slow-healing wounds. Care should be taken to ensure that an adequate area of skin around the incision is exposed to the heat, as thermal sensation in the proximity of a wound is frequently impaired. The presence of metal within the tissues or in the form of metal clips or buttons anchoring a continuous suture is a contra-indication to any form of heat treatment.

Infra-red irradiation has been found to be particularly useful in promoting granulation of the open areas after a radical vulvectomy. Twice-daily treatment, seven days a week, is recommended.

Short wave diathermy for an infected abdominal wound is most easily carried out using a co-planar method with medium sized disc electrodes placed over normal skin either side of the incision. After an initial thermal treatment of 10 minutes, a 20-minute period repeated twice daily seems most satisfactory. Further details and contra-indications are on page 161.

Physiotherapists working on gynaecological wards will find them-selves in a very emotional atmosphere. This emotion may reveal itself in a coarseness and vulgarity which they may find distasteful. At the opposite extreme there may be a reticence and embarrassment that makes it difficult to achieve any satisfactory contact with the patient.

After major gynaecological surgery the second and third postopera-tive days are the most uncomfortable. At this time some patients start to show concern about the effect of the operation on their femininity. This is particularly true of a hysterectomy. On the ninth and tenth days, just prior to her discharge, the patient may become worried about her ability to resume her role as a complete woman and mother.

GYNAECOLOGY IN THE OUTPATIENT DEPARTMENT

Since there are many gynaecological conditions where physiotherapy is not indicated, the role of the gynaecologist is to select those patients who will benefit from the particular skills of a physiotherapist. As some of these skills are only acquired as a result of post-registration training, it is accepted that some stages of the treatments which follow cannot be undertaken by a student. However, a student can learn much by observing an experienced physiotherapist treating a patient and assisting where appropriate.

Treatments are likely to fall into two categories:

1. Restoration of function by re-education of the pelvic floor muscles.
2. Electrical treatments.

Before describing treatments, some aspects of the pelvic floor and its functional relationship to the bladder need clarification.

THE PELVIC FLOOR MUSCLES

These comprise three layers.

1. Superficial (perineal): bands of striated muscles radiating out-wards to the pelvic bones from the central tendinous point of the perineum (perineal body).
2. Middle (urogenital diaphragm): a sheet of fascia filling the triangular space below the symphysis pubis and the pubic rami. It is

pierced by the urethra and vagina and contains some muscle fibres in the urethral portion (compressor urethrae) and below the vagina (deep transverse perineal). The latter are inserted into the perineal body.

3. Deep (levator ani): composite striated muscles containing Types I and II fibres (Gosling et al, 1981). They arise from bone and fascia inside the pelvic brim passing backwards towards the coccyx and insert into the anococcygeal raphe or levator plate. The muscles are thick centrally and thin laterally towards the obturator fascia. The central portions (left and right-pubococcygeus) send fibres to the perineal body and to the anus (puborectalis). Anteriorly they do not meet around the urethra and vagina – the gap being greatest when the muscles are weak. It is to the re-education of these muscles that physiotherapists must direct their attention (Fig. 12/3).

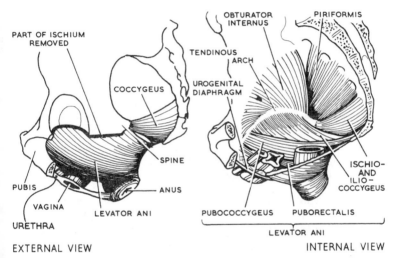

Fig. 12/3   Lateral view of the pelvic diaphragm (external and internal) showing the urogenital diaphragm

Fascia plays an important role in the pelvic floor as it ensheaths the muscles and forms most of their origins and insertions. Surgeons report that the proportion of muscle tissue to fascia is very variable. It is also known that the thinning and loss of muscle fibres laterally is accentuated in obese women and women of advancing age. There is also a correlation of levator muscle mass to general body musculature (Zacharin, 1980).

Comparative studies of the quality of the levator muscles in Occidental and Oriental women have highlighted the greater muscle bulk and less deterioration of the muscles with age in the latter group.

Explanations to account for these changes include adoption of squatting positions for many daily activities, physically hard lifestyle, a diet which discourages obesity and genetic differences (Zacharin, 1977). It is very important to remember that gross stretching occurs in the pelvic floor as a result of childbearing. The effect of this on striated muscles can be resolved by re-education, but overstretched fascia is only corrected by surgery.

Function of the pelvic floor muscles

1. Support of the viscera.
2. Compressive action as part of the closure mechanism of the urethra, vagina and anus.
3. Reflex action in maintenance of intra-abdominal pressure.

Micturition

The bladder is a hollow organ with walls of smooth muscle (the detrusor) and a firm base (trigone). Micturition occurs when the pressure in the bladder exceeds that in the urethra. Funnelling of the bladder neck and relaxation of the levator ani precede the passing of urine (Hutch, 1972) (see Fig. 12/2). The levator muscles then contract, the bladder neck angles are restored and urine that remains in the urethra is milked back into the bladder.

The closure mechanism of the bladder outlet is dependent on a number of physiological factors.

1. The pressure in the urethra is controlled by smooth and striated muscle and has a nerve supply from the autonomic system and not the pudendal nerve as was previously thought (Gosling et al, 1981).
2. Intact angles at the neck of the bladder.
3. The pelvic muscles and fascia.

Urine is normally voided in selected places and at convenient times, each individual having her own pattern of micturition, which can be altered by many factors. When *control* is lost, the person is said to be incontinent and this causes inestimable personal and social problems.

INCONTINENCE

Incontinence is a complex subject and the following information is designed to assist the physiotherapist to distinguish between the various types of incontinence when assessing her patient. It should also help her to understand incontinence when she meets it in other groups of patients, e.g. geriatric patients.

Stress incontinence

This may be a symptom, sign or a condition.

The *symptom* is an involuntary loss of urine on exertion, e.g., coughing or running. The *sign* is the observation of loss of urine from the urethra when coughing or straining, sometimes only when upright. As a *condition* true stress incontinence (as defined by the International Continence Society) is the involuntary loss of urine when pressure in the bladder exceeds maximal urethral pressure in the absence of a detrusor contraction.

True stress incontinence is most amenable to treatment by re-education of the levatores ani as the fault is commonly mechanical, i.e. weakening of the muscles and stretching of the fascia. It is therefore the condition to which the therapist should direct the closest attention.

Frequency

This is usually defined as the passage of urine seven or more times during the day and waking more than twice at night to void. It often presents with other types of incontinence. 'Self-induced' frequency is found in patients who make a habit of voiding regardless of a desire to do so because they are frightened of leaking urine. This habit can be regulated by bladder training (see p. 159).

Urge incontinence

This occurs when the desire to micturate overwhelms the voluntary capacity to control bladder function and spontaneous emptying occurs at any time. It is most easily understood if it is subdivided into motor and sensory categories:

Motor is characterised by detrusor instability and is responsible for about 30 per cent of gynaecological clinic referrals (Frewen, 1978). It is more common in the elderly as it can be secondary to cerebral atherosclerosis. Bladder training is often used to good effect (p. 159). One drug which is commonly used is flavoxate hydrochloride (Urispas).

Sensory is generally related to an acute or chronic infection, urinary calculi or bladder tumour. Treatment is by antibiotics or surgery.

Overflow incontinence

Retention and overflow is caused by an obstruction to the outflow of urine; as the bladder distends and cannot contract properly a leakage of urine occurs at frequent intervals. Impaction of faeces (especially in the elderly) is a common cause, but a large fibroid, an ovarian cyst, a retroverted gravid uterus or a mass in the pelvis can have the same effect. Treatment varies with the cause. Physiotherapy is not indicated.

Continuous incontinence

This may result from a pathological or structural abnormality or be related to major trauma or surgery, e.g. a fistula.

Neurogenic bladder

This is found in a wide range of disorders which affect the brain or spinal cord, including trauma; each requires its own special management. Sometimes termed automatic or reflex bladder.

METHODS OF ASSESSING MICTURITION

In some patients urodynamic, radiological and electromyographic studies have to be used to clarify the problem.

PATIENTS REQUIRING RE-EDUCATION OF THE PELVIC FLOOR

These fall into two groups – postpartum and menopausal. This means that the age of patients being treated may vary from the early twenties to the late seventies. Referrals may come from many sources, e.g. gynaecologists, urologists, general practitioners, postnatal clinics, family planning clinics, health visitors and self-referral by women in the puerperium. The latter is particularly relevant for women who have their babies in hospitals where physiotherapists give them postnatal advice and exercises to combat the effects of childbearing. In such instances, if problems then arise at home in respect of these activities self-referral allows the woman to contact the physiotherapist quickly and receive further advice. Liaison with the general practitioner by the physiotherapist will follow when necessary.

Presenting symptoms

1. Pelvic floor laxity
2. Stress incontinence.

One or both of these symptoms may be present in the menopausal group as a result of progressive oestrogen deficiency. Changes in the vaginal mucosa lead to the hot, dry irritation of senile vaginitis, while in the urethra the mucosa shrinks and allows urine to escape more easily. Oestrogen therapy in the form of implant, oral tablets or topical cream is frequently beneficial.

PELVIC FLOOR LAXITY

When the pelvic floor muscles are stretched and weak the support for the pelvic organs is poor and patients complain of 'heaviness' in the perineal area. Varying degrees of overstretch of the walls of the vagina and urethra (cystocele, rectocele and urethrocele) and uterine supports (1st, 2nd and 3rd degree uterine prolapse) are also found (Figs. 12/4 and 12/5).

Re-education of the levator muscles will relieve these symptoms if they are mild. If there is severe fascial stretching (e.g. gross cystocele or 2nd or 3rd degree uterine prolapse) surgery is required. Pre-operative pelvic floor exercises are worthwhile in most cases.

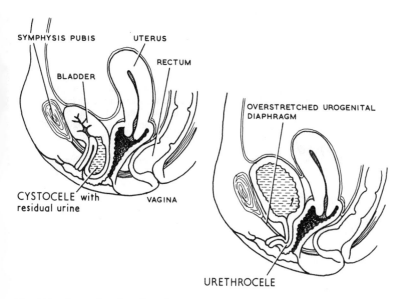

Fig. 12/4   Cystocele and urethrocele

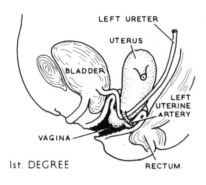

Ist. DEGREE

First degree. Here the uterus descends inside the vagina to, or almost to, the introitus

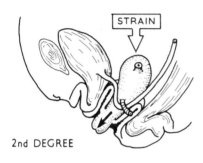

2nd DEGREE

Second degree. Here the cervix projects beyond the vulva when the patient strains

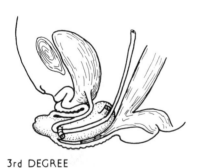

3rd DEGREE
COMPLETE PROCIDENTIA

Fig. 12/5 Degrees of uterovaginal prolapse

Third degree. In third degree prolapse or complete procidentia, the whole uterus lies outside the vagina and most of the vagina is inside out. The cervix may become ulcerated and the acute angulation of the urethra causes difficulty in the initiation of micturition. Hydronephrosis can occasionally be present. It is interesting to note how quickly these severe changes can resolve when the prolapse is reduced. A period of bed rest and vaginal packing generally precedes operative treatment for procidentia

Sexual problems can arise as a result of pelvic floor laxity because the vagina will not be narrowed during intercourse; there will also be difficulty in retaining a contraceptive diaphragm or tampon.

STRESS INCONTINENCE (p. 151)

ASSESSMENT AND TREATMENT OF THE PELVIC FLOOR

Quiet, comfort, privacy and time are essential for the patient's first visit; wherever possible the patient should be seen in a room as curtained cubicles are not acceptable; about 40 minutes should be allowed for the interview.

HISTORY

A chart is a useful way of recording the relevant facts of the patient's history and the results of the vaginal assessment (Fig. 12/6). From the assessment charts it is possible to make comments such as:

1. Patient to be referred to dietician for advice on weight reduction and management of constipation.
2. Advice needed on reduction of smoking to alleviate cough.
3. Pressure gauge readings are noted on chart each visit. Other changes, e.g. decrease in nocturia, frequency and leakage of urine are recorded in patient's notes together with routine for exercises and care at home.

EXPLANATION

This should include simple details about the anatomy of the pelvis with a diagram. Two cupped hands, palms uppermost, hypothenar eminences touching, and a 2.5cm (1in) gap between the little fingers is the best way of illustrating the levator muscles. The compression of the anus, vagina and urethra by the pubococcygeus is shown by bringing the little fingers together and raising them. It is then possible to relate the patient's symptoms to her weak pelvic floor and the need for re-education.

Assessment of the pelvic floor muscles and initial instruction

This is an essential part of the treatment. The muscles are not visible so the therapist must use a digital check or vaginal pressure gauge to assess the contraction.

NAME: MRS A. SMITH   Age: 35   Hospital No: 638 105
ADDRESS: 6 PEMBERSBY LANE
          MARKSTON   Tel: 637
Height: 5 ft. 6 ins.   Shoe size 7   Weight: 12 stone Target: 10½ stone
Occupation: Part time teacher
Description of symptoms and Duration: Leaks urine on exertion — cough
          running and during "keep fit" — since last child
O & G History   (1973) — worse in last 2 years
Parity: 2 + 1

| Date | Delivery | Wt. | Duration | | ? Postnatal pelvic floor ex |
			1st Stage	2nd Stage	
1 1970	♂ Forceps	7lb 6oz	12 hours	1½ hours	—
2 1971	Miscarriage at 11 weeks				
3 1973	♀ SVD	8 lb	3 hours	Fast — 10 mins.	—
4					

Menstruation: ⎫ Pill   Menopause: O
Contraception: ⎭   Coitus: Loss of sensation &
Previous gynae. surgery: D & C 1971   "squeeze"
Medical history:
Other surgery: Tonsillectomy 1960   Other conditions: Obesity
Cough — smoking: ✓ 25/day
        other reasons: O   ✓
Sneeze — allergy: O   Bowels — Loose / normal / constipated

Bladder function:
Nocturia: × 2   Dysuria: O
Frequency: 1—2 hours   Urgency: O
Stress incontinence + unstable bladder: O   ✓
True stress incontinence — mild (occasional) / moderate (every day) / severe (walking) /
Change pants or pads .. 2 or 3 .... times a day

Vaginal examination — ± Effort: ✓
Vaginal prolapse — cystocele / rectocele / urethrocele.   Min / mod / severe / nil
Uterine prolapse — 1 / 2 / 3 / nil ✓
Other symptoms — O

                                    ✓   ✓
Pelvic floor contraction — patient aware / not aware.   Digital — min / mod / strong
Pressure gauge: date .. 7. 7. 82 ....   reading 5 — 3 second hold
                   date .. 11. 8. 82 ....   reading 8 — 5 second hold
                   date .. 27. 10. 82 .... reading 10 — 6 second hold

Fig. 12/6   Assessment chart for re-education of pelvic floor muscles

METHOD

The patient is on a couch in crook lying with knees and feet apart. Wearing disposable gloves and using the thumb and index finger of her left hand the therapist separates the labia and notes if there are signs of vaginal irritation. She asks the patient to cough and then 'bear down', noticing any bulging at the introitus or leakage of urine. Using K-Y jelly she introduces into the vagina the index and middle fingers (or middle only) of her right hand slowly, keeping in mind the direction of the vagina, and locates the fornices and cervix. Keeping her fingers in place, she asks the patient to 'bear down' again – any descent of the base of the bladder, the cervix or anterior vaginal wall will be noted. (If severe fascial stretching is present the therapist's fingers may be pushed out of the vagina.)

The therapist withdraws her fingers until the distal two phalanges are palpating the posterior vaginal wall. On the request 'Don't let me pull my fingers out', the strength of the pelvic floor muscles will be evident by the resultant digital compression if you remember that strong muscles will squeeze the fingers very firmly. The strength of the contraction may be improved by adding closure of the back passage, e.g. 'Close your back passage and front passages, now draw all three up inside – hold for a few seconds and let go slowly'.

When the therapist is satisfied the patient can do this, she concludes the assessment. A vaginal pressure gauge or perineometer is valuable as a teaching aid and over a period of time will demonstrate an improvement in the strength of the muscles as the readings on the gauge increase. (Kegel perineometers, as made by the American gynaecologist A.H.Kegel (1950), are no longer available, but prototype pressure gauges are being tested and it is hoped that they will be in production once preliminary studies are completed.)

Finally, explain to the patient that a definite routine must be followed if the treatment is to be effective.

Routine for exercises

It has been found that a position of sitting or standing with legs slightly apart is most effective, as the weight of the pelvic contents acts as a resistance to the muscles. An effective command is, 'Close the back and front passages, draw them up inside, hold this squeeze and lift for up to six seconds – let go slowly'.

The therapist should check that the patient understands that she should not contract her glutei or abdominal muscles or hold her breath while practising pelvic floor contractions. This is not easy at first, but if she concentrates her attention on the central cleft between her buttocks, she will gradually find she can activate the perineal area alone. As the muscles tire after five or six contractions, the exercise needs to be repeated frequently each day. Discussion with the therapist will ensure that a routine is worked out to suit the patient's everyday activities.

It has been found useful to relate contractions to the clock, e.g. practice on the hour every hour (using an alarm clock or cake timer as an aural stimulus); or linking contractions to activities, e.g. at the sink, having coffee, on the lavatory. Reminders should be given to the patient to brace her pelvic floor (to reduce the downward thrust) whenever she coughs, sneezes or lifts heavy objects. Stopping and starting a flow of urine while micturating is a good 'awareness' test and provides an indication of progress if the stream of urine is stopped more completely, but it should not replace the exercises.

Obesity: If the patient is overweight she needs encouragement to reduce weight or be referred to a dietician.

Persistent cough and sneezing: Chest or allergy clinics may be of assistance. Smoking must be reduced if that is the cause of the coughing.

Follow-up appointments: Patients return for assessment three weeks after the first appointment. Subsequent appointments are at four- to six-week intervals. Those with less severe symptoms will be ready for discharge after about three months (see page 160).

Group therapy

When several patients living near the hospital require treatment weekly exercise sessions as a group can be very beneficial. Patients gain much from contact with others who have similar problems and an element of competition enters for the overweight patients during the weekly 'weigh-in'. The 'pelvic floor group' meets once a week for about 20 minutes. Very little equipment is required; any moderate-sized room is suitable.

Exercises

Pelvic floor contractions are practised in all the variations of lying, sitting and standing, making the positions relate to the patient's daily life. To prevent fatigue of the pelvic floor muscles, strengthening and mobilising exercises for the abdominal and back muscles are interspersed. Posture correction is also taught.

As the pelvic floor muscles increase in strength the contractions can be made more difficult to sustain by practising them while skipping, running or jumping. Coughing, sneezing and lifting with the pelvic floor contracted must also be taught. Duplicated reminder lists of exercises will aid the patient's memory as great emphasis is laid on home practice. The overweight patients are weighed each week and their weight is recorded.

Results

Page 160 shows a retrospective study (1970–76) of 212 patients with stress incontinence who were treated by muscular re-education.

POINTS OF INTEREST FROM RESULTS

1. Initial diagnosis of stress incontinence was made clinically – urodynamics were not used.
2. In all but 16 cases (previous repairs) muscular re-education was the first treatment of choice.
3. Stress incontinence which persists through one or more operations to remove it can frequently be cured by re-education of the pelvic floor muscles.

Bladder retraining

Physiotherapists who are able to teach re-education of the pelvic floor can be involved in bladder retraining. This may be done in the ward or in the outpatient department. Each time the desire to pass urine is felt the pelvic floor is contracted in an effort to delay micturition. If the delay time is slowly lengthened an appreciable improvement in urgency and frequency can be obtained in a few weeks.

Geriatrics

As elderly people become inactive the pelvic floor muscles may atrophy through lack of stimulus of changing intra-abdominal pressure. This leads to difficulty in stopping the act of voiding. It would seem sensible to encourage general activity and attempting to 'stop and start' the stream of urine each time urine is passed. As confidence improves an element of retraining may be possible.

1.	Success (no further stress incontinence)	199	93%
	Failure	13	7%
		212	

2.	Failures – Causes		
	Severe cough	3	
	Gross obesity	1	
	Inappropriate selection in gynaecological clinic (too much utero-vaginal prolapse)	9	
		13	

3.	Duration of successful treatments		
	3–5 months	154	77%
	6–9 months	45	23%
		199	

4.	Pre- or postmenopausal		
	Pre-menopausal	154	72%
	Postmenopausal	58	28%
		212	

5.	Previous failed repairs for stress incontinence (SI), then treated by muscular re-education – 16 out of 212		
	One previous repair for SI	11	
	Two previous repairs for SI	2	
	Three previous repairs for SI	3	
		16 all successful	

6.	Obesity in group of 212		
	*Normal weight	133	59%
	5kg overweight	79	41%

*Standard tables height/weight

Results of a retrospective study (1970–76) (see p. 159)

ELECTRICAL TREATMENTS

Short wave diathermy

The resolution of some gynaecological conditions can be accelerated by the application of heat. The short wave diathermic current is of high frequency and alternating and does not stimulate motor or sensory nerves. It is therefore ideal for heating tissues as deeply placed in the pelvis as the female reproductive organs.

TREATMENT OF INFECTED WOUNDS (p. 147)

PELVIC INFLAMMATORY DISEASE (p. 142)

This responds well to short wave diathermy. It is best treated by the cross-fire method with the patient in lying and side-lying positions on a couch or in a canvas and wood deck-chair. In most cases a thermic initial treatment of five minutes each way followed by treatments of 10 minutes each way daily for two weeks, then three-times weekly for two or three weeks is required. There has been a tendency to stop treatment too early with long-standing pelvic inflammatory disease.

Precautions especially relevant in the treatment of gynaecological patients by short wave diathermy

CLOTHING

The patient should remove all her garments from her waist down to her feet. The skin of the abdomen, buttocks and thighs can then be adequately inspected for scars or other blemishes.

SKIN SENSATION

Every area that is to be treated should be tested for sensation to heat and cold, paying particular attention to any scarred area which may show altered reactions.

MOISTURE

Great care should be taken to see that the perineum and inner aspects of the thighs are dry, as moisture will cause a concentration of the electric field. If the patient is obese a dry Turkish towel could be placed between her thighs.

INTRA-UTERINE DEVICES

These contraceptive devices have been found to lose their shape when subjected to short wave diathermy. Metal devices like the 'Copper 7' concentrate the field.

It is the author's opinion that short wave diathermy is *contra-indicated* for a patient fitted with an intra-uterine device.

MENSTRUATION

It has been the practice not to treat a patient who is menstruating. The author has found it unnecessary to suspend treatment at this time unless the patient has very heavy periods or secondary dysmenor-rhoea. The sanitary protection should be removed before treatment, whether it is a pad or tampon, and the perineum thoroughly dried. The patient can sit on a paper towel if she feels she may soil the towelling. A clean pad or tampon can be replaced after treatment.

PREGNANCY

The effects of short wave diathermy on a fetus are unknown, therefore pregnant women should not be treated. Patients anticipating or suspecting pregnancy should inform the therapist.

LAPAROSCOPIC STERILISATION

If the Fallopian tubes have been occluded by plastic or metal ring clips, short wave diathermy is contra-indicated.

The presence of pacemakers, hearing aids or items of replacement or fixation surgery should be checked by the physiotherapist.

Faradism

If the pelvic floor muscles are very weak patients can experience difficulty in practising exercises; the resultant contractions are so small that the effect on the surrounding tissues and, therefore, the patient's sensation is minimal.

Vaginal or rectal faradism is sometimes used to enhance the contractions, acting as a sensory stimulus, and thus encourage the patient to greater voluntary effort. It can be an uncomfortable treatment which necessitates an internal electrode and a large indifferent electrode on the lower abdomen or sacrum (Scott et al, 1969). The few occasions when the author has used faradism (in women) the internal electrode was placed in the vagina; it is normally in this anterior portion of the pubococcygeus muscles that the contraction needs to be encouraged. Electrical stimuli and active contractions should be interspersed with rest periods. After six to eight treatments the exercises should be continued at home without the faradism.

Electronic stimulators for the pelvic floor muscles, either as implants or vaginal/rectal electrodes connected to batteries worn round the waist are the subject of experiment with indefinite results at present.

Interferential therapy

In the last 10 years many physiotherapy departments have been using this type of current to treat a variety of conditions. Unfortunately there has been little research or clinical studies to guide intending users.

Interferential therapy appears to facilitate healing by utilising a bio-electric effect (De Domenico, 1981). Bio-electric currents occur throughout the body and the majority occur within the same biological frequency and range of 1–100Hz. The most familiar of these to physiotherapists is the electrical activity in nerve and muscle tissue seen in an electromyogram.

The basic physiological effects claimed for interferential therapy are: (a) relief of pain; (b) stimulation of cellular processes (healing effects); (c) autonomic effect (mostly depression of sympathetic activity); and (d) stimulation of motor nerve and striated muscle tissue. The latter is of minimal functional use in the re-education of muscle. The effects vary from a strong tetanic contraction produced by high intensity at 100Hz constant (very painful) to twitch-type contractions at 1–10Hz (rhythmic or constant).

APPLICATION

Urinary incontinence is the most commonly treated pelvic disorder. Many therapists claim success in treating stress incontinence by interferential therapy; it would seem likely that it is detrusor instability (which is present except in genuine stress incontinence) that is being 'damped down' by the autonomic effect of the treatment. However, as the autonomic nervous system also supplies the urethral tissues, including the striated muscle in the walls of the middle of the urethra (Gosling et al, 1981) interferential therapy may have an effect here too.

Treatment details vary; some therapists using a rhythmic sweep from 0–100Hz for 15 minutes thus including the twitch-type contractions at lower frequency and autonomic effect in the range nearer 100Hz. Other therapists separate the upper and lower frequencies by suggesting a rhythmic sweep 80–100Hz for 10 minutes then 5 minutes at 1Hz constant frequency with the patient attempting occasional voluntary contractions.

As this is a non-invasive, relatively comfortable treatment suitable for all age-groups, it could be very useful when evaluated and more precise clinical instructions can be given.

Patients with long-term chronic pelvic inflammatory disease may derive greater benefit from the analgesic and healing effects of interferential therapy as opposed to short wave diathermy.

PRECAUTIONS AND CONTRA-INDICATIONS

Interferential therapy is a relatively safe treatment as there is no heating or mechanical effects in the tissues or electrochemical burns. Consideration should be given to the following:

1. Check condition of skin (avoid or insulate open areas).
2. Skin test for sharp/blunt sensitivity to pain.
3. Avoid febrile conditions, malignancy or pulmonary tuberculosis, or purulent conditions.
4. It is contra-indicated to abdomen and pelvis in pregnancy (effect on fetus unknown).
5. It is contra-indicated in severe cardiac conditions, severe hypotension or hypertension.
6. It is contra-indicated if cardiac pacemakers are in use.
7. Avoid using it on anyone who has comprehension difficulties.
8. Avoid using it in areas of excessive bleeding.

Ultrasound

Ultrasonic energy is a form of mechanical energy with frequencies beyond the range of audible sound, i.e. greater than 20 000Hz. Varying frequencies of ultrasound are used in medicine (Sanders and James, 1980):

Medical usage	Intensity (watts/cm^2)
Surgical	> 10
Therapeutic	0.5–3
Diagnostic	0.001–0.1

Therapeutic ultrasound is widely used in the treatment of recent injuries for its beneficial effect on pain, traumatic and inflammatory conditions and on scar tissue. The immediate effects of childbearing on the perineal area are frequently pain, trauma and inflammation and these respond readily to isonation. Unfortunately that is not the end of the problem; the resulting scar tissue often gives rise to varying

degrees of dyspareunia and distress and thus becomes a gynaecological problem.

New scar tissue will always shorten unless it is repeatedly stretched.
This is due to the property of collagen to gradually shorten when it is
fully formed. This occurs from the third week to the sixth month after
the injury (Evans, 1980). This scar tissue may be superficial as a result
of an episiotomy, or perineal tear, or in deeper tissues, perhaps the
posterior vaginal wall.

TREATMENT

Daily pulsed ultrasound of 3MHz at 0.5 watts/cm^2 pulse ratio 4:1 for
five minutes works well. For deeper areas 1MHz at 0.5 watts/cm^2
pulse ratio 2:1. The transducer is applied in contact and a coupling
agent is used.

Despite the absence of figures from clinical studies it has been
noticed that this is a very successful gynaecological treatment, both in
terms of patient recovery, small number of treatments and economy of
a physiotherapist's time. The softening and stretching of the scar
tissue which follows insonation appears to be permanent. Lehmann
(1965) and Patrick (1978) report this 'softening' effect, but opinions
vary about the efficacy of insonation on scar tissue over six months old.

PRECAUTIONS

Burns: Pain or pins and needles are warning signs – care should be
taken over de-sensitised areas.
Cavitation: A non-thermal effect where bubbles are generated in
sound field – it can be stable or transient. Movement of the transducer
lessens the chance of this occurring (Coakley, 1978).
Overdose: Opinions differ as to a safe dose, but it is generally advisable
to increase duration of treatment rather than intensity.
Damage to crystal: Tests should be carried out in the normal way prior
to treatment. The transducer must remain in contact with coupling
medium while emitting.

CONTRA-INDICATIONS

Deep venous thrombosis
Acute infections
Pregnant uterus (in area to be treated)
Tumours
Radiotherapy to the area requiring treatment (for six months)
Cardiac patients should be treated with care
There are differing opinions as to excluding all patients with
pacemakers from treatment

The role of the physiotherapist does not only lie in the assessment and treatment of the patient's symptoms as mentioned in this chapter.

Prophylaxis must be her aim. Her knowledge of the musculo-skeletal changes in pregnancy, labour and the puerperium should be used to minimise the effects of these processes on women.

Patient care starts during antenatal classes and should include instruction to the student midwives, district midwives and health visitors who have no obstetric physiotherapist working with them. Constant attention should be given to postnatal advice, and particularly exercise schemes and booklets to ensure they are accurate and realistic in teaching self-care to the patients.

Patients in the postnatal ward who have a history of stress incontinence or pelvic laxity should be checked in the physiotherapy outpatient department until they are symptom free. Antenatal, postnatal and gynaecology clinics should have access to a physio-therapist for consultation and referral of patients.

It is by this combination of prophylaxis and active treatment that the physiotherapist can contribute so much to the alleviation of many of the physical problems of modern women of all age groups.

REFERENCES

Coakley, W. T. (1978). Biophysical effects of ultrasound at therapeutic intensities. *Physiotherapy*, **64**, 6, 168.

De Domenico, G. (1981). *Basic Guidelines for Interferential Therapy*, chapter 1. Theramed Books.

Evans, P. (1980). The healing process at cellular level: A review. *Physiotherapy*, **66**, 8, 256.

Frewen, W. K. (1978). An objective assessment of the unstable bladder of psychosomatic origin. *British Journal of Urology*, **50**, 246–9.

Gosling, J. A., Dixon, J. S., Critchley, H. O. D. and Thompson, S. A. (1981). A comparative study of the human external sphincter and periurethral levator ani muscles. *British Journal of Urology*, **53**, 35.

Hutch, J. A. (1972). *Anatomy and Physiology of the Bladder, Trigone and Urethra*. Appleton-Century-Crofts, New York.

Kegel, A. H. (1950). The physiological treatment of urinary stress incontinence. *Journal of Urology*, **63**, 5.

Lehmann, J. F. (1965). *Ultrasound Therapy*. Chapter in *Therapeutic Heat and Cold*, 2nd edition, pp. 321–86 (ed Licht, S.). Williams and Wilkins, Baltimore.

Patrick, M. K. (1978). Applications of therapeutic pulsed ultrasound. *Physiotherapy*, **64**, 4, 104.

Sanders, R. C. and James, A. E. (1980). *Principles and Practice of Ultrasonography in Obstetrics and Gynaecology*, 2nd edition. Appleton-Century-Crofts, New York.

Scott, B. O., Green, V., Couldrey, B. M. (1969). Pelvic faradism: Investigation of methods. *Physiotherapy*, 55, 8, 302.
Zacharin, R. F. (1977). A Chinese anatomy. The pelvic supporting tissues of the Chinese and Occidental female compared and contrasted. *Australian and New Zealand Journal of Obstetrics and Gynaecology*, 17, 1–10.
Zacharin, R. F. (1980). Pulsion enterocele: Review of the functional anatomy of the pelvic floor. *Obstetrics and Gynecology*, 55, 2, 35.

BIBLIOGRAPHY

Garrey, M. M., Govan, A. D. T., Hodge, C. and Callender, R. (1978). *Gynaecology Illustrated*, 2nd edition. Churchill Livingstone, Edinburgh.
Harrison, S. M. and Mandelstam, D. (1982). *The use of exercises in pelvic floor re-education in women. An analysis of technique.* Paper given at the World Congress of Physical Therapy, Stockholm. Included in the Proceedings published by the WCPT, London.
Jordan, J. A. and Stanton, S. L. (1982). *The incontinent woman.* Paper given at a scientific meeting of the Royal College of Obstetricians and Gynaecologists. Included in the Proceedings published by the Royal College of Obstetricians and Gynaecologists, London.
Llewellyn-Jones, D. (1982). *Fundamentals of Obstetrics and Gynaecology*, 3rd edition, Vol 2 *Gynaecology*. Faber and Faber, London.
Mandelstam, D. (ed) (1980). *Incontinence and Its Management*. Croom Helm, London.
Savage, B. (1984). *Interferential Therapy*. Faber and Faber, London.
Soule, S. D. et al (1966). Oral protective enzyme (chymoral) in episiotomy patients. *American Journal of Obstetrics and Gynecology*, 95, 6.
Zacharin, R. F. (1972). *Stress Incontinence of Urine*. Harper and Row, New York.
See also Bibliography on page 140.

SPECIFIC INTEREST GROUP

In the United Kingdom there is a specific interest group – The Association of Chartered Physiotherapists in Obstetrics and Gynaecology. Interested readers may seek further information from the secretary of the Association, c/o The Chartered Society of Physiotherapy, 14 Bedford Row, London WC1R 4ED.

ACKNOWLEDGEMENTS

The author thanks Mr J. Carron Brown, consultant obstetrician and gynaecologist the United Norwich Hospitals, who gave her so much assistance and encouragement with the original chapter. In this revision she has appreciated the help, advice and co-operation from her colleagues in many disciplines at the John Radcliffe Maternity Hospital, Oxford, and from members of the Association of Chartered Physiotherapists in Obstetrics and Gynaecology.

Chapter 13

Head and Neck Surgery

by P. A. DOWNIE, FCSP

This chapter will consider those disorders of the head and neck which the physiotherapist may encounter from time to time. The anatomy and physiology of the head and neck and its contents can be studied in any standard textbook and it is not proposed to describe this except where it is necessary to explain the disorder and its consequent treatment.

BLOCK DISSECTION OF CERVICAL LYMPH NODES

A block dissection of the cervical lymph nodes is frequently carried out when there is malignant disease in the head and neck region. Sometimes it is performed as a procedure in itself but it may well be part of a more radical procedure involving either removal of the larynx, a hemi-mandibulectomy, or glossectomy. It may be bilateral or it may involve only one side. The spinal accessory nerve is almost always divided or excised in the process of dissection; this is because of its anatomical position and also because quite often it is involved in the disease process.

Physiotherapy

The most important requirement for these patients is the teaching of shoulder shrugging exercises before operation and then ensuring that they are carried out postoperatively. The physiotherapist may be asked to treat the chest as well, though this is not required routinely. If however the patient is a known smoker or chronic bronchitic, and many of them are, and if the surgery is more extensive than a straightforward block dissection, chest physiotherapy may be required. Shoulder exercises are the main requirement together with encouragement to move the neck. If exercises are not taught, encouraged and supervised, the trapezii will atrophy and a frozen shoulder will quickly follow. All this is preventable (Downie, 1975).

FACIAL PALSY

Facial palsy is one of the complications of disease of the middle and inner ear. The facial nerve can be compressed or damaged in any part of its course, but as a complication of aural disease it is in its intratemporal course that it will be affected. During this part of the course the nerve, in the narrow bony facial canal, runs from the internal auditory meatus laterally above the labyrinth for a short distance. It makes a right-angled turn back (the genu), then runs down and back in the medial wall of the tympanic cavity (Fig. 13/1)

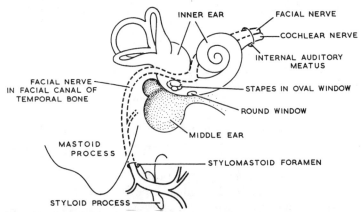

INNER EAR   FACIAL NERVE

COCHLEAR NERVE

INTERNAL AUDITORY MEATUS

FACIAL NERVE IN FACIAL CANAL OF TEMPORAL BONE

STAPES IN OVAL WINDOW

ROUND WINDOW

MIDDLE EAR

MASTOID PROCESS

STYLOMASTOID FORAMEN

STYLOID PROCESS

Fig. 13/1   Lateral view of the intratemporal course of the right facial nerve

and finally passes vertically down in the posterior wall of the cavity surrounded by mastoid air cells. The bony wall of the canal is very thin and may actually be deficient at one or more points.

Due to its position, the canal and nerve may be involved in ear diseases and in surgery, the nerve becoming inflamed, compressed or injured.

Acute infections of the middle ear can involve the sheath of the nerve, especially if an infected mastoid air cell lies just above the nerve in the absence of the bony wall of the canal.

Erosion of the bony wall of the canal is liable to occur in chronic suppurative otitis media, either by infection or a cholesteatoma.

In surgery the nerve may be damaged during the operation or by the displacement of fragments of bone. It may be compressed by haemorrhage or oedema.

In addition to involvement in diseases of the ear the nerve may also be damaged in this part of its course in fractures of the temporal bone. Idiopathic facial palsy (Bell's palsy) can also occur. The cause is unknown and there is no apparent disease of the ear. Groves (1971) postulated the theory that vasospasm results in swelling and ischaemia and consequently compression of the nerve. Such ischaemia could be the result of exposure to draughts and cold.

Types of lesion

The lesion may be a neurapraxia due either to compression by blood or exudate, or caused by bruising. Alternatively, there may be degeneration of the nerve if compression is not relieved or the nerve is damaged during surgery. A combination of both types of lesion is possible.

TREATMENT

A careful assessment has to be made before treatment can be decided upon, in order to estimate the type and level of the lesion. Such assessment includes a test of motor function, nerve conductivity tests and strength-duration measurements, electromyography, and lacrimation, hearing and taste tests. Treatment is then decided upon according to the above tests and the speed of onset and progression of the paralysis.

Facial paralysis developing during acute middle ear infections will usually recover completely without special treatment once the primary condition is treated.

Should the paralysis occur in chronic suppurative otitis media, exploration is usually considered essential. The facial canal is opened and if there is fibrosis and degeneration, the sheath of the nerve is incised, fibrous tissue removed and a nerve graft is carried out. Any cutaneous nerve may be used. Recovery is likely to be slow – some months – and may not be complete.

The onset of facial palsy immediately after aural surgery is likely to indicate that the nerve has been damaged. The surgeon will explore at once and carry out a decompression or graft according to what he finds.

A delayed paralysis following surgery will indicate either too tight packing in the ear, slight contusion of the nerve or, if the paralysis is increasing, bleeding into the facial canal. This will require either removal of the packing or exploration of the facial canal.

Idiopathic facial palsy rarely requires treatment. Many patients recover within two to three weeks without treatment. Some patients recover very slowly, those in whom some nerve fibres have degenerated. A few never gain full recovery and in these there has been total degeneration. Some surgeons treat the patient with adrenocorticotrophic hormone (ACTH) and claim excellent results, others have tried decompression but as yet there is no certain proof that this is effective. Usually treatment is medical and includes reassurance of the patient, care of the eye, exercises for the facial muscles and support for the paralysed muscles.

In all cases general care of the patient as described above for idiopathic facial palsy is essential and physiotherapy is usually ordered.

Physiotherapy

Physiotherapy is usually ordered whatever the type of lesion, since there will be a short or long period before full recovery of the facial muscles. In some cases complete recovery may not occur.

The measures which may be taken include: nerve conductivity tests; strength-duration curves; movement using proprioceptive neuromuscular facilitation (PNF) techniques; infra-red therapy; occasionally ice therapy; occasionally electrical stimulation.

NERVE CONDUCTIVITY TESTS

When facial palsy appears immediately after surgery, a nerve conductivity test may be requested at an early stage, from three to ten days. If the nerve has been completely severed there will be immediate failure in conductivity and no muscle response, whereas if there is a muscle twitch the nerve cannot have been severed.

The usual method of carrying out the test is to have the patient in the lying position. A small button electrode is placed at the exit of the nerve from the stylomastoid foramen and the indifferent electrode on the neck. A pulse of one millisecond is used. The intensity of current needed to obtain a minimal visible contraction on the normal side is compared with that needed on the affected side.

STRENGTH-DURATION CURVES

These are carried out when necessary to determine the type of nerve lesion and the patient's progress (Fig. 13/2).

MOVEMENTS

While there is no ability to contract the muscles the physiotherapist

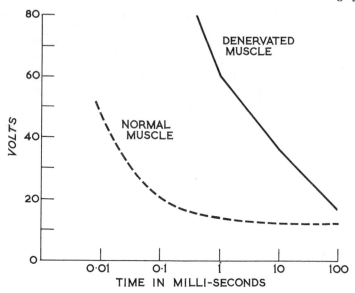

Fig. 13/2   A strength-duration curve

may do the movement for the patient, who is asked to try to 'feel' it and to attempt to hold it. As power begins to return the patient tries to join in and PNF techniques may be used. A spatula can be placed inside the cheek and the patient is asked to pull the cheek in as it is pressed out by the spatula.

INFRA-RED AND ICE THERAPY

The small, delicate facial muscles waste quickly, and can become fibrotic and contracted if recovery is delayed. Stimulation of the circulation and nutrition is therefore valuable, consequently gentle heat is often given before movement. Ice could be used but it has the disadvantage of causing rupture of tiny superficial veins, which is not desirable on the face.

ELECTRICAL STIMULATION

This is rarely used today but occasionally if a patient cannot get the 'idea' of the movement, when paralysis has been present for some time, electrical stimulation can be used until he has acquired the 'feel' and knows what to try to do.

In some patients as the nerve recovers, associated movements tend to occur, for example, as the patient closes the eye the corner of the mouth shoots up. It may be difficult to prevent this but if the patient is shown what is happening he can be encouraged to make an effort to control it.

The physiotherapist will encourage the patient to take care of the eye, stressing that he should not go out without covering it. If trouble does occur she must report it at once.

HYPOPHYSECTOMY

This is the surgical removal of the pituitary gland (hypophysis cerebri). It may be performed on patients who have multiple bone mestastases resulting from a primary carcinoma of breast, prostate or occasionally thyroid. It is known that some of these tumours are hormone dependent and although bilateral oophorectomy and/or adrenalectomy are more frequently performed, some units prefer the operation of hypophysectomy.

The results of this operation can be quite dramatic particularly in the relief of pain if that has been the predominant feature.

Hypophysectomy may be carried out by a neurosurgeon, or an ear, nose and throat (ENT) specialist. If surgical removal is considered undesirable, ablation of the gland may be achieved by the implantation of yttrium rods in the pituitary fossa. This latter will be carried out under radiographic control by a radiotherapist. Surgical removal of the gland or radiation ablation is normally carried out using a transsphenoidal approach and under general anaesthesia. Two other approaches may occasionally be used, the transfrontal or trans-ethmoidal.

Following surgery the patient will require replacement drug therapy for the rest of life; this will include steroids, thyroid extract and occasionally Pitressin.

Physiotherapy

Breathing exercises should be taught pre-operatively and it should be carefully explained to the patient that as he will be nursed in a recumbent position postoperatively, these exercises are very important. He must also be told to avoid blowing his nose, and to reduce coughing to a minimum so that a cerebrospinal fluid leak is avoided.

If the metastatic bone disease has affected the vertebral column it is not uncommon to find that these patients are in a spinal jacket and in which case breathing exercises are even more vital.

Bed exercises should be taught and encouraged and mobilisation and general rehabilitation will need to be assessed and graded according to the patient's condition and capabilities.

JAW SURGERY

Increasingly, the physiotherapist is being more involved in the treatment of patients who undergo jaw surgery for malignant disease. Maxillo-facial fractures are dealt with in Chapter 15, likewise the plastic surgical repair following extensive tissue excision for malignant disease. This short section will confine itself to hemi-mandibulectomy, maxillectomy and partial glossectomy.

Many cancers involving the jaw are considered curable but often the surgical excision has to be radical. For both these reasons rehabilitation is important.

Hemi-mandibulectomy

If the operation entails the resection of other than the mandible or part of the mandible it may be known as a commando procedure. Technically this description covers the excision of part of the tongue, the buccal area, a unilateral or bilateral block dissection of cervical nodes in addition to the affected mandible. Whether the operation is a simple hemi-mandibulectomy or the more extensive procedure breathing exercises should be taught pre-operatively and jaw movements as well as neck movements should be checked.

Following a simple hemi-mandibulectomy, the postoperative physiotherapy will be straightforward. Once the drains are removed the patient should be encouraged to open and close his mouth; these movements should be carried out in front of a mirror so that the mouth is opened symmetrically. Provided the excision does not include the mandibular symphysis there should be no problem, and function should be rapidly restored (Figs. 13/3a and b).

If the symphysis is excised there is nearly always a tendency to drooling, which makes eating and drinking both messy and difficult. Intensive exercises to the lips with finger assistance or resistance may help in the retraining. A prosthesis is almost always inserted either at the initial excision or as a secondary procedure.

Social rehabilitation, i.e. enabling the patient to take his place in society once more, is almost the most important aspect. This can mean seeing that he is able to mix with people, go into shops etc; the physiotherapist should be prepared to help in this.

Following maxillectomy and glossectomy, breathing exercises should be encouraged. If general classes are held, all these patients should be encouraged to partake and extra head and neck exercises should be incorporated for them. If a block dissection of the cervical

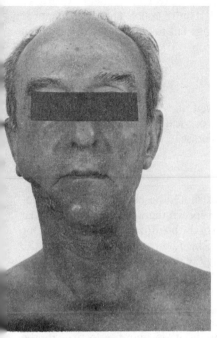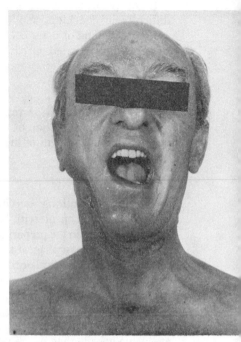

Fig. 13/3(a) A patient who has undergone right hemi-mandibulectomy and block dissection of lymph nodes. (b) The range of movement following surgery

lymph nodes is carried out at the same time the special requirements discussed on page 168 should be noted.

CARCINOMA OF THE LARYNX

Cancer of the larynx accounts for 1 per cent of all cancers diagnosed and the incidence is higher in men than in women. Smoking and an excess intake of alcohol are said to be contributory causes.

Primary treatment for the disease will be either radiotherapy or cytotoxic drugs thus allowing the voice to be preserved. Many of these patients are elderly and the physiotherapist may be asked to treat the chest of some of those undergoing radiotherapy. Very occasionally the larynx becomes extremely oedematous during radiotherapy and an emergency tracheostomy may need to be performed. These patients will certainly need treatment. If postural drainage is felt to be necessary to aid the adequate clearance of sputum, this is usually possible but the physiotherapist should first ask the prescribing doctor.

If the recurrent laryngeal nerve is involved, patients will have difficulty in coughing, and will require much encouragement. If radiotherapy and/or cytotoxic drugs fail to control the disease then surgery will be carried out.

Laryngectomy

The entire larynx will be removed and if necessary a bilateral or unilateral block dissection of the cervical lymph nodes – this will be dependent on the extent of the disease.

Physiotherapy

Pre-operative breathing exercises should be taught and the physiotherapist should consult with her speech therapist colleague to learn how she can help in the preparing of the breathing control required for the teaching of oesophageal speech. The patient will have had the operative procedure explained by the doctors and will know that he will have a permanent tracheostomy. The physiotherapist should be prepared to reassure the patient that this 'hole in the neck' will in no way affect his daily activities.

Postoperatively, breathing exercises and vibrations and shakings are usually all that is required: it is more effective if the physiotherapist combines with a nurse who will suck the secretions out, while the chest is vibrated. As his condition improves and if secretions continue, the patient can be taught to suction himself. Postural drainage is *not* advocated for the first three to four days, because it is very uncomfortable for the patient. If necessary he can be put down on his side either flat or with two pillows.

These patients are up very quickly and unless they were in poor condition pre-operatively or had to undergo very extensive surgery, they should not present problems. Shoulder joint and girdle movements should be encouraged and likewise neck movements, once the drains are out. Later, these patients should be encouraged to dress and be taken out and about in the hospital grounds and the street, prior to discharge.

MÉNIÈRE'S DISEASE

This is a disease first described by Prosper Ménière in 1861, in which there is an increase in the quantity of endolymph in the labyrinths. It is characterised by sudden attacks of vertigo, nausea and vomiting, tinnitus and deafness. The attack may last less than an hour, several hours or longer and there may be premonitory signs such as a dull ache in the ear or there may be no warning. Some patients have a history of tinnitus and increasing deafness in one or both ears, but otherwise the ears are normal.

The actual cause is unknown though many theories exist. One fairly widely accepted theory is that there is spasm of the blood vessels supplying the labyrinth, resulting in ischaemia. This theory is reinforced by the fact that vasodilator drugs and cervical sympathectomy appear to bring about an improvement in the condition. It is also found that attacks are sometimes precipitated by stress and anxiety and exposure to cold. The attacks are slightly more common in men than women and first occur before the áge of 50.

Once an attack has occurred the patient tends to become tense and depressed. This is partly due to the tinnitus and partly because the patient is frightened of how this condition may affect his everyday life. An attack may be so severe that the patient may fall and be quite unable to walk and such an attack might be serious in his work or, for example, when driving a car. The vertigo may not be as severe or prolonged as this and after one or two attacks the condition may never occur again. Attacks can usually be controlled by conservative treatment.

Medical treatment

This is directed towards the reduction of the hypertension of endolymph, relief of fear and depression, and control of symptoms. During a severe attack the patient should lie flat in bed with the head supported by pillows. The nausea is controlled by drugs such as prochlorperazine maleate, and sedatives; tranquillisers will relieve anxiety. Between attacks salt and water restriction and vasodilator drugs such as nicotinic acid and tolazoline hydrochloride are often valuable.

If this treatment does not prove effective, conservative surgical treatment or radical surgery in the form of total destruction of the labyrinth may prove necessary.

Surgical treatment

This may be conservative in the form of surgical sympathectomy, decompression of the labyrinth or selective destruction of the labyrinth by placing the tip of an ultrasound applicator on one end of the lateral semicircular canal.

Ménière's disease may also be treated by total destruction of a labyrinth by withdrawing the membranous lateral semicircular duct through an opening in the bony capsule or by removing the utricle through the oval window.

These operations are followed by vertigo, particularly severe after total destruction, but usually lessening gradually over a period of several weeks. When there has been selective destruction the patient is warned that he may suffer from mild attacks of vertigo for about three months. During this time vertigo is controlled by drugs but physiotherapy is often helpful.

Physiotherapy

Occasionally vertigo persists and physiotherapy may then be ordered. The giddiness is aggravated by any change of position and is particularly bad on sudden movements of the head or eyes. For this reason the patient tends to hold the head and eyes still and to move the trunk slowly and carefully. The neck and shoulder muscles therefore become tense and often remain so, long after the giddiness has permanently disappeared.

The object of physical treatment is to gain relaxation of tense muscles and to overcome the fear of giddiness, until it completely ceases and the patient is capable of carrying out normal activities with normal self-confidence. If these aims are not achieved, the tenseness continues and activities are limited through fear of the unpleasant sensation of vertigo.

The exact routine of exercise varies. It is common to begin with eye movements, first slowly, then quickly, and then a combination of both. The use of long and short focus is also valuable. Provided that the head is supported, head bending forward and rotation may also be given. Head backward bending is often avoided as it seems to produce more vertigo. On the next day, the same movements may be practised in the long-sitting position and head rolling and head extension may be added, performed first with the eyes open and then with eyes closed. These movements should also be performed slowly at first and then quickly, and then changing rapidly from one speed to another. Shoulder movements to gain relaxation are now added and slow trunk movements. The patient can then join a class of other patients, so that the spirit of competition may enter into the treatment. Exercises in sitting, stressing trunk and head flexion and extension, are given, and standing, trying to gain steady balance, is added. Progression is made daily by adding exercises in standing and by using changes of posture, first with the eyes open and then closed. Ball throwing makes a useful exercise to obtain balance and co-ordination. Ball work may be developed in standing and walking so that moving about freely is encouraged. Later balance walking, walking round objects and passing other people should all be used.

Patients vary in their progress and exercises must be chosen accordingly. The mental make-up of the patient has a great deal to do with the rate of recovery. The treatment should be pressed to the limit of tolerance of the individual, and encouragement given in order to restore confidence. The patient has to learn that a movement which makes him a little giddy has no untoward effects, and the next day that same movement may well fail to produce giddiness.

NASAL SINUSITIS

This is an inflammation of the mucous membrane lining the nasal sinuses (Fig. 13/4). It may be acute or chronic. The maxillary sinus is most often affected.

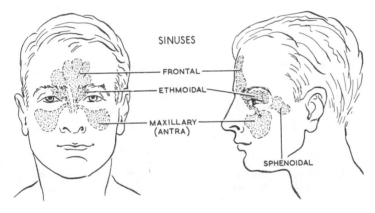

Fig. 13/4   The nasal sinuses

Acute sinusitis

Acute sinusitis is most often caused by the virus of the common cold. It also results from chronic dental infection, trauma or infected tonsils and/or adenoids. Infection is especially likely to occur if there is partial obstruction of the opening from the nose to the sinus, such as may be present when there is a deflected nasal septum, enlarged adenoids or an allergic state of the nose causing swelling of the nasal mucous membrane. Sinusitis is also often associated with chest infections.

The inflammation is characterised by swelling and exudate with increased secretion of mucus. If the organism is virulent, the patient's resistance low or the exudate cannot drain adequately, due to blockage of the opening, the exudate may become purulent. Symptoms are general and local. There is a slight rise in temperature, a feeling of general malaise and headache. Pain is usually present, sometimes with tenderness on pressure. If the maxillary sinus is affected pain is felt in the cheek in the region of the upper teeth; in frontal sinusitis it is just under the upper margin of the orbital cavity; in ethmoidal sinusitis at the upper part of the side of the nose.

Nasal discharge is mucoid at first in most patients, but after a few days may become purulent. Once adequate drainage is established, relief of pain may be expected and within a few days the condition may be cleared and discharge ceases.

Chronic sinusitis

Chronic sinusitis often develops insidiously following either an acute attack which fails to resolve completely, or repeated colds or tooth infection. Permanent changes take place in the lining membrane of the sinus and sometimes in the bony walls. The mucous membrane becomes thickened and fibrotic, cilia disappear, mucous glands hypertrophy and a thick sticky mucus is difficult to move. The secretions therefore stagnate and become infected.

Constant absorption of toxins and swallowing of infected material upsets the general health and causes chronic gastritis so that the patient is likely to complain of headache, tiredness and digestive disturbances.

Local symptoms are mucopurulent nasal discharge and pain in the face, worse in the morning since secretions have accumulated during the night. A postnasal drip is often very worrying to the patient.

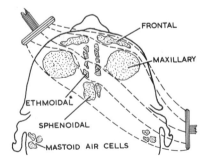

Fig. 13/5   Cross-fire technique for short wave diathermy to the nasal sinuses

Physiotherapy

If physiotherapy is ordered it will probably take the form of short wave diathermy. Chronic sinusitis can respond quite dramatically to short wave diathermy which should be applied using the cross-fire technique (Fig. 13/5). Very mild doses of short wave diathermy of short duration should be given so that the circulation and vitality of the mucous membrane is stimulated without increasing tissue metabolism and the activity of micro-organisms. If there is an increase in symptoms, particularly pain, treatment MUST be stopped. Very occasionally, short wave diathermy is prescribed for acute sinusitis; in this case it must be given with even greater care.

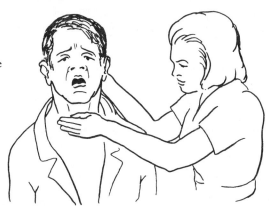

Fig. 13/6 Support for a patient following thyroidectomy while he coughs. One hand on the occiput, the other over the incision

THYROIDECTOMY

Surgery of the thyroid gland can take the form of a partial, hemi- or total thyroidectomy. Total thyroidectomy is rare, except in the case of malignant disease when it may be combined with a bilateral block dissection of the cervical lymph nodes.

More often a partial or hemi-thyroidectomy is performed and is carried out through a collar incision (p. 91). Pre- and postoperative chest physiotherapy may or may not be given. If it is, particular attention should be paid to the upper lobes of the lung, for it is these that are most likely to develop atelectasis. Because of the close proximity of the recurrent laryngeal nerve to the thyroid gland, it may be bruised at operation thus making coughing more difficult, as well as giving the patient a degree of hoarseness of speech. Many patients are very frightened about coughing and one method of support is shown in Figure 13/6. Clips are normally used to close the incision and will be removed very quickly – probably half on the first postoperative day and the remainder on the third day. Following thyroidectomy, patients are mobilised rapidly and can be discharged on the sixth postoperative day, unless after-treatment is required, e.g. radiotherapy or chemotherapy in the case of malignant disease.

Occasionally, a patient presents with a retrosternal thyroid and if this necessitates the splitting of the upper part of the sternum, then the physiotherapy care will be a modification of that given for a thoracotomy. Again, emphasis will be on the upper lobes of the lungs.

With any surgery in the neck region, patients are apprehensive about moving their heads. The physiotherapist should encourage head and neck movement and see that a correct posture is rapidly regained. The positioning of pillows is important and the physiotherapist can teach the nurse the best way to give maximum comfort and a good head position by the judicious placing of them.

REFERENCES

Downie, P. A. (1975). The rehabilitation of patients following head and neck surgery. *Journal of Laryngology and Otology* **LXXXIX**, 12.

Groves, J. (1971). *Facial paralysis*. Chapter included in Vol 2 *Scott-Browne's Diseases of the Ear, Nose and Throat*, 3rd edition (jt eds Ballantyne, J. and Groves, J.). Butterworths, London.

BIBLIOGRAPHY

Downie, P. A. (1978). *Cancer Rehabilitation: an Introduction for Physiotherapists and the Allied Professions*. Chapter 8. Faber and Faber, London.

Stell, P. M. and Maran, A. G. D. (1978). *Head and Neck Surgery*, 2nd edition. William Heinemann Medical Books Limited, London.

Tait, Vera (1978). *Has Voice – Will Speak*. Obtainable from the author, Old Coastguards, West Appledore, Bideford, Devon EX39 1SB.

Chapter 14

Skin Conditions

by B. V. JONES, MA, MCSP, DipTP

Few patients are referred to physiotherapy departments for the treatment of skin disease. The range and efficacy of other methods of treatment (drugs and dressings) have reduced the need for physiotherapists to spend their time in treating these conditions. However, a small number of patients are still referred. This usually occurs where drug treatment alone has proved inadequate to alleviate the condition, or where drug treatment is more effective if combined with ultraviolet irradiation.

In order to treat these patients effectively, the physiotherapist needs to have an appreciation of the methods of treatment available to her and a knowledge of the skin conditions concerned. She should also appreciate that the skin is frequently a mirror of the mental state of the patient. As in all other conditions she should therefore treat the patient as a whole rather than confining her attention exclusively to a localised area.

METHODS OF TREATMENT

Relaxation

If the patient is being treated by tranquilliser drugs, instruction in relaxation techniques may be of great benefit as an adjunct to treatment. Many physicians now believe that the ability of the patient to relax without recourse to sedative drugs (which may become addictive) is of prime importance. Because of this more patients who find it difficult to relax may be referred for instruction in the future. Physiotherapists should ensure that they are skilled in communicating the art of relaxation and should use this in the treatment of skin conditions, if the condition is related to mental stress (see Chapter 10). Training in relaxation is also important where the skin condition causes itching, e.g. eczema. The patient's natural desire to scratch will cause further skin irritation and the ability to relax will be of great benefit in controlling this.

Ultraviolet irradiation

The beneficial effect of natural sunlight and the improvement seen in many skin diseases during the summer months, is sufficient indication of the value of ultraviolet light. Physiotherapists have traditionally used artificial sources of ultraviolet rays in the treatment of skin diseases. Dosage can be varied from the sub-erythemal dose, that is, 75 per cent of a first degree (E1) erythema dose, through all the degrees of erythema according to the desired effect. In clinical practice the effect aimed for is most likely to be increased cell production leading to thickening of the skin, increased desquamation, increased blood supply to the skin or increased pigmentation. Irradiation of the whole body is said to have a tonic effect. The usefulness of ultraviolet irradiation on areas denuded of skin, e.g. infected wounds, is doubted by many. It seems to be more logical and effective to culture the bacteria and apply the appropriate antibiotic. However, in a few cases, use of the abiotic rays of the spectrum may be appropriate.

When applying treatment the most appropriate ultraviolet source must be used. Treatment given with an air-cooled source of ultraviolet may be either from a mercury vapour lamp or fluorescent tubes. The spectra of these differ. The mercury vapour lamp gives rays from 184.9nm to 390nm (1849 Å–3900 Å) while the fluorescent tube gives rays from 280nm to 390nm (2800 Å–3900 Å). Where an erythema reaction is desired, irradiation from a fluorescent source will probably be the best choice as there is a higher percentage of the longer wavelengths. The initial choice of source is important as the same lamp must be used at subsequent treatments.

DEFINITION

The nanometre is now the official Standard International Unit of wavelength and has replaced the Ångström.

1 Ångström   = one ten millionth of a millimetre.
1 nanometre = 10 Ångström
1 nm   = 10 Å

Prefix nano
Symbol n

Heat

The physiotherapist may also find that the application of mild heat has beneficial effects in the treatment of localised skin infections, such as boils, carbuncles or infected wounds. Heat may be applied superficially using infra-red rays or more deeply by short wave diathermy or microwave diathermy. The rationale underlying the use of heat is that increased metabolic activity and increased blood supply will aid the local tissues to combat the infection. The heat should be directed to the area of blood supply rather than towards the infection, so that the rate of bacterial growth is not stimulated (for example, heat could be applied to the forearm in the case of an infection of the hand). This type of treatment should be given in association with localised and systemic antibiotics.

Cold

An effective erythema can be obtained by massaging the local area with an ice cube. This may be preferable to the use of dry heat and is useful in the treatment of an area of skin which threatens to break down into a pressure sore.

Tissue mobilising techniques

Where the skin condition has led to fibrosis and thickening of the tissues, with the possibility of contracture and deformity, the mobility of the tissues must be maintained, and deep localised massage, with active movements, ultrasound and possibly passive stretchings, may be appropriate.

ASSESSMENT AND RECORDING

In this field no less than in other areas of physiotherapy, the preliminary assessment of the patient's condition is essential. Careful observation of the affected skin area should be made and the extent, type and severity of the eruption should be noted. Standard diagrams of the anterior and posterior aspect of the body are useful, so that the affected areas can be outlined and the pre-treatment record kept with the patient's treatment card.

A careful scrutiny of the patient's notes will be made in order to determine relevant points in the history of the condition, especially so that the type of medicaments being given can be known. Some of these may be sensitisers, e.g. coal tar, which will alter the patient's reaction to ultraviolet radiation. The patient's skin reaction to sunlight should be tested if the treatment prescribed includes ultraviolet irradiation. The result of this test and the other findings should be carefully recorded on the patient's treatment card. A special note should be made concerning the extent of the area treated so that at subsequent treatments the possibility of overdose because of altered screening is avoided.

In the treatment of most skin conditions re-assessment of the affected area should be made at each attendance, and the treatment should be based on the findings. A careful recording of the day-to-day condition and the consequent modifications to treatment is therefore of prime importance. Objective evidence such as a tracing of a wound, or the extent of an active area of acne, should be recorded rather than subjective assessments such as 'patient improved'. The physiotherapist should be in a position to base her reports to the dermatologist on factual evidence rather than optimism.

SKIN CONDITIONS REFERRED FOR PHYSIOTHERAPY

Acne vulgaris

This is a chronic inflammatory disease of the sebaceous glands. The condition most commonly affects those parts where the glands are large, i.e. the face, chest and upper back, and is seen in adolescents and young adults primarily, though very occasionally the condition may persist into later life. The essential lesion of the condition is the blackhead, or comedo, a firm mass of keratin which blocks the follicular pore. This may cause inflammation of the surrounding tissues or it may become secondarily infected with eventual fibrous tissue formation and unsightly scarring.

In mild cases no treatment other than careful skin toilet is required. Severe cases respond well to a prolonged course of a tetracycline antibiotic. The few patients who are referred for physiotherapists to treat are those who have severe acne which is not responding well to other forms of therapy. The rationale underlying this referral is that cases of acne improve in the summer months and therefore ultraviolet irradiation from an artificial source can be used to supplement the effects of natural sunlight. Exceptions to this are patients who have fair or sensitive skins, as they are often made worse by local ultraviolet radiation.

The affected skin should be washed with soap and water prior to treatment and gently dried with a clean towel and then irradiated by an air-cooled mercury vapour lamp. A first degree erythema is given to improve the condition of the skin and this is repeated when the reaction has died down. A first degree erythema is preferred to a second as the aim of the treatment is to stimulate skin metabolism rather than produce desquamation. The technique of ultraviolet irradiation will vary with the area being treated. The physiotherapist must ensure that her screening techniques are such that there is no possibility of 'overlap' dosage. In the interests of the patient it is as well to screen to the natural bony features of the body, such as the jaw line or the clavicular line. A more acceptable cosmetic effect can be obtained by allowing a natural fade-off of irradiation, but this can only be done where screening is not essential.

Psoriasis

This condition affects approximately 1–2 per cent of people with white skin. The cause is unknown but the abnormality results in unduly rapid cell division within the epidermis. Normally the cells reproduce at such a rate that the epidermal turnover takes approximately 28 days. In psoriasis the turnover rate is seven times as fast, i.e. every four days. The amount of skin area affected varies from trivial to extensive. Characteristically, initial lesions are on the extensor aspects of elbows and knees and in the scalp, or over the sacral area. Severe cases may have total skin involvement, although the face is usually spared. The condition appears to be adversely affected by mental stress, although the course of the condition is typically unpredictable and exacerbations cannot always be attributed to this factor.

The affected area shows a slightly raised red plaque, with a sharp margin between it and healthy skin. The plaque is surmounted by dry silvery grey scales. If the scales are removed the underlying skin bleeds easily.

Medical treatment for psoriasis is usually by the administration of local or, very occasionally, systemic agents which contain a toxic substance to slow down the rate of cell division. Where these fail, or in the case of a patient whose condition is becoming rapidly worse, admission to hospital may be advised. It is in the intensive treatment of patients with psoriasis that the physiotherapist is most likely to become involved. The usual treatment is a modification of the Ingram regime. The patient bathes first thing in the morning in a tar bath and scrubs off his psoriatic scales. He then attends the physiotherapy department for general ultraviolet irradiation from a fluorescent source. As the irradiation is given daily, no more than a first degree erythema should be achieved and some authorities believe that a sub-erythemal dose only should be given. The lesions are then covered with dithranol paste and with a suitable dressing until removal the next day prior to bathing. Removal of the paste can be facilitated by the use of liquid paraffin. This treatment is effective in nearly all cases though many relapse again.

PUVA

Ultraviolet light has been used in the treatment of psoriasis for many years using minimal erythema reaction in conjunction with various preparations. Recent developments in the treatment of this skin condition have changed the approach in the management of psoriasis. It has been found that irradiation by long wave ultraviolet rays plus the oral administration of psoralens inhibits epithelial DNA synthesis. Psoralens (8-methoxypsoralen) given two hours before irradiation results in a photochemical reaction in which the psoralens bind to the DNA thiamine bases. Psoralens can also intercalate with two base pairs and give interstrand cross linkages (Pathak and Kramer, 1969; Cole, 1970; Dall'Acqua, Marciani and Ciavatta, 1971); this inhibits DNA synthesis and cell division.

SOURCE OF IRRADIATION

Special fluorescent tubes have been designed to produce wavelengths between 320nm and 390nm – the psoralens being activated by wavelengths of 365nm. These burners are housed in a hexagonal shaped cubicle and the patient stands inside the cubicle and receives a general irradiation. This new technique is called PUVA which stands for psoralens and long wave ultraviolet.

MEDICAL AND PHYSIOTHERAPY TREATMENT

Before commencing PUVA treatment the doctor's examination should include an eye examination and laboratory tests which will be repeated at 6 and 12 months and yearly thereafter.

Three, four or five tablets of 10mg each (the number prescribed depends on kg body-weight), are taken two hours before irradiation. If, on evaluation, the patient complains of nausea, the tablets should be taken at 15-minute intervals. The treatment must be prescribed by a consultant or other competent doctor.

INSTRUCTIONS FOR PATIENTS HAVING PUVA TREATMENT

1. Take the amount of tablets prescribed two hours before the ultraviolet treatment.

2. Tablets should be taken with food or after eating. Do not take them on an empty stomach.
3. Polaroid sunglasses must be worn from the time of taking the tablets until 12 hours after.
4. Avoid exposure to sunlight for 12 hours after the ultraviolet treatment. Should exposure to sunlight be unavoidable, e.g. driving or any outdoor activities, the skin should be protected with clothing, a hat or the use of sun-screening agents.
5. It may be necessary to use oils or lubricating lotions on your skin since the treatment tends to make your skin dry.
6. Topical treatments such as tars and cortisone creams should not be used during PUVA treatment unless prescribed by your consultant.
7. It is recommended that birth control measures are used while on PUVA treatment.
8. It is important to attend each month after completion of treatment to keep a check on the skin.

DURATION OF TREATMENT

This depends on the individual's reaction to ultraviolet light:

1. Red-headed people who freckle are started at five minutes and progress by one minute up to 15 minutes.
2. People who redden and then tan are started at six minutes and progress by two minutes up to 20 minutes.
3. People who tan but do not burn are started at seven minutes and progress by three minutes up to 25 minutes.

The purpose of the treatment is not to produce an erythema reaction: if one should occur a suitable interval must elapse to allow it to subside before further treatment is given. Attendances are therefore limited to two or three times a week and should be spaced so that any reaction from the previous time would have become apparent before the next irradiation. This regime takes about six to eight weeks but the actual duration of the treatment is variable and will alter according to the time it takes for the lesions to clear.

MAINTENANCE DOSAGE

Each individual patient will be assessed. A possible maintenance scheme might be:

Once a week for four treatments, then once a fortnight for four treatments, followed by once in three weeks for four treatments and finally once a month for four treatments. The patient stays at the interval necessary to control the psoriasis.

PRECAUTIONS

The patient must always wear a pair of goggles and if there is no psoriasis on the face, a towel should be used to completely cover the face. The physiotherapist should remain within calling distance. The patient is instructed to take off the towel and goggles and leave the cubicle should he feel faint and to call the physiotherapist immediately.

Alopecia areata

This is a relatively common condition in which patches of baldness appear spontaneously. There is no evidence to suggest that any type of physiotherapy will increase the rate of regrowth of hair in the affected areas, although high frequency stimulation and ultraviolet irradiation have been tried. Complete recovery of the affected patches usually occurs but may take from three months to two years. If ultraviolet irradiation is requested, a second degree erythema should be given to the affected area of scalp after careful cleansing with spirit to remove grease. Subsequent treatment would be given when the erythema of the previous dose has died down. The new growth of hair frequently lacks pigment but this is gradually developed.

Vitiligo

This is a condition in which there is a patchy loss of melanin pigmentation. Areas of the body show irregular patches of skin lacking in pigment. The cause of the condition is unknown but it is sufficiently widespread to affect 1 per cent of the population. Recent advances in the treatment of this condition have shown some success in re-pigmentation after treatment of the affected areas with trimethylpsoralen lotion followed by exposure to sunlight. The drug should be applied to the skin or alternatively taken by mouth approximately two hours before ultraviolet irradiation. The dose should be sub-erythemal and repeated not more often than every five days. The course should be prolonged, extending over a period of three to four months. During this time the affected patches should show evidence of re-pigmentation. If there is no response in this time the treatment is discontinued. However, if improvement is occurring treatment is continued for many months. Unfortunately the re-pigmentation may not be permanent and relapses occur frequently.

SKIN INFECTIONS

Furuncle

A furuncle or boil is an acute staphylococcal infection of the hair follicle. The infection discharges through the hair follicle after a series of inflammatory changes in which necrotic tissue is broken down into liquid pus. Any area of the body can be the site for a boil but areas of friction such as the back of the neck are the most likely. A series of boils affecting different parts of the body is known as a furunculosis.

The patient is first aware of pain and an area of redness is visible over the site of the infection. This becomes a raised area which quickly shows a yellow centre. After a short while the skin over this central core breaks down and pus is discharged onto the surface. Frequently a solid core of unliquefied pus is also discharged. The affected area is quickly repaired by fibrous tissue and a scar is left to mark the place where the boil existed.

A single boil is very often left to run its own course. Patients who are obviously prone to this kind of skin infection may be treated with appropriate antibiotics, such as penicillin. Only a few patients will ever find their way to a physiotherapy department. The treatment for those who do will depend upon the stage in which the boil presents itself. In the early stage before the boil has started to discharge mild co-planar short wave diathermy should be given. This aims at providing heat to the base of the boil, and the electrodes should be positioned so that the field passes deep to the boil. The treatment by heat accelerates the metabolic processes and encourages discharge of pus. Once discharge has occurred, the localised area may be treated by a more superficial type of heat such as infra-red radiation in order to aid the healing process. Boils which do not drain freely or do not discharge their contents completely may be treated by local ultraviolet irradiation using the sinus applicator.

Carbuncle

If the infection spreads subcutaneously to affect a group of hair follicles a large area of skin may break down to reveal a deep slough which may take a long time to heal. This kind of skin infection requires the administration of antibiotics. The patient may be referred to the physiotherapy department when the objects of physical treatment will be to aid the rapid breakdown of slough and assist in the healing of the affected area.

Treatment will be along the lines already indicated for a boil except that initially there is a wider breakdown of the skin and the area of infected tissue thus revealed should be treated by ultraviolet irradiation using a fourth degree erythema or double-fourth degree erythema to the affected area. The surrounding tissue should of course be carefully screened. Following irradiation the site may be dressed using a proteolytic enzyme such as Trypure. Both the irradiation and the enzyme will aid the breakdown of slough. When the area is clean the aim is to stimulate rapid re-epithelialisation and this may be done by the administration of heat, or a first or second degree erythema dose of ultraviolet irradiation to the wound and surrounding area.

Hidradenitis axillae

The apocrine sweat glands of the axilla are occasionally the site of a severe chronic bacterial infection which may be confused with furunculosis. The condition is more severe and may run a chronic course over 10 to 15 years, during which time there is severe scarring with possible contracture of the fibrous tissue.

The condition appears first as multiple red tender nodules which eventually break down and suppurate. Spread of infection occurs with increasing involvement of all the apocrine glands until these are ultimately destroyed.

Treatment is by local and systemic antibiotics and in order to encourage free drainage surgical interference may be necessary. Scrupulous cleanliness of the area is essential in order to combat the superficial spread of the infection. The patient may be referred to the physiotherapist for mild short wave diathermy to the axillary region in order to encourage the free evacuation of the infected material by the application of heat. It is also important to ensure that the patient understands the need to maintain a full active range of movement in the shoulder joint to prevent contracture of the axillary tissue.

Pressure sores

A sore is a popular term for almost any lesion of the skin or mucous membrane. A local impairment of the circulation caused by sustained pressure can result in a pressure sore. The damage to the tissues is the result of a temporary reduction in the blood supply. The changes can be observed at various stages. At first the skin appears erythematous and it is important to note the colour changes as the part has a livid hue just before the skin breaks down. Once the skin has broken down it becomes an open wound which may easily become infected.

PREVENTION

In order to prevent the occurrence of pressure sores, patients who are immobile should be encouraged to relieve pressure from weight-bearing areas at frequent intervals either by moving themselves into a different position or, if they are in bed and immobile, they should be turned frequently. They may be nursed on medical sheepskins, ripple mattresses, sorbo packs or in a Roto-rest bed. Strict hygiene should be observed and local massage over the area of pressure may be carried out.

If the area shows signs of redness over the pressure area, frequent mild thermal doses of infra-red may be given to improve the circulation. In addition, massaging the local area with an ice cube may be performed.

SKIN BREAKDOWN

If the skin breaks down, a first degree erythema dose of ultraviolet using the longer wavelengths may be given to stimulate growth and increase the skin resistance. The circulation is maintained by infra-red irradiation on alternate days. If the part becomes infected then stronger erythema reactions will be required to combat the infection by making use of the bactericidal effects of ultraviolet.

Infected wounds

A wound is an injury to the body caused by physical means with disruption of the normal continuity of the body structures. An open wound is one that has a free outward opening. An open wound which has become infected may be treated with ultraviolet. The surrounding skin should be protected and a local irradiation given. The degree of erythema depends on the condition of the wound; if there is pus a fourth or double-fourth dosage is used initially, and is reduced as the infection clears. As granulation tissue appears the dosage should be reduced to a third or second degree, possibly protecting the area of granulation or using a blue uviol filter or cellophane to filter out the shorter abiotic rays. The surrounding skin may be given a first degree erythema using the Kromayer lamp at a distance or an air-cooled mercury vapour lamp.

CLEANING AND DRESSING THE WOUND

The wound will need to be cleaned before treatment and afterwards dressed with the appropriate medication using a strict aseptic technique.

SINUSES

If there is a sinus involved then a suitable quartz applicator should be used with the Kromayer to enable healing of the sinus from below upwards.

PHYSIOTHERAPY AS AN AID TO DIAGNOSIS IN SKIN CONDITIONS

Occasionally physiotherapists are asked to assist in the diagnosis of skin conditions. By using a Wood's filter in association with a Kromayer ultraviolet light source, certain types of tinea of the scalp (ringworm) can be shown as a bright blue-green fluorescence. Similarly, erythrasma gives a coral red fluorescence. This condition usually affects the groins, toe webs and the perianal region.

Photosensitivity and photopatch testing are used in the diagnosis of conditions where the skin has become hypersensitive to light. Such conditions may arise as the result of systemic or local exposure to a sensitising substance. There is a wide range of possible sensitisers including drugs (sulphonamides, chlorpromazine, tetracycline), soaps, antiseptics, and silver and gold salts. In other cases no direct cause for the hypersensitivity can be found. Because the tests require the use of an ultraviolet light source, physiotherapists may be asked to assist with them. A Kromayer lamp with a filter of ordinary window glass is used for the test. This eliminates rays below 320nm (3200 Å). The minimal erythema dose (MED) for the lamp without the filter is calculated using a normal skin.

Photopatch testing is carried out in the following way. Patch tests of the suspected sensitiser are applied to both sides of the back or other suitable skin surface (one side then acts as a control). The patches are removed and the skin cleaned after 24 hours. The control areas are then covered with black paper to obscure the light. The test areas are irradiated by the Kromayer lamp with the filter using the minimal erythema dose. The areas are inspected 24 hours later. A positive reaction is shown by a reproduction of the photo allergy and the sensitising substance can then be identified. A comparison with the control side will show the degree of photosensitivity.

REFERENCES

Cole, R. S. (1970). Light induced cross-linking of DNA in the presence of a furocoumarin (psoralen). *Biochimica et Biophysica Acta*, **217**, 30.

Dall'Acqua, F., Marciani, S. and Ciavatta, L. (1971). Formation of interstrand cross-linkings in the photoreactions between furocoumarins and DNA. *Zeitschrift für Naturforschung (B)*, **26**, 561.
Pathak, M. A. and Kramer, D. M. (1969). Photosensitization of skin in vivo by furocoumarins (psoralens). *Biochimica et Biophysica Acta*, **195**, 197.

BIBLIOGRAPHY

Barton, A. and Barton, M. (1981). *The Management and Prevention of Pressure Sores*. Faber and Faber, London.
Current status of oral PUVA therapy for psoriasis. (1979). *Journal of the American Academy of Dermatology*, **1**, 2.
Rook, A., Wilkinson, D. S. and Ebling, F. J. G. (1979). *Textbook of Dermatology*, 3rd edition. Blackwell Scientific Publications Limited, Oxford.
Sneddon, I. B. and Church, R. E. (1976). *Nursing Skin Diseases*, 3rd edition. Edward Arnold (Publishers) Ltd, London.
Sneddon, I. B. and Church, R. E. (1983). *Practical Dermatology*, 4th edition. Edward Arnold (Publishers) Ltd, London.
Wilkinson, D. S. (1977). *The Nursing and Management of Skin Diseases*, 4th edition. Faber and Faber, London.

Chapter 15

Plastic Surgery

by S. BOARDMAN, MCSP and P. M. WALKER, MCSP

The term plastic surgery was used by the Germans at the beginning of this century to describe surgery concerned with 'moulding of tissues.'

The first recorded reconstructive surgery was performed in India 600 years B.C. where amputation of the nose was a common punishment, and forehead skin was used to construct a new nose. Tagliococci, an Italian surgeon, reconstructed noses using an arm flap in the 16th century. The recorded use of free skin graft dates from the 19th century when new techniques were described by Jacques Reverdin, Ollier and Thiersch in Paris, and Wolfe in Glasgow. The challenge of mutilating injuries during the First World War stimulated the development of plastic surgery and it became a specialty in its own right. The pioneer in the UK was Sir Harold Gilles. During the Second World War, surgeons such as Gilles, Kilner, MacIndoe and Mowlem laid the foundation of the specialty as it is now known.

Much of the present day plastic surgery is concerned with the replacement and reconstruction of soft tissues. This can include skin, subcutaneous tissues, nerves, tendons, blood vessels, the main object being to restore and improve function.

THE SKIN AND ITS FUNCTION

It should be remembered that skin is not just a collection of epithelial cells, but a composite organ of epidermis and dermis (Fig. 15/1). The epidermis is stratified and is made up of five layers of cells, the deepest of these, the stratum germinatum, being the cell producing layer.

The dermis is made up of two layers. In the upper layer lie the capillary loops, the smallest lymphatics and nerve endings, including touch corpuscles, while the deeper layer consists largely of fibrous tissue with an interlacing of elastic fibres, and this rests directly on

Fig. 15/1 The structure of the skin

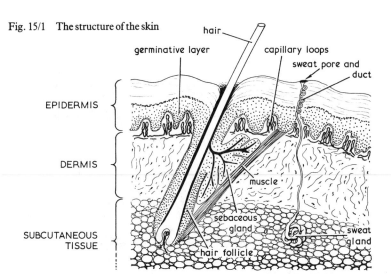

subcutaneous tissue. This latter consists of bundles of connective tissue interspersed with fat cells. The glandular parts of some of the several glands and deep hair follicles lie in this area. This subcutaneous layer serves to support blood vessels, lymphatics and nerves and protects underlying structures.

The skin is the largest organ of the body, representing about 16 per cent of the total weight of the normal adult. It has many functions, but the two most important when considering skin loss, are protection against invasion by bacteria, and prevention of fluid and protein loss from the body.

If primary healing does not take place, surgery may be required to provide skin cover.

There are two methods of skin transfer:

1. Free skin grafts, which are without a blood supply for up to 48 hours after transfer.
2. Skin flaps, which are joined to the body by a functioning arterial and venous flow.

METHODS OF SKIN REPLACEMENT

Free skin grafts (Fig. 15/2)

These may be split skin or full thickness.

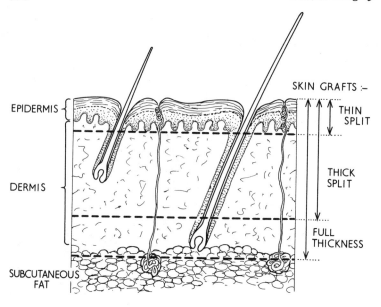

SPLIT SKIN

These can vary from the very thin to three-quarter skin thickness.
They are cut with a knife or dermatome. Such grafts are used in the
grafting of burns. After cutting, they are spread on Tulle Gras for ease
of handling and applied to the raw areas.

The donor sites heal within 10 to 12 days. The grafted area may be
nursed exposed or with dressings, according to the wishes of the
surgeon. The recipient area must always have a good blood supply and
be free from necrotic tissue and infection (particularly haemolytic
streptococcus).

For the first 48 hours, a split skin graft survives on the exudate from
the underlying granulating tissue. By 48 hours, capillaries will have
grown into the graft and vascularised it. Haematoma or tangential
movement of the graft will prevent vascularisation and the graft will
fail.

Following skin grafts, exercises may be commenced at about five to
seven days. Joints not directly involved in grafting may be moved, but
movements of these must not cause friction on newly applied skin.
Once the grafts are well established, the application of a bland cream
to soften scars is desirable, e.g. lanolin or hydrous ointment may be
used. This should be *gently* kneaded in; heavy-handedness must be
avoided otherwise blistering occurs.

Split skin grafts often contract considerably, and may have to be replaced or released at a later stage, more split skin or full thickness grafts being added, or skin flaps used.

FULL THICKNESS GRAFTS

Wolfe grafts: These are small full thickness grafts of skin excluding fat, usually taken from the post-auricular or supraclavicular area to repair facial defects, such as eyelids. The donor site will not regenerate and must itself be closed by a split skin graft or direct suture. Full thickness skin graft contracts less than a split skin graft and so is the graft of choice for releasing contracture of the eyelids which can lead to corneal ulceration.

Skin flaps and pedicles

These consist of skin and subcutaneous tissue.

They take their own blood supply, and can be used to cover areas where the blood supply is poor, or non-existent, as over cortical bone, cartilage, joint and bare tendon. Flaps do not contract so can be used to prevent or correct deformities. In order to maintain the viability of the flap, transfer of skin can sometimes only be done in stages. In some flaps, there is a 'random' supply of blood vessels. Other flaps are designed to include at least one sizeable artery or vein; the latter type can be much longer. Examples of these arterial or axial pattern flaps are the forehead and delto-pectoral flaps.

The principal types of flaps are:

1. Transposition flaps
2. Pedicle flaps
3. Direct flaps
4. Free flaps – due to the advent of microsurgery.

TRANSPOSITION FLAPS (Fig. 15/3)

These are used to replace defects by transposing skin and subcutaneous tissues from an adjacent site, the donor site being covered by a split skin graft or sutured directly. They are often

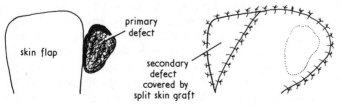

skin flap

primary
defect

secondary
defect
covered by
split skin graft

Fig. 15/3   Transposition (rotation) flap used to cover a defect

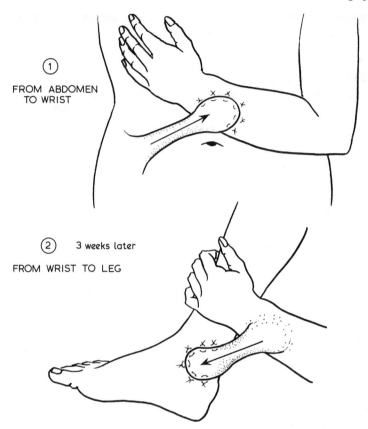

① FROM ABDOMEN TO WRIST

② 3 weeks later FROM WRIST TO LEG

Fig. 15/4 A pedicle flap. (1) The abdominal pedicle is raised and attached to the wrist (2) The abdominal end of the pedicle is detached and re-attached to the ankle area

employed in the grafting of pressure sores, and in themselves demand little treatment from the physiotherapist.

PEDICLE FLAPS

Pedicle flaps raised and sometimes tubed are used most often for the replacement of traumatic defects of the face and neck; (nowadays they are less commonly used). From a physiotherapy point of view the acromio-thoracic and abdominal pedicles are important ones to mention. Pedicles may be raised from the upper chest wall, the lower end being swung into position to repair the nose or chin defect, and held in place for three weeks. This will necessitate a mild side flexion and rotation of the neck. They may also be raised from the abdomen and transposed either to the face and neck or a limb via an intermediary (Fig. 15/4), e.g. a pedicle raised on the abdomen can be attached to a wrist and after three weeks it is detached from its base and carried by the wrist to the lower leg as replacement skin.

DIRECT FLAP

These are open, their undersurface remaining raw throughout their attachment period.

CROSS-LEG FLAPS (Fig. 15/5)

The cross-leg flap is perhaps one of the most common in use, one leg being the donor for the other. A flap is raised; one end is attached to

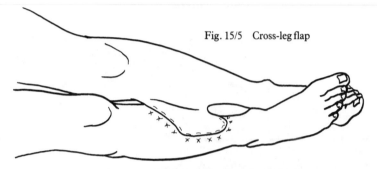

Fig. 15/5   Cross-leg flap

the recipient site, and the other remains attached to the donor site. The donor site itself is then resurfaced with a split skin graft. The position is maintained for three weeks, during which time the physiotherapist supervises joint care and muscle function. Some of these repairs entail acrobatic positions and often lead to discomfort in the joint involved, and muscle spasm. Such tension and consequent pain may be relieved by the application of heat or ice and massage to the muscles and joints involved. Extreme care must be taken to prevent damage to the flap by heat, for the circulation is reduced and burning and destruction may ensue. It must be remembered that the area is anaesthetic and the patient may be unable to give adequate warning of excess heat. Deep kneading can relieve spasm and discomfort in a matter of a few days. Exercises too are given in the form of static muscle contractions and movements of joints wherever possible.

More recently, with constant use of microsurgery and improved techniques, the cross-leg flap has been largely superseded by the use of free flaps in the UK.

Other examples of direct flaps are: abdominal, delto-pectoral and groin flaps.

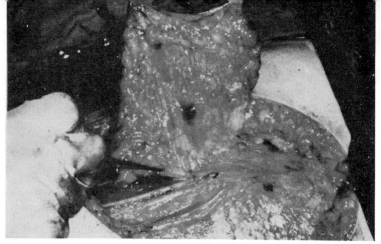

Fig. 15/6   Free flap. *Stage 1*: Lifting the flap from the abdomen

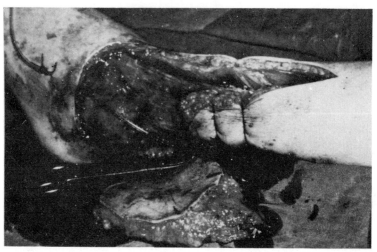

Fig. 15/7   Free flap. *Stage 2*: The area on the lower leg to be covered by the flap

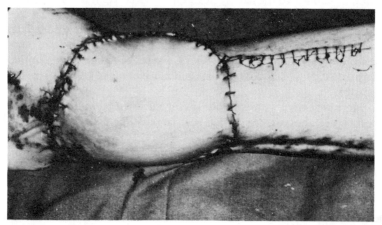

Fig. 15/8   Free flap. *Stage 3*: The flap in situ

Pedicle and direct flaps are both means of 'making good' one area, by robbing another. They can be transposed from one limb to another via an intermediary, e.g. a flap or pedicle raised on the abdomen can be attached to the wrist, and after three weeks it is detached from its base and carried by the wrist to the lower leg as replacement skin. Incidentally, un-united fractures are often encouraged to heal when the compound site is given good skin cover.

FREE FLAPS (Figs. 15/6, 15/7 and 15/8)

This is a flap which is completely detached from the donor site and transposed directly to the recipient area. Using a microscope, the blood vessels are dissected out (at least one large artery and vein) and anastomosed with vessels in the recipient area.

Now that the microscope is widely used in surgical procedures, free flaps are often used in place of those previously mentioned. As the operation necessitates the dissection and anastomosis of vessels, pre-operative arteriograms and venograms are required.

An example of this flap is one based on the superficial circumflex iliac artery. The skin flap is raised together with the underlying artery and accompanying veins. The flap and vessels are placed over the recipient area where the vessels are anastomosed to those in the local area and the flap sutured in place. It must be remembered that this is a full thickness flap and therefore the donor site has to be covered by a split skin graft or, if possible, sutured directly.

Postoperatively the blood flow through the flap is monitored by a photo-electric plethysmograph. As there are no intermediate stages to this procedure the time factor is reduced and unlike previous flaps the patient is not subjected to uncomfortable positions which often cause joint stiffness.

As this operation is a lengthy procedure the patient is anaesthetised for several hours and chest complications could occur. Pre- and postoperative exercises are essential. General exercises may be given but the pre-operative condition (e.g. un-united fractures) must be taken into consideration. The flap must not be put under any tension.

The length of time on bed rest is governed by the site of the flap, i.e. a patient with a flap sited in the head and neck region may be up in a chair within two or three days whereas the patient with a flap on the lower limb may be confined to bed for 14 days.

THE USE OF PLASTIC SURGERY

Conditions seen in the plastic surgery unit may, for simplicity, be divided into those requiring:

1. Head and neck surgery
2. Hand surgery
3. Trunk and limb surgery
4. Cosmetic surgery.

HEAD AND NECK SURGERY

This entails radical surgery dealing with such conditions as carcinoma of the jaw, tongue, bony and skin structures of the face.

Having undertaken radical excision of the malignant area, it will be necessary to perform reconstructive surgery, which could include

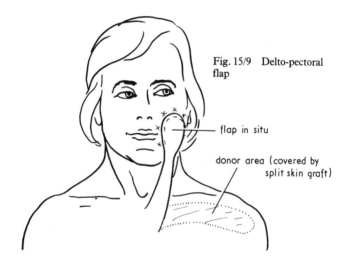

Fig. 15/9   Delto-pectoral flap

— flap in situ

donor area (covered by split skin graft)

raising of pedicles, delto-pectoral, forehead flaps or free flaps to replace the soft tissues (Fig. 15/9).

When bony structures such as the mandible and maxilla are excised, reconstruction may be carried out by the use of bone grafts or artificial prostheses.

PHYSIOTHERAPY

Pre-operative physiotherapy may include an explanation of the procedures to be undertaken, including the possible necessity of tracheostomy, difficulty in speech, eating and general discomfort. Breathing exercises must be taught. They are usually carried out in the half-lying position as grafts may be applied at the time of surgery, and the least amount of movement during the first few days is desirable to prevent skin loss. Leg exercises are taught for the prevention of thrombosis.

Postoperatively on return from theatre, the patient may have a tracheostomy and is nursed in a half-lying position – flaps or pedicles may have been used for the soft tissue reconstruction and bone grafts for bony reconstruction. Breathing exercises to clear the chest are carried out, maintaining the half-lying position. Patients with tracheostomies receive regular suction. Leg exercises must also be performed.

Special attention is paid to pedicles and flaps to prevent (a) kinking, and (b) torsion. Either of these could cut off the blood supply and lead to necrosis.

If the patient develops a chest condition, treatment for this must take preference over the reconstructive surgery, in which case the patient may be tipped, turned and moved for postural drainage.

It should be noted that radical head and neck surgery can lead to psychological problems and patients need constant reassurance and aid with communication which may include speech therapy. Ultimately, they will need help to adjust to society at large.

Facial fractures

Patients with facial fractures are admitted to a plastic surgery unit as they often have severe lacerations as a result of going through a windscreen. (Since the wearing of seat belts was made compulsory facial lacerations are seen much less frequently.) Other factors causing these injuries include direct blows, e.g. punches.

The most common fracture sites are:

1. Mandible
2. Maxilla
3. Zygoma
4. Nose.

NB: The first aid treatment in dealing with facial fractures must be noted:

Patients should *never* be laid on their backs, because the tongue can fall back and obstruct the airways.

FIXATION

A mandible is fixed by interdental wiring or cap splints. The maxilla and zygoma are usually fixed by interdental wiring and external splintage (Fig. 15/10).

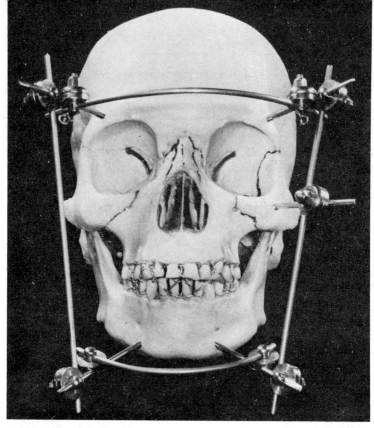

Fig. 15/10   Interdental wiring and external splintage following fracture of both maxilla and zygoma

The nose is immobilised by (a) plaster of Paris splint; (b) two small metal plates on either side of the bridge or (c) Orthoplast.

Fractures involving the zygoma may lead to trismus, i.e. difficulty in opening the mouth.

PHYSIOTHERAPY

Most of these patients present as emergencies. When first seen wiring and splintage may be present and the nose may also be packed.

Breathing exercises are carried out because the patient may have a considerable amount of blood in the mouth and back of the throat which could lead to chest complications. As the teeth are wired together, difficulty may be experienced in expectorating. Suction is carried out via the gap in the interdental wiring. Packing of the nose will exclude nasal suction.

After the splintage is removed, if trismus is still present, short wave diathermy to the temperomandibular joint is given, using low dosages.

Jaw osteotomies are performed for abnormal bite and/or cosmetic reasons and are treated as a fractured jaw.

Cleft lip and palate

Any combination of cleft lip and palate may be present:

(a) Unilateral cleft lip
(b) Bilateral cleft lip
(c) Unilateral lip and palate
(d) Bilateral lip and palate
(e) Palate only.

First, the cleft lip is repaired at about three months, or earlier, according to the surgeon. If it is bilateral the second side is repaired six weeks after the first side.

At nine to twelve months the palate is repaired, i.e. before the child commences speech.

Just before the child starts school, revision of scars and correction of any nasal deformity are undertaken.

PHYSIOTHERAPY

Chest physiotherapy may be necessary as some children become undernourished, due to feeding difficulties, and therefore are more prone to chest infections. This will include postural drainage, turning and vibrations, both pre- and postoperatively.

Facial palsy

This may be congenital or acquired, causing great distress to the patient. The face symmetry may be improved with surgery. The most common operation is the fascial sling. Fascia may be taken from the tensor fascia lata and attached to the zygomatic arch and the zygomaticus muscle, thereby hitching up the sagging muscles.

In some cases nerve grafts are being used as an alternative approach.

HANDS

Hand surgery and rehabilitation must aim towards producing maximum function, cosmetic appearance being of secondary importance.

One of the major problems following hand surgery is stiffness. Some causes of stiffness are (a) oedema, (b) pain, (c) immobilisation, or (d) scar tissue.

The more the above problems are reduced to a minimum, the more chance the patient has of regaining good function.

Crush injuries of hands

Following crush injury there is gross swelling, due to the presence of excess tissue fluid and also excessive bleeding. The patient is taken to theatre and the tissue is decompressed by the evacuation of blood and fluid. Dead tissue should be excised to prevent infection occurring.

Fractures are reduced and if unstable are fixed with Kirschner wire. Nerves and blood vessels are repaired and skin loss made good by split skin grafts or full thickness flaps. *The hand is elevated to minimise oedema.*

PHYSIOTHERAPY

Immediately after the operation physiotherapy is commenced and shoulder and elbow exercises are carried out.

It may be possible to carry out hand movements in the early stage if a skin graft has not been applied; should it be applied movements are deferred for five days. From the commencement of treatment, joint range should be measured at frequent intervals.

Oedema is controlled by massage, exercises in elevation and a pressure bandage.

At the earliest opportunity, active exercises are commenced to each individual joint, and the hand as a whole, as well as accessory movements.

When the incision has healed and skin grafts settled, a bland cream is massaged into the scars to soften them. At a later stage, if the scars have become adherent, ultrasound may be used.

It must be remembered that gross hand deformities may also cause psychological problems, with which the patient may need some help. If these deformities prevent him from returning to his former work, a hand assessment should be carried out and a meeting with the disablement rehabilitation officer (DRO) should be arranged in order to find the patient more suitable work.

Tendon repairs

PRIMARY REPAIR

This is the surgery of choice where possible, suturing the two ends together soon after the injury has occurred.

After the repair, the patient is treated in a Kleinert-type splint

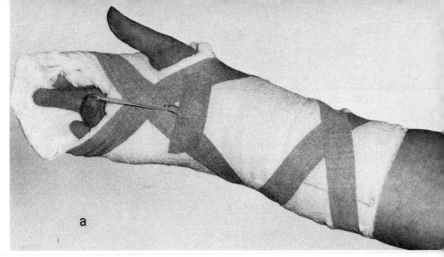

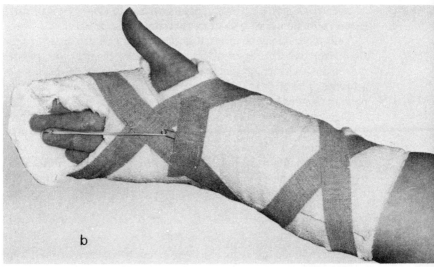

Fig. 15/11   Kleinert-type splint. (a) The resting position. (b) Extension of the finger

(Figs. 15/11a and b). This splint allows for active movement in all the joints, including those affected by the tendon repair.

Flexor tendons: Extension of the finger is allowed within the limits of the splint. Following this, the patient relaxes the finger and the elastic band will return to its former position of flexion, thereby offering resistance to the antagonists and giving reflex relaxation of the agonists.

Extensor tendons: The finger is held in maximum extension to prevent the tendons becoming slack as the patient begins to mobilise the finger.

In both cases, the splint is removed after three weeks.

PHYSIOTHERAPY

Immediately postoperatively, the patient is instructed to exercise within the Kleinert splint, actively extending the finger and allowing the elastic band to flex it.

After three weeks the plaster of Paris is removed and gentle active exercises are commenced. Massage with a bland cream may be given to the scar. Passive stretching may be required at eight weeks as the tendons often become adherent within the flexor sheath and thus there may be difficulty in extending the finger. At eight weeks a dynamic splint to aid extension may be applied.

SECONDARY REPAIR

Flexor tendon graft: If the surgeon is unable to carry out a primary suture, a tendon graft will almost certainly be necessary.

A silastic rod may be inserted for about six weeks in order to keep the flexor sheaths open while the patient regains full passive movement, which may be lost due to inactivity since the time of accident. The graft is then inserted. This is usually taken from the palmaris longus or extensor digitorum brevis tendons.

Kleinert splinting is again used and the splint removed after three weeks when active physiotherapy is commenced.

Following tendon grafts and repairs, the aim must be to regain full range movements and it must be impressed upon the patient the need to exercise frequently when at home. It will require maximum effort and co-operation on his part to obtain a good result.

Mallet finger

This is a common injury in which the extensor tendon is avulsed from its attachment at the base of the distal phalanx (Fig. 15/12).

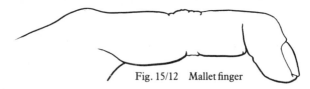

Fig. 15/12   Mallet finger

TREATMENT

The finger is splinted for at least six weeks with the distal interphalangeal joint hyperextended. Following this gentle mobilisation commences, with instruction given on the wearing of the splints during activities likely to cause recurrences of the injury.

Dupuytren's contracture

This is a condition affecting the palmar aponeurosis in which thickening, fibrosis and contracture occur.

TREATMENT

Surgery is performed removing the affected tissue and skin may be transposed from the dorsum of the finger to repair the defect or a skin graft used. Some surgeons leave the wound of the palm open and encourage early movement.

Physiotherapy commences immediately postoperatively, to prevent stiffness of those joints not involved in surgery.

Recently, mobilisation of the affected joints has been commenced at two to five days, the hand being placed in a polythene bag or silicone oil.

Once healing has occurred, massage and ultrasonics may be given to soften the scars.

Rheumatoid arthritis

Prophylactic synovectomies

These may be performed with the hope of preventing further damage. The hypertrophic synovium is removed and active exercises are commenced after five to ten days in order to regain function.

Common deformities seen in rheumatoid arthritis are:

1. Ulnar deviation
2. Subluxation of the metacarpophalangeal joints
3. Swan neck deformity (Fig. 15/13)
4. Boutonnière deformity (Fig. 15/14)

A *replacement arthroplasty* may be used to correct deformities of the metacarpophalangeal joints. This is performed using silastic joints, e.g. Swanson's.

PHYSIOTHERAPY

Immediately postoperatively, the patient is mobilised within the retraining splint. (This is a lively-type splint to prevent ulnar deviation recurring.) Gentle passive movements may also be given to these new joints. After three weeks, when supervised by the physiotherapist, the splint may be removed for treatment, although the patient is encouraged to wear the splint for about three months (Figs. 15/15a, b, c.).

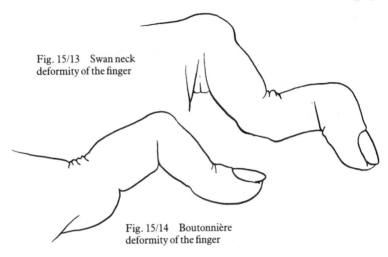

Fig. 15/13   Swan neck
deformity of the finger

Fig. 15/14   Boutonnière
deformity of the finger

Correction of deformities

Deformities involving the interphalangeal joints, such as Boutonnière and swan neck, are corrected by Harrison pegs. These are small, angled, polypropylene pegs inserted into the medullary cavity of the phalanges and which, in effect, arthrodese the joint in a functional and stable position.

TREATMENT

This being a form of arthrodesis, mobilisation of the affected joint must *not* be undertaken. As the patient has been immobilised in plaster of Paris, it may be necessary to mobilise the other joints.

Ulnar styloidectomy

This is performed either because of pain, or to prevent rupture of the extensor tendons. Little physiotherapy is required.

Syndactyly

This is the condition where two or more digits are joined by a skin web. Occasionally bony continuity may be present.

Fig. 15/15 (*opposite*)   (a) Rheumatoid arthritis of the hands. (b) Following surgery, the patient wears a retraining splint. (c) The hand, with the splint removed.

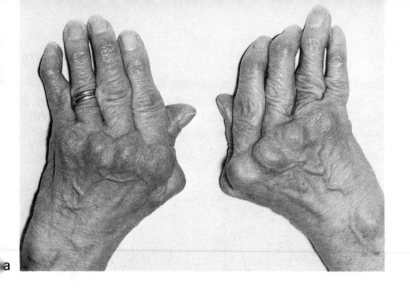

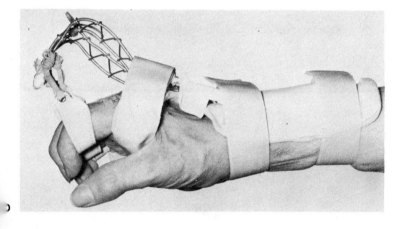

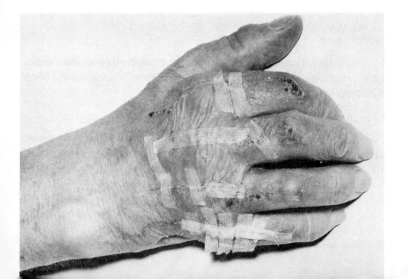

TREATMENT

The fingers are separated surgically and a skin graft may be inserted (Fig. 15/16). Once the skin grafts have settled, physiotherapy in the form of active movements is commenced.

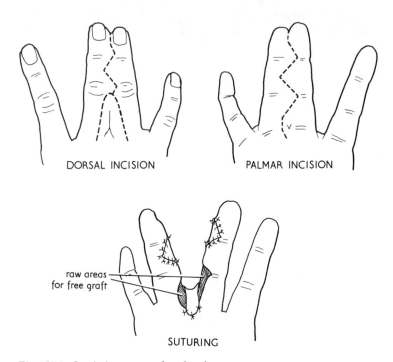

Fig. 15/16   Surgical treatment of syndactyly

Pollicisation

This is an operation devised to replace the thumb using another digit. This is transferred with intact vessels and nerves, and implanted on to the thumb metacarpal.

PHYSIOTHERAPY

This is commenced when the plaster is removed, i.e. when bony union has occurred. It must be noted that the new joint and skin sensation of the thumb continues to be that of the transposed digit, therefore re-education should be directed with this in mind.

Toe and thumb transfer (Figs. 15/17, 15/18, 15/19 and 15/20)

An alternative method of pollicisation is the free transference of a toe to take the place of the thumb. In the authors' unit the second toe is used. The surgical technique is as follows:

1. Amputation of the toe at the metatarsophalangeal joint together with the dorsalis pedis artery and veins, digital nerves and tendons.
2. Fixation of bone at the level of the metacarpophalangeal joint with the use of bone grafts, wiring or pegs.
3. Anastamosis of vessels, tendons and nerves:
   (a) Dorsalis pedis to radial artery
   (b) Vein to cephalic vein
   (c) Extensor tendon to extensor pollicis longus.
       Flexor digitorum profundis to flexor pollicis longus
   (d) Volar digital nerve to the digital nerve of the thumb.

No movement should occur at the *point of arthrodesis*, but active exercises may be commenced at three weeks to encourage flexion and extension of the terminal joint and apposition using the carpometacarpal joint.

Replantation

In the past, severe injuries of the hand have often led to amputation but now replantation has been made possible by the use of the microscope in surgery (Figs. 15/21 and 15/22).

The term *replantation* is used *only* when the part is completely severed and is sewn back. *Revascularisation* is the term used if even a fragment of skin or other tissue is intact with the proximal portion.

In one unit the following surgical procedures usually occur:

1. The bone is approximated and held with either K-wires or interosseus wiring
2. The extensor tendons are repaired
3. The veins are anastomosed
4. The flexor tendons are repaired
5. The arteries are anastomosed
6. The nerves are sutured.

The hand is immobilised by a loose plaster of Paris shell for approximately 10 days: if the replant appears healthy gentle exercises may commence. These patients may be on treatment for several months; the usual precautions because of anaesthesia of the part being taken as for tendon and nerve repairs.

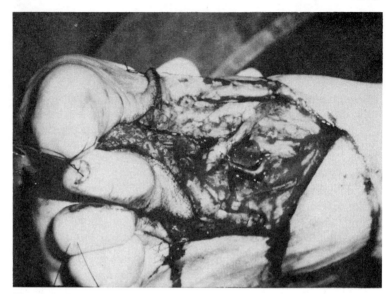

Fig. 15/17   Removal of the toe

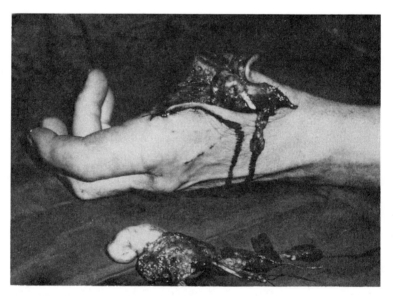

Fig. 15/18   The toe prior to suture to the thumb site

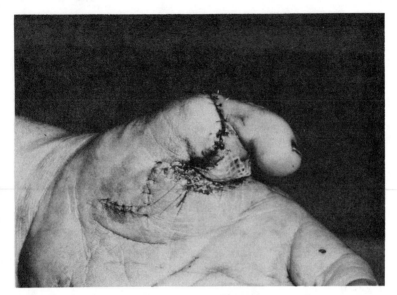

Fig. 15/19   Toe in situ as the thumb

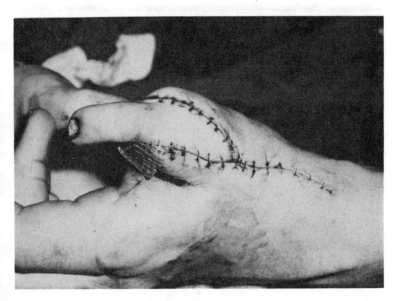

Fig. 15/20   Toe in situ as the thumb, at end of operation

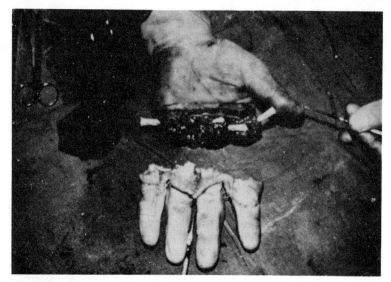

Fig. 15/21   Complete severance of fingers

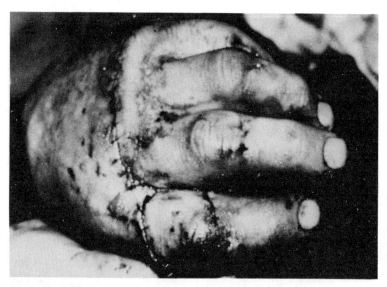

Fig. 15/22   Fingers replanted

TRUNK AND LOWER LIMB

Pressure sores

If pressure sores fail to heal, it may be necessary to excise the sore and any underlying necrotic tissue including bone, and cover it with skin. This is usually performed by the use of a transposition flap and most commonly to the sacrum, ischial tuberosity and/or greater trochanters.

Transposition or rotation flap: This is a rectangle or square of skin and subcutaneous tissue which is rotated around a pivot into an immediately adjacent defect. The donor area is covered by a split skin graft (Fig. 15/3). When, or if, possible the patient is nursed on a low air loss bed (see p. 234), the flap being exposed and free from pressure.

PHYSIOTHERAPY

Breathing exercises to prevent chest infections are given and wherever possible active movements to all joints. Care must be taken to ensure that there is no stress on the flap which would endanger the circulation. It should be remembered that many of these patients have neurological conditions, such as paraplegia and multiple sclerosis. It is, therefore, most important to carry out passive movements in order to prevent contractures. Total rehabilitation must be planned to suit their condition.

When the flap is stable and circulation satisfactory, this is at approximately three weeks, the patient is allowed up for short periods. The length of time is gradually increased as the circulation in the flap continues to improve. A careful watch must be kept and if the flap shows signs of breaking down, the patient must be returned to bed and the pressure removed.

Malignant melanoma

This is a malignant, pigmented tumour which often presents as a dark mole which grows rapidly and later becomes irritable and occasionally bleeds. Wide excision and skin graft is the treatment of choice. Approximately 7cm either side and 10cm towards the proximal lymph nodes is removed and a split skin graft used to cover the defect. Block dissection of the proximal lymph nodes may also be undertaken.

PHYSIOTHERAPY

As this condition can affect any part of the body, physiotherapy is given accordingly.

Lower limb: The grafted area is immobilised and if a block dissection of the groin nodes has been performed, the patient is nursed with the hip in flexion. Movements are given to the distal joints to maintain circulation, prevent thrombosis and stiffness in the limb. Movements are given to the other limb.

After two weeks, gentle mobilisation to the hip joint is commenced followed by walking at about three weeks. A double thickness layer of Tubigrip is applied for ambulation, and it may be necessary to wear this for many months. Swelling may occur because of interference with the lymphatic drainage.

Upper limb: If this condition occurs in the upper limb, and a block dissection of the cervical nodes has been performed, it is essential to give postoperative breathing exercises. The patient's chest condition must always be noted and, if necessary, treated.

Lymphoedema

This may be congenital or acquired. Oedema is due to a blockage of lymphatic vessels. Acquired lymphoedema often follows surgery where excision of lymph nodes has been undertaken; in the tropics, filariasis can be a cause.

TREATMENT

1. *Thompson operation – or buried dermal flap*: In this operation fat and lymphoedematous tissue is excised, usually from groin to ankle or wrist to axilla around half the circumference of the limb. One of the resulting two flaps is de-epithelialised and then sutured between the muscle bellies (Fig. 15/23). This establishes a communication between the usually patent deep system of lymphatics which subsequently drains the more superficial layers. The remaining flap is sutured over the de-epithelialised area and a pressure dressing applied. The patient is nursed in bed with the leg elevated for 10 days or until the wound has healed.

PHYSIOTHERAPY

Chest physiotherapy and ankle exercises to prevent thrombosis are carried out. At 10 days, if the wound has healed, a Bisgaard (red/blue-line) bandage or a layer of Tubigrip is applied and the patient swings the leg over the side of the bed. At 10 to 12 days,

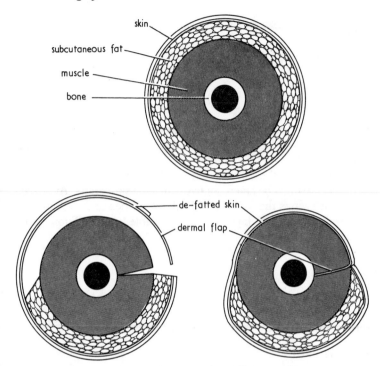

Fig. 15/23 Thompson operation for lymphoedema (diagrammatic)

weight-bearing commences followed by walking re-education, as the patient has often been in bed for two to three weeks and the wound is extensive.

2. *Charles operation*: In this operation the skin and lymphoedematous tissue is excised down to deep fascia, from knee to ankle, the skin being separated and used to cover the defect.

PHYSIOTHERAPY

The leg is immobilised until the skin graft has become established. After seven days, gentle active movements are commenced and weight-bearing allowed at 10 to 12 days with a double layer of Tubigrip being worn for support.

Ulcers and lacerations with skin necrosis

These conditions usually occur in older patients and those patients with impairment of blood supply or who through the use of drugs and radiotherapy develop paper thin or fibrotic skin.

Ulcers

The patient is admitted for bed rest, elevation of the leg and cleaning of the ulcer. Once clean and healthy looking a split skin graft is applied to close the defect.

PHYSIOTHERAPY

Pre-operatively, maintenance exercises to increase circulation, prevent thrombosis, decrease oedema and prevent joint stiffness are carried out.

Postoperatively the patient will continue the maintenance exercises, but care must be taken not to disturb the skin grafts. At 10 days the patient swings the leg over the side of the bed and walking may commence at 12 to 14 days, wearing a double layer of Tubigrip for support.

Lacerations

Skin necrosis may be caused by lacerations and failure to heal after suturing. The laceration may be jagged and surrounding tissue necrotic. In this case a skin graft is used to cover the defect.

PHYSIOTHERAPY

Postoperatively physiotherapy is carried out as for ulcers.

Compound fractures

The fractures most commonly seen on a plastic surgery unit are compound fractures of the tibia and fibula, where skin loss is evident. A fracture will not unite if there is inadequate skin cover, and if infection occurs serious problems such as osteomyelitis may ensue.

The aim of treatment is to provide skin cover as soon as possible, by the use of a skin graft. The quality of skin must then be improved so as to prevent further breakdown and, consequently, frequent hospital admissions. A free flap is applied but if this is impossible a cross-leg flap or tube pedicle will be used.

There are several ways of dealing with the management of these fractures while providing skin cover:

1. The patient may be nursed in an above-knee plaster cast with a window over the site of the skin loss, or
2. In traction with a Steinmann pin through the calcaneus, or
3. With external fixation (Fig. 15/24).

PHYSIOTHERAPY

Exercises may be carried out on the affected limb but with particular precautions being taken not to disturb the fracture site or skin graft.

Maintenance exercises are carried out as for orthopaedic patients; sandbags, springs, etc being used to maintain the strength of the good leg and arms.

Breathing exercises are carried out if necessary, but as the majority of these patients are young men, chest complications are rare. If, however, patients present with multiple injuries, e.g. fractured ribs, sternum or mandible, breathing exercises then become a necessity.

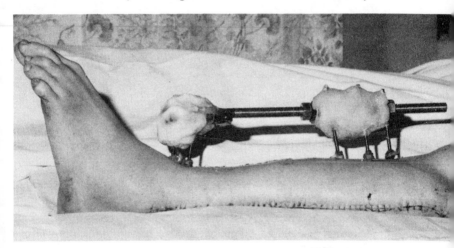

Fig. 15/24 External fixation for compound fracture of tibia (*note*: the screws are protected by plastic)

As soon as skin cover has been achieved, patients are often referred back to the orthopaedic surgeon and therefore the final rehabilitation is carried out from the orthopaedic ward.

COSMETIC SURGERY

Rhinoplasty

This is an operation to improve the appearance or function of the nose. It is undertaken for congenital or post-traumatic deformities and is often a two-stage operation consisting of: (1) sub-mucal resection, and (2) in-fracture, i.e. the nasal bones are separated from the maxilla, thus allowing them to be mobilised and the correct position attained. Immobilisation is carried out by the use of plaster of Paris.

Face lifting

This is to eliminate wrinkles; an incision being made in front of the ears, the skin undermined and pulled tight. This may also be accompanied by eyelid reductions.

Dermabrasion

This is used to flatten irregularities of the skin such as are caused by acne. Sandpaper or wire brushes are used to perform the operation.

Port wine stains

These are congenital birth marks. They may be excised and skin grafted.

Abdominal lipectomy

This is performed to remove excess fatty tissue from the abdomen. It is also known as an apronectomy.

Mammaplasty

This is carried out to reduce or augment breast tissue.
Mammary hypoplasia: This is lack of breast tissue which may be congenital or acquired. Augmentation is achieved by the insertion of a silicone prosthesis.
Mammary hyperplasia: This is an increase in breast tissue which is again congenital or acquired and surgery may be carried out to remove this excess tissue.

Bat or prominent ears

The operation is usually performed on school children who are often teased about the condition. This is corrected by the excision of some post-auricular skin and alteration of the cartilaginous tissue of the ears if necessary.

PHYSIOTHERAPY

Little physiotherapy is carried out for any of the above conditions unless the patient has an underlying chest condition. In the case of mammaplasty, breathing exercises may be required as tight strapping around the chest impedes lung expansion.

OTHER CONDITIONS

Scar revision

Disfiguring scars, i.e. those following trauma, must be allowed to settle before further surgery is contemplated. The most simple procedure is to excise and resuture. Ultrasound may be used on any scars to soften the area.

Z-PLASTY (Fig. 15/25)

This is an operation whereby the course of the scar is altered, i.e. to try to allow the scar to blend in with the surrounding tissue by, wherever possible, lying in the same direction as the skin lines.

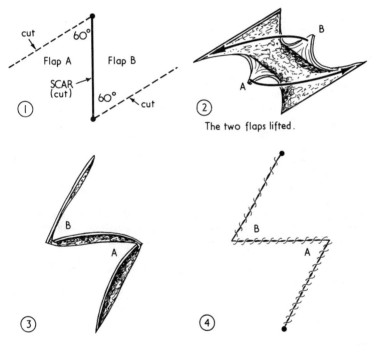

Fig. 15/25   Diagrams to show the mechanics of a Z-plasty. (Cut one out for yourself on paper)

Hypospadias

This is a congenital deformity whereby the urethra opens on to the undersurface of the penis or perineum. The aim of surgery is to move the opening forward to the tip of the penis. This is done by:

1. Releasing the chordae
2. Creating a gutter through which the urethra may pass and inserting a temporary catheter
3. Skin grafting around the catheter.

As this is mostly performed on young children, little or no physiotherapy is needed.

BIBLIOGRAPHY

Burke, F. D. (1983). Microsurgery in the upper limb. *Physiotherapy*, **69**, 10, 346–9.

Conolly, W. B. (1980). *A Colour Atlas of Hand Conditions*. Wolfe Medical and Scientific Publications, London.

Grabb, W. C. and Smith, J. W. (1973). *Plastic Surgery: A Concise Guide to Clinical Practice*, 2nd edition. Little, Brown and Co, Boston.

Jackson, I. T. (ed) (1981). *Recent Advances in Plastic Surgery – 2*. Churchill Livingstone, Edinburgh.

Jones, B., Smith, P. and Harrison, D. (1983). Replantation. (Leading article.) *British Medical Journal*, **287**, 1–2.

Lister, G. (1977). *The Hand: Diagnosis and Indications*. Churchill Livingstone, Edinburgh.

McGregor, I. A. (1980). *Fundamental Techniques of Plastic Surgery and Their Surgical Applications*, 7th edition. Churchill Livingstone, Edinburgh.

O'Brien, B. (1977). *Microvascular Reconstructive Surgery*. Churchill Livingstone, Edinburgh.

Reid, C. D. A. and Gossett, J. (eds) (1979). *Mutilating Injuries of the Hand*. Churchill Livingstone, Edinburgh.

Watson, N. (1983). Dupuytren's contracture. *Physiotherapy*, **69**, 10, 353–4.

Wynn Parry, C. B. (1981). *Rehabilitation of the Hand*, 4th edition. Butterworths, London.

Chapter 16

Burns

by S. BOARDMAN, MCSP and P. M. WALKER, MCSP

A burn is a lesion caused by heat or any substance which has a cauterising effect on the skin. For an understanding of the skin and its function see Chapter 15, pages 196–7.

All age-groups may be affected but children and the elderly are at risk, similarly psychiatric and epileptic patients are particular risk groups. Many burns result from accidents in the home, most of which are preventable.

Types

FLAME BURNS

These occur when there is actual contact with flames, i.e. clothing catching fire.

They are predominantly full thickness burns.

SCALDS

These occur when there is contact with steam, hot water, etc; the depth being variable depending on the heat and type of fluid involved.

CONTACT

Contact with hot bitumen, hot presses and bars of an electric fire (where no shock is felt) produce burns which are often full thickness but may be of any depth.

FLASH

Explosions causing a flash produce superficial or partial thickness burns.

ELECTRICAL

When a current, either AC or DC, passes through the body a full thickness burn occurs.

CHEMICAL

The application of acid or alkali on the skin causes a burn of any depth dependent on the concentration of the chemical.

Effects

In any burn, particularly if it is extensive, the immediate and serious effects are shock, severe fluid and protein depletion, and the chance of gross infection if every possible care is not taken.

SHOCK

Shock is the first hazard to be combated or, better still, prevented. Crile has stated that 'the best treatment for shock is prevention' and since shock is anticipated in burns it can be counteracted by early treatment. In burns, shock is delayed and results from the fluid and protein loss from the blood due to the increased permeability of the vessel walls. Due to this loss, the viscosity of the blood is increased. The compound effect of decreased circulatory volume and increased viscosity leads to a fall in blood pressure based upon decreased venous return to the heart. When fluid loss is allowed to continue vasoconstriction takes place, eventually affecting the blood supply to the viscera and alimentary tract, sometimes resulting in kidney and liver damage.

In partial thickness burns, blisters occur due to seepage of fluid between the layers of the epidermis. Together with loss of fluid into the tissues, again due to the increased permeability of vessel walls, this gives rise to gross oedema (Fig. 16/1).

INFECTION

Infection is another serious complication in burns. Organisms embedded in hair follicles and sweat glands can survive the sterilising effect of excess heat and provide sources of infection. Further infection can occur from contamination from outside sources. This is why the isolation and treatment of these patients are carried out under the strictest conditions. The necrotic skin and constant oozing provide the ideal host for receiving and growth of bacteria, and where this is not adequately combated general toxic effects are produced. Local infection complicates surgery, for obviously where there is infection there will be an inability to accept grafts.

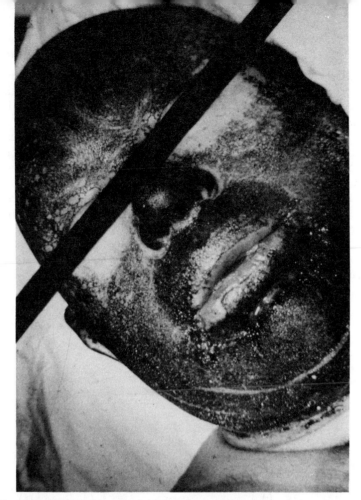

Fig. 16/1   A patient with a severely burned face showing the gross oedema

Classification

Under this heading we must consider the depth, the size and the position of the burn in assessing its severity. Burns fall into two categories, partial thickness and full thickness. In the former, the epithelium and superficial layers of the dermis only are involved and healing can occur by first intention. In full thickness burns the dermis is totally destroyed and with it the epithelial lining of the sweat glands and hair follicles so that no regenerative islands are left and healing can occur only from the wound edges, resulting in unstable scarring and underlying contractures.

It must be borne in mind that the assessment of depth of some burns is not easily definable in the first 48 hours, and even then the difference between partial and full thickness burns can by no means be correctly defined. What appears to be deep may prove to be partial, and what is partial thickness may indeed become deep due to further destruction of partly damaged cells by pressure or infection.

Partial thickness burns may be acutely painful since the nerve endings are damaged, whereas in full thickness burns the nerve endings are totally destroyed, and therefore the acute pain and immediate systemic effects from it are often less severe. Burn areas, of course, are invariably of mixed partial and full thickness involvement.

The depth of the burn is dependent on the temperature to which the area is exposed and the duration of the exposure.

In assessing the extent of the area involved the 'rule of nine' is useful to remember (Fig. 16/2). The percentages of the total body area in adults are as follows:

head and neck	9%	arms	9% each
front of trunk	18%	legs	18% each
back of trunk	18%	perineum	1%

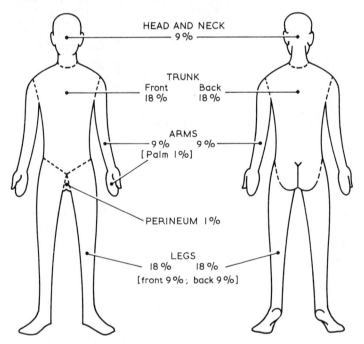

Fig. 16/2   The 'rule of nine' for assessing the extent of the burned area

It is of interest to note that the palm of the hand is 1 per cent. As a rule 20 per cent burns in adults and 15 per cent in children necessitate intravenous fluid replacement. No one area gives rise to greater fluid loss than another but it is stated that there is greater loss in superficial than in deep burns.

With regard to the position of burns, wherever hands, feet, face and joints are involved, these should be regarded as major burns. It is the obvious functional importance of hands and feet that place them in this category. Burns of the feet, because of their weight-bearing function, are major burns. It has been stated that the hands are, next to the brain, man's greatest asset and when they are burnt it must be remembered that man is robbed of a large quota of his independence.

Joints fall into this major burn concept because their flexor surfaces, so often involved, tend to contract, thus producing accompanying ligamentous tightening and, if neglected, resultant joint changes. As far as the face is concerned, apart from the cosmetic importance of treating it as a major burn, burns of the eyelids can produce contracture. This in turn, because the result is inadequate coverage of the eyes, can lead to corneal ulceration. It must also be remembered that facial burns are often associated with inhalation burns and involvement of the respiratory tract, when intubation and ventilation may be necessary.

From the point of view of infection some areas are known to be much more prone to pseudomonas than others, e.g. the trunk and the inner side of the thighs.

The severity of burns is not estimated only by their extent, depth and position. The age and general condition of the patient must also be taken into consideration. The elderly and the very young are at much greater risk than other age-groups, the former due often to their lower resistance to infection and their relative immobility resulting from possible secondary disability such as heart and lung conditions or arthritic joint changes. The more elderly the patient, the lower the percentage of burn that may prove fatal.

In children it is generally accepted that they are at great risk because the relationship between their total body surface and their circularised volume is such that they lose comparatively more essential constituents of the body through a burn of given extent than an adult.

General treatment

The majority of patients with severe burns are usually admitted to the casualty department of district general hospitals, where treatment should be commenced before transfer to a burns unit.

More and more specialised units are being established, and early transfer within the first 24 hours is ideal. These units provide the specialised care that is urgently required and, by their construction, equipment and management, are geared to minimise the chance of infection which is so very prevalent in burns. In most units patients are nursed in individual rooms where the temperature can be controlled and the patient receives all the intensive care that is necessary following such severe trauma.

PRIORITIES ON ADMISSION

1. Ensure a clear airway
2. Exclude other serious injury
3. Provide adequate analgesia
4. Fluid replacement
5. History of injury, e.g. burn, date, time, circumstances, temperature, duration of contact and first aid measures
6. Medical history, e.g. alcoholic, drug addict, psychiatric
7. Social history
8. Examination of the burn

The airway should be checked. In cases of pulmonary complications endotracheal intubation or tracheostomy with pulmonary ventilation may be needed.

The replacement of fluid loss is of prime importance to counteract 'burns shock' but care is necessary to avoid under or over transfusion. Urine output is carefully monitored and a urinary catheter allows hourly estimation.

Before the burns are dressed they are cleaned and the blisters are de-roofed. Patients with superficial burns have them covered with paraffin gauze dressings and left for one week. Deep dermal or full thickness burns are dressed with silver sulphadiazine, chlorhexidine or similar preparations; the dressings are changed daily.

Superficial burns should heal by natural intent in about 12 days. Deep dermal and full thickness burns will require surgical intervention.

Over the years the time factor has been reduced for the excision of dead tissue, and in many cases the operation can be performed between two and five days after the initial injury. This is clearly beneficial as mobility and function may be quickly regained and the length of stay in hospital reduced. Where this is not possible because of the patient's general condition, surgery is delayed for three weeks during which time the slough will begin to separate. When patients sustain mixed thickness burns which are difficult to assess, dressings using silver sulphadiazine for three weeks are of infinite value, as they allow the depth of burn to declare itself. Any superficial and partial thickness burns will by this time have practically healed. When possible, the defect is covered by autografts, i.e. the patient's own skin.

The ideal environment for the treatment of burns is one where infection can be readily controlled. Patients are therefore isolated and this isolation can lead to difficulties in management. Many patients suffering from burns find it depressing and frightening to be alone, and in some cases they may already have psychological and social problems, such as alcoholism, depression, or epilepsy; these problems need very careful assessment and treatment with the help of psychiatric and social workers. In making plans for future rehabilitation this aspect must not be disregarded.

In such an environment of isolation, treatment can be easily carried out, room temperatures can be controlled to individual needs and a strict aseptic routine can be followed at all times.

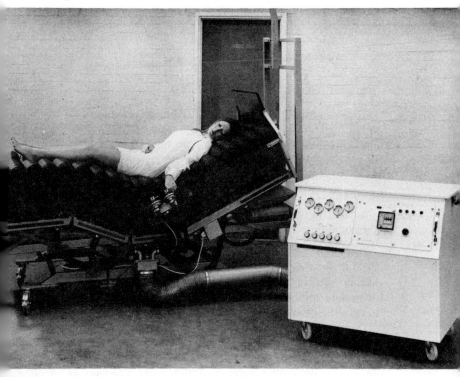

Fig. 16/3   The low air loss bed

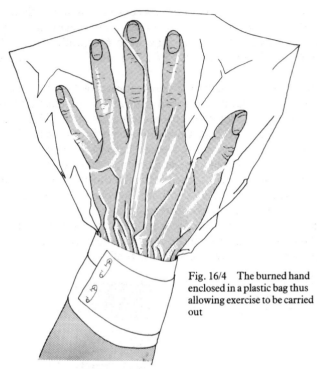

Fig. 16/4 The burned hand enclosed in a plastic bag thus allowing exercise to be carried out

Ideally in the early stage, patients with extensive burns are nursed on low air loss beds (Fig. 16/3). This is an air displacement system. The bed consists of five sections each adjusting to the body contour, the pressures of which can be individually controlled to suit the needs of the patient. Nursing care with this type of bed is simplified by:

1. The elimination of pressure areas.
2. Lifting and turning the patients is reduced to a minimum.
3. Changing of bed linen is reduced as only a top sheet is required.

Physiotherapists find that the tipping mechanism is easily controlled which is an asset in the treatment of the chest. However, they do criticise the fact that patients have difficulty in moving themselves around the bed and for this reason it is necessary to transfer the patient to a hospital type bed as soon as possible.

The hands should be elevated to prevent oedema; to prevent contractures hands are covered with silver sulphadiazine or silicone oil and placed in plastic bags or gauntlets so that exercises can be carried out easily and mobility maintained (Fig. 16/4). The bags are changed daily or as required.

Saline baths used to be employed a great deal for the badly burned but in some units their popularity has waned, because of the dangers of cross-infection. However, when they are used, they can be invaluable in facilitating early movement and easing the removal of dressings. Patients can be immersed gently in tanks containing normal saline, diluted 1 : 20, at body temperature. The patient may be initially apprehensive but exercises under these conditions can be more comfortably carried out. These baths are given every two or three days and they are discontinued for at least five days after grafting. If the baths are not given, showers are of great value.

Physiotherapy in the treatment of burns

AIMS OF TREATMENT

1. To prevent chest complications
2. To maintain mobility and prevent contractures

In extensively burned patients, breathing exercises is the earliest treatment given. Many of these patients suffer inhalation of hot and poisonous gases or steam, and the mucous membrane linings of the respiratory tract become inflamed and oedematous thus making intubation and ventilation a possibility. Only on rare occasions is tracheostomy performed. This carries with it the danger of infection if it is not managed correctly. Suction should be carried out with the greatest possible care using a 'no-touch' technique. If the patient is ventilated, the physiotherapist may be asked to carry out vibrations while the doctor bag-squeezes, and the nurse uses suction.

After the patient has been extubated, an intermittent positive pressure breathing machine, such as the Bird or Bennett is often used. These machines are also of infinite value on patients who have an underlying chronic chest condition present prior to their burns.

It should be noted that children with burns of the face and trunk easily develop acute chest symptoms, but respiratory complications often take 24 hours or more to develop.

If the patient has chest burns but no obvious respiratory complications, care must be taken; expansion only should be checked and vibration and percussions not given, as further trauma to already burned tissues may result in superficial burns becoming full thickness.

If burns are full thickness and circumferential, the patient will be encased in a tight armour of eschar (burn scab). The surgeon may perform a longitudinal incision or escharotomy in order to allow chest expansion and thereby prevent lung collapse.

Positioning of the patient is most important and a close watch must be kept on this by the physiotherapist as well as by the nursing staff. Burns overlying the flexor aspect of joints give rise to contracture. These must be prevented. Splints are ideal though with severe burns they are difficult to apply effectively. Plaster of Paris with Kramer wire, Plastazote, Polyform and Orthoplast are all used in an effort to support and maintain good functional positions of joints including the cervical spine. Here it must be stated that some contractures are not completely preventable, but it is still important that every effort is made to minimise them. The use of boards and splints to prevent foot drop are essential and knees should be maintained as straight as possible. The head and neck should be supported in a mid- and extended position. Since oedema is very prevalent in burns, hands in particular should be elevated by fixation to suitable apparatus beside and above the bed and sometimes upon well-placed pillows.

All movements can be encouraged from the time the patient is admitted to hospital. However, when autografts are applied, the grafted areas must not be mobilised for at least five days when the first dressing takes place. This does not prevent physiotherapists giving movements to ungrafted areas and it is indeed essential that they should continue them.

Movements can be commenced between five and seven days.

A feature of burns illness is a mental surrender to apathy – often aggravated by necessary isolation. Combined with this is a suppression of intellectual and aesthetic interests and a withdrawal from personal relationships. The physiotherapist's daily, or twice daily, visits give these patients a regular and closer contact with the outside world and this in turn demands of the physiotherapist a great understanding and the ability to provide mental stimulation. In some units complete isolation is maintained only during the pre-grafting period, then, after grafting, the patient is transferred to a three- or four-bedded ward where the encouragement and company of others is undoubtedly an added incentive to recovery.

The treatment of burns is extremely time-consuming for the physiotherapist. When burns are extensive it is necessary to encourage specific and general mobilisation; it must be remembered that these patients tire easily and must be allowed frequent rest periods. Time must be spent in encouragement, endeavouring to give confidence to patients who, due partly to their isolation and largely to the severity of their injuries, need maximum reassurance and come to look on their physiotherapist as a source of special contact with the rest of the medical team.

AMBULATION

This varies from unit to unit, but from the authors' experience it has been found that early ambulation is desirable. Red/blue-line bandage or Tubigrip is used as support bandaging and patients with severe leg burns may also be walked before grafting.

It is advisable to swing the well-bandaged legs over the side of the bed before commencing weight-bearing. Following surgery, blistering of newly grafted areas can occur due to the inadequacy of newly established circulation to the grafted areas and therefore weight-bearing may not commence for seven to ten days. Standing around is *not* permitted, and when sitting out the lower limbs should be elevated. Crêpe bandages, Tubigrip or elastic stockings will have to be worn for several weeks by those with grafted legs, to prevent oedema. The adapting of footwear may be necessary where there is need to compensate for contracture (e.g. tight calf contractures may need a heel-raise) or to relieve specific pressure areas. This can be done with foam rubber or Plastazote.

The patient should attend the physiotherapy department at the earliest possible opportunity and this is often the patient's first contact with the outside world following the burn. Here supportive therapy and great encouragement is required because the disfigurement caused by the burn is often demoralising. Helping patients to surmount and overcome their natural self-consciousness is something in which the physiotherapist can play a very helpful role (see Chapter 17).

THE HAND

The hand is a perfect piece of mechanism on which man is constantly dependent. As such it is considered necessary to dwell a little on its individual treatment.

Hands are common sites for burns, not only through direct involvement, but also because they are so often used in a reflex action to protect the face. There are more dorsal than palmar burns, partly due to the thick palmar skin.

Once again the maintenance of a good functional position is essential. The wrist should be extended, the metacarpophalangeal joints flexed, the interphalangeal joints extended and the thumb in abduction and slight flexion. If the patient is unable to maintain full active movements, or is unco-operative, splinting may be applied, and thus the typical burns deformity of the hand, i.e. dropped wrist, hyperextended metacarpophalangeal joints and flexed interphalangeal joints, is prevented (Fig. 16/5).

After healing sensation is not entirely normal, and patients must be warned of the dangers of coming into contact with direct heat, e.g. hot plates, radiators, etc, as well as against exposure to sun for at least 12 months. Once the grafts are healed and skin becomes more stable, the patient attends the rehabilitation department where the physiotherapist gives the patient hand exercises. Warm water baths can also be of value but no direct heat in the form of infra-red lamps or wax

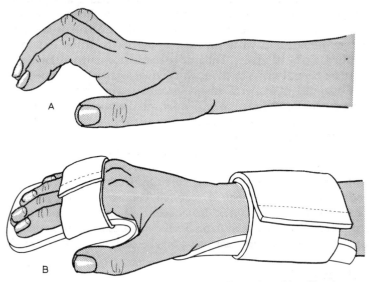

Fig. 16/5   (a) The contractures of a burned hand. (b) Correction achieved by adequate splinting

should be given. Massage with hand cream such as lanolin is given in order to soften the scar. These treatments are usually carried out in conjunction with the occupational therapy department.

Advances, which originated in the USA, are still being made in the prevention of hypertrophic scars after burns. One method adopted in this country is proving most successful. It consists of the use of precisely-measured pressure garments, such as gloves and stockings, made of an elasticated mesh material. The wearing of such garments can start at about two weeks after the burned or grafted areas are healed (Fig. 16/6). It has been found necessary to insist on these being worn 24 hours a day for 6 to 18 months, except for brief periods to enable washing, etc (Fig. 16/7). These garments are often used in

Fig. 16/6 A patient with a healed burned and grafted chest

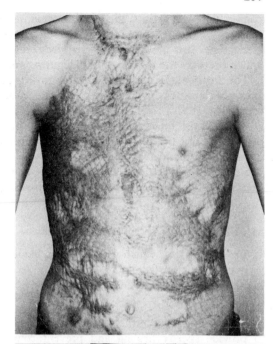

Fig. 16/7 The same patient as in Figure 16/6 wearing a precisely measured pressure garment to prevent the development of hypertrophic scars

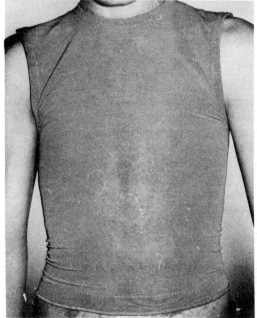

conjunction with splints, the latter maintaining pressure in the axilla or neck where pressure from the elasticated mesh would be inadequate. It is the exact and even pressure of these two materials which prevents the formation of disfiguring and disabling scars.

The theory of the success of such methods is that the application of pressure elongates the fibroblasts, thus preventing raised and bumpy scar tissue.

Watch must be retained over patients thus treated after their discharge until the pressure can be safely removed, i.e. until the hypertrophic tendencies are overcome.

Sometimes cortisone is injected into the scars. If primary healing does not take place, surgery may be required to provide skin cover.

METHODS OF SKIN TRANSFER

1. Free skin grafts which are without a blood supply for up to 48 hours after transfer.
2. Skin flaps, which are joined to the body by a functioning arterial and venous flow.

In the treatment of burns, split skin grafts are most commonly used to provide speedy healing and prevent complications caused by infection.

At a later stage when reconstructive surgery takes place skin flaps may be used.

SPLIT SKIN GRAFT

These can vary from the very thin to three-quarter skin thickness and are cut with a knife or dermatome. Such grafts are used very largely in the surgery of repair and particularly in the grafting of burns. After cutting, they are applied to the raw areas with a backing of Tulle Gras. The donor sites heal within 10–12 days.

The patient may be nursed exposed or with dressings, according to the wishes of the surgeon. The recipient area must always have a good blood supply and be free from necrotic tissue and infection (particularly haemolytic streptococcus).

For the first 48 hours a split skin graft survives on the exudate from the underlying granulating tissue. By 48 hours capillaries will have grown into the graft and vascularised it. The formation of haematoma or tangential movement of the graft will prevent vascularisation and the graft will fail.

Following skin grafts, movements can be commenced after five to seven days. Joints not directly involved in grafting can be moved, but movement of these must not cause friction on the newly applied skin. Once the grafts are well-established, the application of a bland cream, e.g. lanolin, is desirable, to soften the scars. This should be gently kneaded in – 'heavy handedness' must be avoided, otherwise blistering occurs.

Full thickness burns require split skin grafting in order to gain a skin cover; however, this often contracts considerably and may either have to be replaced or released at a later stage with further split skin, full thickness grafts, or skin flaps being used.

It must be remembered that split skin grafts contract for several months and therefore it is very important for the patient to continue his exercises under the care of a physiotherapist at the local hospital or, in severe cases, at a rehabilitation centre.

If contractures do occur, the patient will have to be admitted for further surgery; if release of the contractures with the use of further split skin graft or a Z-plasty is not satisfactory, flaps may be necessary. (See page 225 for Z-plasty technique.)

FULL THICKNESS GRAFTS (WOLFE GRAFTS)

These are small and of full thickness skin, excluding fat. They are usually taken from the post-auricular or supraclavicular areas to repair facial defects such as eyelids. The donor site will not regenerate and must itself be closed by a split skin graft or direct suture.

In burns of the face, eyelids are often involved and since their contraction can lead to corneal ulceration it is important to apply a graft at the earliest opportunity. The Wolfe graft contracts less than a split skin graft and this is therefore the graft of choice.

See Chapter 15, pages 199–202 for details of other types of flaps.

Following major burns, extensive rehabilitation is essential as scar tissue continues to contract for many months after the burn. This needs the co-operation of the whole team, including physiotherapist, occupational therapist, social worker and other medical staff. Consideration must be given to the type of aids, splints, etc which the patient may require.

As many burns units cover a large area, the patients often live many miles away. It is essential, therefore, that good follow-up physiotherapy treatment is established in their local hospitals and the physiotherapists must make themselves responsible for setting up adequate lines of communication in order that the patient receives the best possible treatment.

BIBLIOGRAPHY

Bernstein, N. (1976). *Emotional Care of the Facially Burned and Disfigured*. Little Brown and Co. Boston.

Cason, J. S. (1981). *Treatment of Burns*. Chapman and Hall, London.

Laing, J. E. and Harvey, J. (1972). *Management and Nursing of Burns*, 2nd edition. English Universities Press, London.

MacAllan, E. S. and Jackson, I. T. (1971). *Plastic Surgery and Burns Treatment*. William Heinemann Medical Books Limited, London.

Muir, I. F. K. and Barclay, T. L. (1974). *Burns and Their Treatment*. Lloyd Luke (Medical Books) Limited, London.

ACKNOWLEDGEMENTS

The authors thank Mr Brian Morgan FRCS, consultant plastic surgeon to University College Hospital and Mount Vernon Hospital, Northwood, for his help, advice and encouragement in the revision of these two chapters. They also thank Mediscus Products Limited, Wareham, Dorset, for providing Figure 16/3 and for permission to use it in Chapter 16. They thank Mr R. Blake, medical photographer Mount Vernon Hospital for his help with the photographs, and finally they thank Marie Louise Autin for typing the chapters.

Chapter 17

A Patient's Viewpoint of Physiotherapy Following Severe Burns

by JAMES PARTRIDGE, BA (Oxon), MSc

The role of the professional in medical care and rehabilitation is now the subject of substantial literature. Medical and paramedical students are expected to digest some of the insights gained from sociological studies: 'the sick role', 'the doctor-patient relationship', 'the professionalisation of illness' – these and similar terms are now familiar. Books such as Ivan Illich's *Medical Nemesis* are required reading.

Such sociological debates are vitally important to enhancing the self-awareness of health care workers and of medicine as a whole. But they are almost exclusively generalised in tone and content. They do not, for example, discuss the specific problems associated with burns and plastic surgery. The student professional will find it difficult to glean much of practical usefulness from these academic discussions. This was brought home to me very forcefully when I was asked to talk to a lecture room full of student nurses (at St Thomas' Hospital) about my experiences with severe burns. I had nervously envisaged myself giving a lecture – which didn't seem right at all! Very quickly it became apparent that my audience was positively bursting with bottled-up questions about pain, hospitalisation and recovery – 'How had I *felt*?' For these quite experienced student nurses this was their first and possibly only chance to articulate their personal anxieties about how they related to their patients.

I hope that the presence of this chapter in an otherwise technical textbook will help physiotherapists to appreciate more fully the special circumstances and problems of being severely burnt and undergoing extensive plastic surgery. My successful recovery owes much to the work of physiotherapists and I have done my best in this chapter to explain why. The art of surgery is finely displayed in operating theatres – but surgery alone will not get a patient back into active life.

LOOKING BACK

It is now eight years since I left the plastic surgery wards of Queen Mary's Hospital, Roehampton. In the preceding four years I had received intensive and exhaustive treatment there for severe burns to my face, hands, legs and body sustained when a Land Rover I was driving overturned and caught fire. Now I am a dairy farmer in the Channel Islands, married with two children.

The fact that I am now living at all is miraculous enough – 40 years earlier I would have had little chance in a similar accident. That I am now leading a full and exceedingly active life is just one of the many success stories that should inspire all who work with the severely burnt and disfigured. Often patients lose touch with the hospital and the staff who were responsible for their treatment – as I have – and it may be tempting to put that loss of contact down to the difficulties and anxieties experienced in the aftermath of such serious injuries. Equally, no news may herald good news.

Nonetheless recovery and rehabilitation after facial and other burns is an agonising business. I soon learnt that no amount of even the most brilliant and ingenious surgical manoeuvres can heal the deep psychological scarring that accompanies this kind of personal disaster. The physical pain and restriction of numerous operations, of thick bands of keloid scars, and of highly sensitive skin is bad enough, and can be an hourly and daily trial for years after the initial injury. But the mental process of appreciating what has happened and the life-long struggle to come to terms with disfigurement – and, most of all, of other people's reaction to it – require greater strength than the simple physical demands of recovery.

Physiotherapy in the public mind is seen as synonymous with physical exercises. Surely therefore facially damaged patients like myself do not need physiotherapy? My own experience suggests otherwise. Although my limbs definitely needed 'exercise' so did the mess which was, and is, my face. My physiotherapists duly administered the daily torture of standard exercises for bedridden cases, but they did much more than that. They became daily visitors often more able than other staff to listen. They won my respect. And, most important, they contrived to convince me that I could be mobile and strong again.

I frequently reflect on the strange irony that I am now employed in one of the most demanding physical and manual jobs. 'Single-handed farming' might literally describe it because my left hand actually has only one functional finger. But the fact is that this very hand was rescued from extinction (in other words amputation) by hours of painstaking work by surgeons and physiotherapists – and me! Not that my physios were miracle workers; they were simply people experienced in and dedicated to retrieving depleted bodies and minds from the brink.

I have divided my account of my recovery into three parts: the initial stage of skin replacement after being burnt, the process of plastic surgery, and the aftermath. Although I learnt some technical jargon in the course of treatment, I make no claim to know the details of operations and what follows is therefore decidedly non-technical.

ACCIDENT AND HOSPITALISATION

I was just 18 when the accident happened, a fit, sporting and not unintelligent character. My sights were fixed on going to university. I had only very rarely set foot in a hospital. 'It'll never happen to me' was my happy-go-lucky attitude to hospitals and injuries on the rare occasions when I thought about them. That illusion was suddenly shattered on a winter's night in Wales in 1970. The Land Rover I was driving was completely burnt out – my four friends escaped practically unscathed but I had been lying in the blazing cab for a few fleeting seconds before I had found the energy to escape – another minute and I would have been incinerated. I thought I must be badly singed – my face seemed to be swelling fast. I supposed I ought to go to hospital for a check-up; I was conscious of people at the scene wanting to rush me to one nearby and then we went by ambulance to Chepstow hospital. I hobbled into the operating theatre there, lay down and lost consciousness, completely oblivious to the fact that I was in acute danger of kidney failure.

For the next four and a half months I was hospitalised and bed-bound. An initial medical estimate of my likely recovery time had been a cleverly optimistic three weeks. My parents and friends arrived or sent their best wishes for a speedy recovery – and I confidently believed that my 'minor burns and scalds' would not stop me taking up a job at a Canadian ski resort in the next month.

Ten days in intensive care gave me little indication of the truth. Then I was transferred to Roehampton and informed on arrival by a very affable doctor that I had 33 per cent third degree burns. Still I did not understand. The following day I was lowered into a deliciously warm saline bath. The heavy bandages on my legs and arms were removed and I started to realise: huge areas were just raw meat. A shiver of horror shot down my spine but I cheerfully laughed it off. Only later back in my bed did the devastating impact of it all hit home. I still had no idea what my face looked like – no mirrors available.

The operations soon started and I was introduced to the mysteries of plastic surgery: skin grafts, donor sites, 'strep and staph infections', keloid scarring, barrier nursing, pre-meds and post-op inspections of treated areas (sometimes undertaken after I had been injected with a drug called ketamine producing in me a series of weird and scary hallucinations). My memory of detail in the next three months is sketchy: every week I seemed to be either undergoing operations or trying to recover from one. At times infection raged and skin grafts simply slid off, but gradually the flesh returned.

I had had vague pretensions to being a reasonable athlete at school. I was certainly fit and healthy. So when a woman came in one morning soon after I had arrived at Roehampton and said she was the physiotherapist and suggested I should do a few exercises I did not anticipate any difficulties. How wrong I was! In the space of a fortnight my muscles had become flabby and depleted, my limbs were stiff and I had no strength at all. Pat, as I came to know her, had seen similar cases – 'It is bound to hurt' she would say.

It did hurt. It was agony, no more, no less. I think agony is worse than pain: I can still recall that agony, but not the pain. Sore, semi-healed, semi-raw areas are not meant to be touched, let alone moved, I thought. 'Just a little bit more . . . Well done. Again. Push . . . Good. Rest. Pull . . . OK. Rest. We'll try some more this afternoon.' These commands – or rather the coaxing – remain etched in my mind to this day. They sum up my initial response to physiotherapy which was not very favourable!

Pat, I know now, was not being sadistic. In those early days she was carefully assessing my pain thresholds. By daily visits, however brief, she was observing what motivated me. We didn't talk at all about end-results; if I asked some futile question about the future, she would simply point to the progress so far. She didn't want to give me false hopes – but she said just enough to allow me to set my own private targets: 40 double knee-bends, holding a pen, playing a game of draughts left-handed, and the ultimate goal – walking.

The saturation treatment of those months left me with little energy for much else. Even the strangeness of the routine, the dreariness of the food (Complan with every meal), the frustration of only seeing people's eyes above their surgical masks, all paled into insignificance. I had no choice but to resign myself to them. Would I ever get out? The contours of the cracks on the ceiling became a dream-like landscape of hills and rivers, sun and shade. Dejection was setting in. Each day Pat came in – always keen to get me out of my apathy. And indeed the gentle moving of muscles did shake me out of my lethargy momentarily. She didn't achieve much – she probably knew from the medical staff that I was fairly weak: all my energies and body-weight were being expended on healing. I lost four stone and grew an inch just lying there for three months. But at last the patching up of raw areas was nearly complete.

At this point physiotherapy became important. And by then Pat had got to know me: the groundwork had already been done. She had bothered to come in every day. She had listened to my grumbles and often done something effective about them. She had told me much of the possibilities of plastic surgery, information which I could not obtain from other staff and which many patients never receive, and this was particularly valuable to me. Uninformed often means uninspired and this is probably especially true in the case of plastic surgery for facial damage.

Towards the end of my initial skin replacement treatment it was a physiotherapeutic aid which inadvertently opened up a whole new set of problems for me. Pat's efforts were concentrated partly on getting my legs used to being vertical again (with the support of pink elasticated bandages) and partly on straightening out the fingers on my left hand. Three of these fingers proved to be unresponsive to treatment, due to the tendons being burnt through, and I eventually had the fingers amputated to the first joint. Amazingly, however, my middle finger had some chance of being functional. A shiny metal-coated splint was strapped to it to increase the pressure and stretch the tendons. Until then I had seen no mirror since the accident but that shiny surface allowed me my first blurred view of my horribly damaged face. Inspecting my face as closely as possible with the splint was a good preparation for the shock when I eventually plucked up courage to ask for a real mirror.

But fortunately I was soon distracted by my earnest and long frustrated desire to walk. My legs had shrivelled to matchsticks and the right thigh, being almost completely burnt had taken an age to heal. I badly wanted to walk again. The days of waiting had created such a strong ambition, one that overshadowed all other feelings – including those about the facial damage. Pat had been working on strengthening my calf and thigh muscles sufficiently and, most important, she had given me the confidence to know that I would walk again.

On the very day the world watched as Apollo astronauts walked on the moon for the second time, my recovery in a little insignificant ward in a London hospital also took a major leap forward. For the first time in four and a half months my feet touched the ground and I stumbled a few steps in a circle round my bed. Walking was the signal for me to leave the burns unit: all the skin I had lost on my face, hands, legs and body had been replaced and at last I could be discharged. My hands served very few functions, my legs allowed me to walk for 30 seconds at a time, and my face was a contorted mass of scars and inflamed skin – but at last I was out.

The elation of that moment of leaving was only slightly tinged with apprehension. The targets which I had set had all so far been achieved. I think all the hospital staff shared my joy: Pat certainly did. Although it was her job to do what she could for me, she had managed in a meaningful personal way to 'stay with me' throughout the treatment. 'Staying with me' meant visiting even when it was apparently pointless, gaining my respect and trust, realising how to motivate me, setting realistic aims for recovery and sharing in the thrill of achievement. That list sounds like an ingredients list for successful physiotherapy and in a way it is. But what is crucial is that each patient reacts differently and that the physio has to take a personal interest and understanding in each case. Moreover, physios should understand their critical role in psychological recovery: with their whole-hearted help patients can take full advantage of the opportunities opened up by their surgical treatment.

Keloid scarring is a good illustration of this. In common with many young burns victims, I suffered greatly from keloid scarring from the outset of my treatment. Thick bands of hard intractable scars on hands and legs are extremely debilitating, and they contort the face grotesquely; the resultant pulls and stresses on neighbouring skin are excruciatingly painful. Frequently the scarring was setting in before the wounds or grafts had healed. The physio is in an awkward position here: on the one hand she can encourage movement very soon after an operation, and thereby risk damaging the recently-replaced skin, in an attempt to forestall the keloiding. Alternatively she can delay exercise until healing is complete by which time it may well be too late. This dilemma was immensely frustrating for me and Pat and I spent considerable time discussing the pros and cons with the medical staff. Her willingness to get involved in the issue was perhaps the first instance of a good two-way relationship forming between us – not, I stress, a heavy emotional involvement but simply a mutual understanding and respect.

PLASTIC SURGERY

The four and a half months of skin replacement was finally completed and I was gladly discharged for a few weeks' recuperation at home. I was a changed person: the brash self-confidence of six months previously had given way to a somewhat more thoughtful but nervous disposition. I had learnt a lot about life and about myself in hospital – a totally alien environment at the start of my treatment but now one which offered considerable security and support. My joy at being discharged and at being at home again was tempered by my realisation that I was totally unprepared for the outside world.

It wasn't just that I looked on the world somewhat differently. People looked at me, even stared at me, with a mixture of curiosity, pity, suspicion, sometimes with fear and anxiety. Looking at myself each morning in the mirror confirmed what I now saw in the eyes of others: my face was seriously disfigured and likely to be so for the rest of my life. The first occasion when this uncomfortable fact was vividly brought home to me was an unexpected visit to a pub with an old friend. Whereas in hospital the reactions of staff and other patients to me were, I perceived, normal and untainted by the association of disfigurement with mental abnormality, the reception I met in the pub was quite otherwise. While my friend bought drinks, I tried my best to fend off the stares, the whispering behind my back, a few hostile remarks, and the general air of curiosity that gripped all the drinkers as soon as I walked through the door. This episode not only convinced me that I should start facial reconstruction, but it also forced me into considering how I would deal with public responses to my injuries.

Two or three times a week during my period at home I went to hospital to have my dressings changed and to visit the physiotherapy department. Now that I was out of the confines of the ward new forms of exercise could be tried: weight training (at first very light indeed!) strengthened my legs and hands as well as generally tuning up other depleted muscles. I badly wanted to make big strides in fitness at this stage but soon learnt that strained and aching muscles resulted from excessive work. Slowly and patiently was the message.

My relationship with the physios was broadening out. During the skin replacement stage, Pat and her colleagues had been one of the key motivating forces in my recovery. From this point on, however, I took a much more active part in the treatment. The targets were no longer as straightforward as in the earlier phase (like walking). I was now developing more complex objectives, some to do with returning to a reasonably athletic state, others relating to mental progress. Physiotherapy was not just the general physical back-up to surgery, it became the sounding board for ideas and plans.

One major issue in those first months out of hospital was whether or not I should take up a place at university in the coming autumn. A meeting in late May with one of the surgical staff had put doubts in my mind. He wondered whether I should take a year off and get myself thoroughly ready for the ordeal. Up until then I had confidently assumed that I *would* be fit enough and was inwardly preparing myself. I was thrown into turmoil. I knew that a great deal of surgery had to be done in the next few years but this suggestion seemed to be questioning my ability to follow a normal life.

Since my fitness seemed in doubt I naturally consulted Pat. Knowing me far better than did the junior surgeon, she immediately realised his mistaken approach: the surest way to halt my return to 'a normal life' was to suggest that I was physically incapable of taking up where I had left off. The accident and my injuries had to be viewed as incidental; if blown up into an insuperable barrier, my self-confidence would be further shattered. How glad I was of Pat's interest and support.

Embarking on my course of plastic surgery which was to last intermittently for three and a half years gave me the opportunity to quiz my surgeon on the chances of regaining my lost appearance. First, he said, my hands needed attention: continued physiotherapy would, with luck and hard work, gradually rejuvenate my right hand, but my left was proving unresponsive to that kind of treatment. Only the middle finger functioned efficiently. I had to decide whether I wanted the other fingers pinned straight (they were bent down towards the palm and immovable). I was sure the fingers would be even less use in that position but agreed to continue physiotherapy and reach a decision later. After one term at university I concluded that drastic action was needed: I could pick up only the lightest load with the hand as it was. What would happen, I asked Pat, if the useless bits of finger were amputated? Her experience suggested that as long as a pad of skin was surgically made to protect the knuckle stumps, the half-fingers could be very efficient. And thus it turned out.

Dealing surgically with my hand presented relatively straightforward options, and although my surgeon had never suggested finger amputation, he was pleased when I reached that conclusion on my own. I would never have believed that I could actually sign a form to have my fingers amputated, but one morning I did, and apart from the occasional phantom limb sensation early on, have never regretted it. Without the redundant ends, the fingers (or stumps) on this hand found new life. I could now pick up weights though my arm as a whole was puny. Gradually the strength returned to my fingers – many exercises were prescribed and after much painstaking work the whole hand and arm became useful instead of an awkward encumbrance.

My facial disfigurement posed an entirely different and more complex set of problems. From the outset my surgeon was at pains to stress that he could not promise miracles. Contrary to popular myth, plastic surgeons cannot use plastic to stick on to re-create lost looks! Every operation, he emphasised, was bound to be a gamble. A satisfactory result could not be guaranteed after one operation, or two or three or four. . ., but as long as I was fit and healthy and able to withstand the physical demands of treatment he would persevere on one condition: that I *wanted* him to do so. That was a most important proviso. In the early days of plastic surgery I had no qualms: every operation seemed to take me a little closer to an acceptable facial appearance. But as time went on, after over 50 operations, my willingness and resilience were weakening. Moreover, as I learnt more about the technical possibilities and the limitations of surgery, so I realised that additional operations would achieve less and less. Thus, although I could have persisted for years, I reached saturation point. I will briefly outline what was done.

Full thickness (Wolfe) skin grafts were applied to my nose, my eyelids (upper and lower) and my top lip, the skin coming first from behind my ear and then from the inside of the upper arm. Because of the keloid pulls exerted by my chin and distorted neck, my eyelids required repeated operations to achieve a decent result. After the third of these had failed (very demoralising after the excruciating pain of having 50 or 60 little stitches all around the eye), attention shifted to my chin. This was a real patchwork quilt of grafts and scars, and after one unsuccessful attempt to salvage it with a thin skin graft discussion started on more radical measures. As I had been using every university vacation for surgery of some kind, I could not envisage what other treatment could still be contemplated.

One afternoon in the physio department I was working off some excess energy on the weights and saying how frustrating it was not to be able to get my eyes right. A group of physios gathered and started debating the options. The difficulty I experienced – in common with many other patients – of discussing treatment options with the surgical staff was raised. I asked for a clear description of what skin flaps were and what they could achieve. I discovered that a pedicle flap could be raised elsewhere on one's body and then transferred to completely cover a scarred area. As it happened, a woman recovering from a small flap was in the department that afternoon and I was allowed to see the smooth end-product. This was not the first or last occasion when physios with experience helped me to make sense of a problem which seemed unresolvable in the confines of the ward.

My surgeon was fascinated by the whole idea: I would take a year off university, travel a bit to start with, then come in to hospital to have a pedicle flap raised and eventually spread over my chin and neck. In the event, a back pedicle was used because my stomach area was scarred. This was very convenient as there was no need for an arm attachment stage. I was extremely lucky: the 12-inch tube was healthy from the start and was moved in four stages to replace my chin very successfully. It was a long process, taking six months to complete.

My sanity remained intact principally because I could escape from the hospital regularly. With the help of physios a thick foam back support was designed which I strapped round my chest enabling me to sit with my back against a seat. This contraption allowed me to drive a car while the flap developed and became healthily established. In addition, many visitors and regular jaunts to the physio department kept my morale and fitness in trim. By July 1974, the new chin was in place and my pleasure was shared by all who had made it possible. The tensions around my eyes and nose were released and I could now rejoice in the knowledge that I looked at least tolerably socially presentable!

AFTERWARDS

Probably the most difficult aspect of burns and plastic surgery concerns the psychological impact of facial burns on the unfortunate victim. Although not strictly or solely the province of physiotherapists, helping patients to come to terms with facial disfigurement must be very clearly on their agenda, as indeed it must be for medical, nursing and ancillary staff alike. I am not making a plea here for some extra investment in pity by physios (or other staff); nor am I suggesting that physios are hard-hearted or insensitive! Rather I shall describe briefly my own experience of facing up to facial disfigurement and hope to strike one or two useful themes which will enable the reader to understand a little more about what a burns victim is going through.

Facial damage is first and foremost damage to one's own self-image. The mirror and the eyes of others tell the same tale: one's appearance is severely tarnished. For me, any pretensions to handsomeness were lost forever. For a woman the sense of loss may be even more traumatic and long-lasting.

In itself, the loss of good looks would not be so intolerable were it not for the disquieting fact that bad looks in the public eye are associated with a series of pejorative attributes. At a simple level (but a highly influential one) children's films frequently depict the baddies as ugly (sometimes disfigured) men, in marked contrast to the normal-looking handsome goody. It is not therefore surprising that the bearer of the mask of disfigurement carries with him or her a stigma which imposes itself on any relationship or contact with other people.

To be more specific, my facial damage has been assumed by others to be variously the result of my mental (or even moral?) ineptitude, abnormality from birth – do I have the right to survive at all, they wonder? or some other personal failure. I have been assumed to be rather stupid, probably illiterate, possibly mentally ill, even violent; protective parents have shielded their children from me (yet ironically it is often children who are most wonderfully naive and natural and able to ask me direct questions without embarrassment). The abnormal behaviour I have witnessed would fill a book in itself – people staring fixedly, trance-like at me; others rushing up to ask if they can help me over the road or carry my bag; and once at a restaurant a woman left her table, unable to finish her expensive meal. At the other end of the scale people seem to think I must be some sort of hero – am I a racing driver like Niki Lauda, or perhaps an RAF veteran?

The hardest thing about stigma is that one imputes those same pejorative attributes to oneself as others are prone to. The social impact of facial damage can be seen in the everyday lives of some victims: living alone, bereft of friends (especially relationships with the opposite sex), often unemployed, these victims are suffering from the worst effects of stigma. Society is adding insult to injury. Not until I completely and positively accepted my looks did I start to organise an effective counter to this attitude. To resign oneself to one's looks is inadequate. One has to realise that the scars are now an integral part of 'being me'. How I reached that point of positive acceptance is far less easy to describe. A combination of support from my family, friends, hospital staff and many others, and my own refusal to see the accident as the end of meaningful life probably sums up my own recovery, but other burns cases will reach that point by other routes.

Before I reached that stage, however, I think I strove to deflect any stigmatising attitudes by an extravagant show of superficial over-confidence. Inside I was full of nervousness and acute awareness as to how I was being received by others. I recall my first days at university mostly in this light, trying manfully to deny to all around that I had anything wrong with me at all. Gradually – and it was a long process – a *modus vivendi* became established. I no longer worried about the stares, the occasional hurtful remark, the schoolgirl giggling or the awkwardness when people met me for the first time. I hope I became easier to be with, less concerned with myself and how others saw me, and more just an ordinary and an active member of society. But it took a long time and even today there are moments of anguish.

In a way the physiotherapists and the nurses who dealt with me, Pat and her colleagues, represented my first female audience and my first new friends since the accident. But more importantly, they took the trouble to understand the predicament of facial damage. As long as physios and other staff (not least the surgical staff themselves) are sensitive to the deep psychological scarring that goes with facial burns, and as long as a strong family and social network exists outside the hospital, burns victims have every chance of healing those emotional scars in time.

REFERENCE

For those readers who have been as impressed with this chapter as myself, the following paper describing the techniques used for the re-fashioning of James Partridge's face will be of interest (editor).

Evans, A. J. (1981). Cosmetic surgery of burns. *British Journal of Hospital Medicine*, June issue, 547–50.

Chapter 18

Amputations

by C. VAN DE VEN, MCSP

Amputation of a limb performed for vascular disorders when other treatment has proved ineffective, or amputation as a result of trauma, malignancy or deformity should be accepted as a positive form of treatment, thus relieving the patient of a painful, useless, dangerous and often infected extremity.

After amputation has been performed, the patient can be rehabilitated to a fully independent life, return to work, and in time become as active as he was prior to amputation, depending upon his general condition.

The amputee needs time and help to overcome the psychological shock resulting from the loss of a limb. He realises that he is different from other people and, more important, that this difference will be apparent. He will be uncertain of his future and will need encouragement from all members of the rehabilitation team: the surgeon, nursing staff, physiotherapists, occupational therapists, social workers, the medical officer at the limb fitting centre, prosthetist and his general practitioner. All these people must work in close co-operation with one another.

Rehabilitation is one continual process from the time the surgeon decides to amputate until such time that the patient is independent with his definitive prosthesis. This may take weeks, although the patient is unlikely to remain in hospital for the whole of this period.

Amputations of upper and lower limbs involve differences in cause, age-group and rehabilitation, and so will be considered separately. The ratio of lower limb to upper limb amputees is of the order of 20 : 1.

LOWER LIMB AMPUTATIONS

This is the larger group of amputees and these patients are seen in greater numbers by physiotherapists.

Indications for amputation

The causes of lower limb amputation together with the approximate percentage of cases are as follows:

Cause	%
Peripheral vascular disease	62.9
Diabetes	19.9
Trauma	10.2
Malignancy	4.8
Congenital deformities	1.0
Others	1.2
	100.0

It can be seen that peripheral vascular disease and diabetic gangrene, both diseases associated with the elderly, account for the majority of lower limb amputations, and accordingly in any one year 75 per cent of new lower limb amputees are over the age of 60. These patients often have many of the other problems associated with the elderly: cardiac involvement, low exercise tolerance, arteriosclerosis of the cerebral vessels causing possible hemiplegia and diminished mental ability, poor respiratory function, reduced visual acuity, poor healing, osteoarthritis and neuropathy.

Traumatic amputations more commonly affect the younger age-groups and are mostly necessitated by road traffic accidents and industrial injuries. Malignant disease is also a reason for amputation in patients in the younger age-groups. Amputations for congenital deformity and limb length discrepancies are usually performed on children and young adults. This is best delayed until the patient is old enough to decide for himself that he wishes to have the operation performed.

The Limb Fitting Service

Before discussing the treatment of the amputee, it is important to understand something of the prosthetic service available to the patient. This obviously varies in different countries, but in the United Kingdom a uniform and comprehensive service is offered to all amputees.

There are 30 limb fitting centres throughout England, Wales and Northern Ireland which are administered directly by the Department of Health and Social Security (DHSS). There are also seven centres in

Scotland for which the Scottish Home and Health Department (SHHD) is responsible. The patient is referred to his nearest centre by the surgeon at the hospital at which he had his amputation. There he is seen by a medical officer who will be responsible for his limb fitting programme and prosthetic rehabilitation. The patient is examined, assessed and usually measured for his temporary prosthesis on his first visit.

The patient remains under the care of the Artificial Limb Fitting Service all his life, for he will, from time to time, require repairs and replacement of his artificial limb. He will be supplied, as necessary, with sufficient woollen, cotton or nylon stump socks, bandages, walking aids and other appliances. Should the patient move to another part of the country he can be transferred to his nearest regional limb fitting centre.

All artificial limbs are made by independent manufacturers under contract to the Department of Health and Social Security.

Surgery and levels of amputation

Whatever the pathology predisposing to amputation, there are various factors which will influence the surgeon in his selection of level of amputation. As well as the pathology, he will consider such things as surgical techniques, viability of tissue, prostheses and, not least, the patient's particular needs, taking into account his occupation, importance of good cosmesis, age and sex.

HINDQUARTER AMPUTATION

This amputation is performed almost solely for malignancy as a life-saving procedure and here, obviously, the pathological factors are of prime importance. The surgeon has no choice but to remove the entire limb and part of the ilium, pubis, ischium and sacrum on that side, leaving peritoneum, muscle and fascia to cover and support the internal organs.

HIP DISARTICULATION

This procedure is commonly performed in cases of malignancy; it may also be necessary following extensive trauma but is seldom done for vascular insufficiency. The limb is disarticulated at the hip joint and the bony pelvis is left intact, thus producing a good weight-bearing platform.

MID-THIGH AMPUTATION

This is the amputation which is perhaps most commonly found in the elderly group of patients. In the patient with vascular disease, an above-knee amputation is one in which primary healing occurs more readily than the through-knee or below-knee amputation. However, compared with these other levels, the above-knee amputee will have more difficulty in learning to control his prosthesis and in achieving a good gait and, in the case of the elderly patient, the attainment of total independence will be more of a problem. Proprioception from the knee joint will be lost and the patient must bear weight on the prosthesis at the ischial tuberosity. Hip flexion contractures occur very easily unless care is taken to prevent them, the shorter stumps tending to become flexed and abducted (due particularly to the strong pull of tensor fascia lata). The longer above-knee stumps by contrast tend to become flexed and adducted (there will be more of the adductor group intact and these muscles have a mechanical advantage over the pull of the short tensor fascia lata).

The surgeon makes the above-knee stump as long as possible, but must leave 11.5–12.5cm (4½–5in) between the end of the stump and the knee axis in order to allow space for the knee control mechanism to be put into prosthesis. If there is a hip flexion contracture, a long stump is a disadvantage, as the end of the long stump magnifies the contracture and the prosthesis will be very bulky to accommodate this.

Surgeons use the myoplastic technique or a myodesis in which muscle groups are sutured together over the bone end or attached to the bone at physiological tension. The muscles therefore retain their contractile property, circulation to the stump is improved, and the stump will be more powerful in the control of a prosthesis.

AMPUTATION AT KNEE JOINT LEVEL

This includes disarticulation of the knee and the Gritti-Stokes amputation. In the former, the tibia together with the fibula is disarticulated at the knee joint. The patella is retained and the patellar tendon is sutured to the anterior cruciate ligament, the hamstrings are sutured to the posterior cruciate ligament and so act as hip extensors. A strong powerful stump results with no muscle imbalance, and full end-bearing is possible on the broad expanse of the femoral condyles. Most of the proprioception of the knee joint is retained.

In the Gritti-Stokes technique, the femur is sectioned transversely through the condyles and the condyles are trimmed down medially and laterally. The articular surface of the patella is shaved off and the patella positioned at the distal end of the femur. Bony union should occur and weight is taken on the patella.

Full end-bearing is possible on the knee disarticulation, but due to the relatively smaller weight-bearing surface in the Gritti-Stokes amputation, this is often not possible and a certain amount of weight must be taken through the ischial tuberosity. The Gritti-Stokes amputation necessitates smaller skin flaps with better vascular nutrition and therefore primary healing is more certain.

BELOW-KNEE AMPUTATION

If at all possible, the surgeon will elect to perform a below-knee amputation. The great advantage is that the normal knee joint with its proprioception is retained and therefore balance and a good gait pattern will be more easily attained, particularly if the patient is able to wear a patellar tendon bearing prosthesis which leaves the knee function unrestricted (Fig. 18/1). The optimum level is 14cm (5½in)

Fig. 18/1   Two patients with below-knee amputations, wearing patellar tendon bearing prostheses. Note that control of these prostheses depends entirely upon the hip and knee joints and muscles, particularly the quadriceps and hamstrings

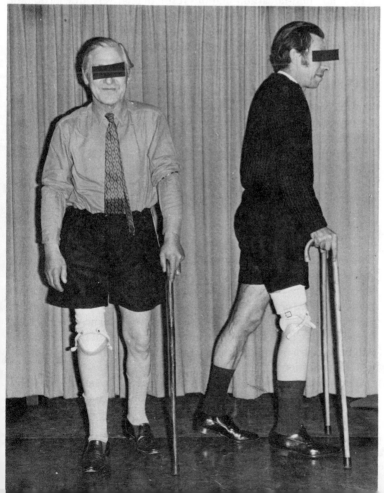

below the tibial plateau, although a patient with a slightly shorter stump would still achieve good function with a prosthesis.

The fibula is sectioned slightly more proximally than the tibia, and the end of the tibia is bevelled to avoid a prominent bone end. A myoplastic technique is used, resulting in the advantages previously described.

SYMES AMPUTATION

This involves disarticulation at the ankle joint and removal of the medial and lateral malleoli to the level of the articular surface of the tibia. This amputation is usually not done in vascular conditions, as a higher level will often be necessary due to insufficient blood supply. Good end-bearing is possible, the heel pad being sutured into position over the distal end of the tibia and fibula.

FOOT AMPUTATIONS

Trans- and mid-tarsal amputations result in relatively little locomotor difficulty, the main problem being that of the provision of satisfactory footwear. Other amputations, e.g. the Chopart and Lisfranc, will require special prostheses, provided by limb fitting centres.

PHYSIOTHERAPY

The physiotherapist's role in the rehabilitation of the amputee can be considered in three stages: pre-operative, postoperative (pre-prosthetic), and prosthetic.

Again, it must be emphasised that rehabilitation is one continual process, the final goal for the patient being independence on his definitive prosthesis and a return to normal activities, within the limitations of his age and condition.

Pre-operative stage

Treatment at this stage is most applicable to the patient with vascular disease, and in these cases a pre-operative exercise programme is valuable. Many of these patients have been at home or in hospital confined to bed or to a chair because of a lesion of the foot, gangrene or ischaemic pain. If the patient has been walking at all he will only have been hobbling from one room to another, the joints of the affected leg will be held in a position of flexion (the reflex response to pain) and his general condition will be poor.

The physiotherapist must assess the patient's physical abilities and also take into account his mental attitude and home conditions. On the basis of this assessment she will commence and progress the physical treatment programme, at all times with reference to the surgeon, nursing staff and other members of the rehabilitation team.

During the pre-operative stage, the patient begins to adapt to his changing circumstances, learns to know the staff who are concerned with his rehabilitation, and perhaps meets other amputees who are progressing towards independence. At this stage the therapists and social worker should be finding out about the patient's home situation, if possible meeting close relatives and involving them in the patient's programme of rehabilitation. The psychological aspect is very important and the physiotherapist can do much to help and motivate the patient at this stage.

Depending upon the time available and the general condition of the patient, the following should be included in the treatment programme:

1. Strengthening exercises for the upper trunk and upper limbs to facilitate transfers and for moving up and down the bed.
2. Strengthening and mobilising exercises for the lower trunk, necessary for all activities, rolling, sitting up, walking.
3. Strengthening exercises for the unaffected leg for crutch walking, standing, transferring.
4. Exercises for the affected leg to increase the range of movement and improve stability of those joints which will remain after amputation.
5. Walking if possible. Patient should have protected footwear on the affected leg with a heel-raise if flexion deformities are present.
6. Maximal independence including ability to move about the bed using the unaffected leg, rolling, prone lying.
7. It is important to teach wheelchair activities even though it is hoped that the patient will ultimately achieve independence on a prosthesis. Many elderly patients will require a wheelchair on a permanent basis as a second method of mobility. This wheelchair should be correctly assessed by the occupational therapy or physiotherapy department.

Postoperative stage

The aims of treatment at this stage are:

1. Prevention of joint contractures.
2. To strengthen and co-ordinate the muscles controlling the stump.
3. To strengthen and mobilise the unaffected leg.
4. To strengthen and mobilise the trunk and retrain balance.

5. To teach the patient to regain independence in functional activities.
6. To control oedema of the stump and commence early ambulation.
7. Re-education of sensation in the healed stump.

Physiotherapy will be commenced the day following operation. It should always be remembered that most of the patients undergoing amputation for vascular reasons have been heavy smokers for many years, therefore chest complications are not uncommon. Routine postoperative breathing exercises should be commenced on the first day.

The majority of amputees experience stump pain postoperatively. Occasionally this is often directly proportional to the amount of pain present pre-operatively. The physiotherapist must be aware of the problem as severe pain may limit the rehabilitation programme. Pain can be due from a number of reasons which must be assessed and recognised: (a) ischaemic pain due to incorrect level of amputation; (b) non-healing stump due to infection; (c) nerve pain, which may be referred back or hip pain; and (d) phantom sensation or phantom pain.

PREVENTION OF CONTRACTURES

Attention should be given to the position of the patient in bed. The stump should lie parallel to the unaffected leg with the joints extended. There should be no pillow under the stump and there should be fracture boards beneath the mattress. Both physiotherapists and nursing staff should keep a check on the patient's position. The patient should understand its importance and be encouraged to maintain it.

A routine of prone lying, with all joints in as much extension as possible, is commenced as soon as the patient can tolerate it, ideally for 15 to 20 minutes, three times daily (Fig. 18/2). If the patient is unable to lie prone because of cardiac or respiratory problems, he should lie supine for as long as he can tolerate it, again two or three times a day. Again it is essential to maintain a correct position.

Providing the patient is medically fit, he should be encouraged to transfer out of bed, into a wheelchair on the first or second postoperative day. This can be organised by the occupational therapist or physiotherapist who will ensure that a suitable wheelchair is used. It is essential that a stump board is supplied to support the stump and help reduce oedema.

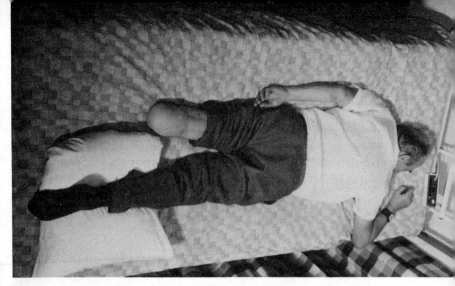

Fig. 18/2 Prone lying. Note position of patient's head turned towards the side of the remaining leg, thus maintaining hip and knee extension of the amputated side. The remaining leg is supported to prevent damage to the foot, and a 'call button' is positioned correctly in case of distress

STRENGTHENING OF THE STUMP

Isometric work for the muscles of the stump is started postoperatively. As the wound heals, manually resisted isotonic work can be given and gradually progressed. It is inadvisable, particularly when the myoplastic technique has been used, to give strong resisted work immediately, as there will be much suture material in the wound and care must be taken not to pull on this.

The physiotherapist must at all times watch for any muscle imbalance and pay particular attention to the weaker groups, which will most likely be the extensors of the hip and knee and possibly the hip adductors, in fact, those muscles necessary to oppose a potential contracture. Stability of all joints of the stump will be essential in the effective control of a prosthesis.

STRENGTHENING AND MOBILISING THE UNAFFECTED LEG

Strong isometric 'holds' with the hip and knee in extension are useful in helping to retain the supportive function of the leg, and this isometric work together with resisted isotonic exercises can be started the day following operation. During the next few days, as the patient's general condition improves, these exercises are progressed. Providing the stump is supported by a bandage or firm dressing, standing and walking in the parallel bars and on crutches may be possible, emphasis being placed on hip extension. This must be done with great care so as not to increase oedema in the stump. Not all patients, particularly the elderly, are capable of this.

TO STRENGTHEN AND MOBILISE THE TRUNK

'Bridging' exercises (Fig. 18/3) and rolling exercises (Figs. 18/4 and 18/5) can be commenced on the first day, and when the patient is able to sit on the edge of his bed, resisted sitting balance work is given (Figs. 18/6 and 18/7). As soon as the patient is able to go to the physiotherapy department, resisted trunk exercises are progressed on mats together with reciprocal leg activity. The use of the wobble board

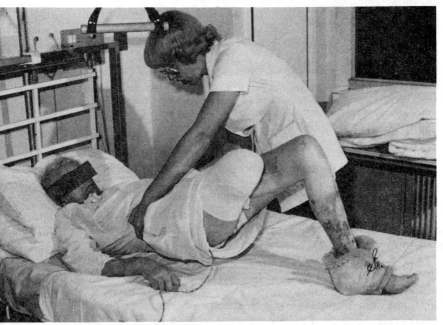

Fig. 18/3   Bridging exercises. Note the condition of the remaining leg, with protection for the ischaemic foot using a sheepskin bootee

can also improve sitting balance (Fig. 18/8). Attention is also given to the upper trunk and upper limbs, and weight and pulley systems are useful for this (Figs. 18/9 and 18/10). Group work can be of value although elderly patients benefit more from individual treatment sessions, and two of these sessions daily in the physiotherapy department, with occupational therapy as well, is usually an adequate programme for these patients.

INDEPENDENCE IN FUNCTIONAL ACTIVITIES

At all times the patient must be encouraged to be as independent as

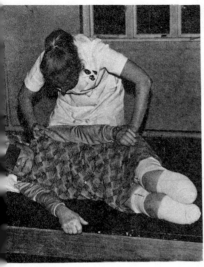

Fig. 18/4

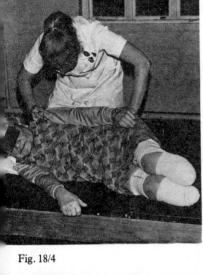

Fig. 18/5

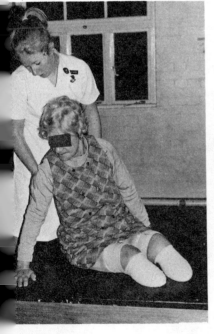

Fig. 18/6

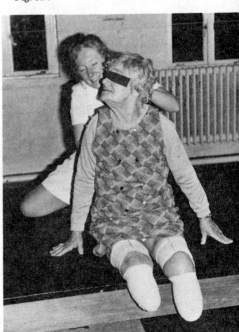

Fig. 18/7   Resisted sitting balance

Figs. 18/4, 18/5, 18/6 demonstrate a rolling to sitting sequence with guided resistance

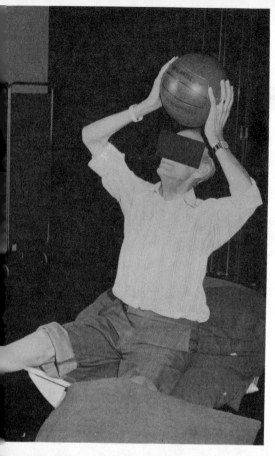

Fig. 18/8   Use of the wobble board. Note pillow protection of new amputation stump, also pillows placed behind the patient as a safety precaution

Fig. 18/9   Bilateral arm patterns: strengthening both upper limbs and trunk. Note extension of both lower limbs

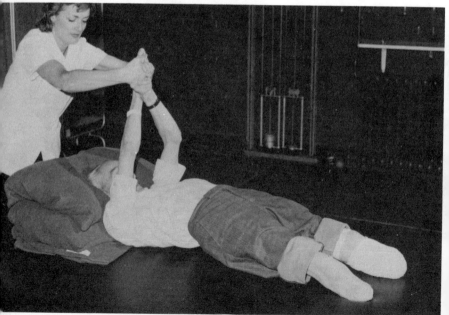

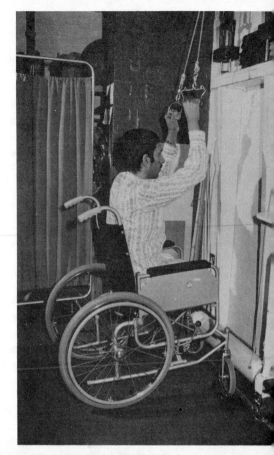

Fig. 18/10 Using weight and pulley system to strengthen upper limbs

Fig. 18/11 Amputee practising dressing with the occupational therapist helping. Note the importance of bridging

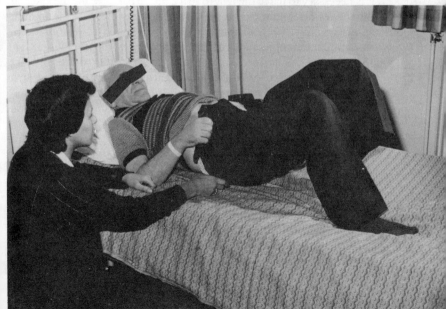

possible. His treatment programme should progress in the physiotherapy department as soon as he is fit enough to leave the ward,
usually about the fourth day. He should dress himself in the morning
(sometimes it is necessary for the occupational therapist to give
dressing practice (Fig. 18/11)), and he should wear a good walking
shoe on the unaffected leg. Basic wheelchair independence is taught
including transfers from bed to chair and from chair to lavatory, and
he should be able to wheel himself around the ward and if possible to
the physiotherapy department.

CONTROL OF OEDEMA AND EARLY AMBULATION

Controlling oedema is essential and it must be reduced as quickly as
possible. Wound healing can be delayed by excessive oedema, and it is
important that the stump assumes its ultimate size quickly, so that the
limb fitting programme can be commenced.

There has been much discussion concerning the methods of oedema
control, and probably good bandaging is the best known. The purpose
of bandaging is to disperse the terminal oedema which is usually
present in all new amputation stumps. Bandaging will also condition
the patient to the constant all-round pressure which will be present
when wearing a prosthesis. It also encourages the patient to become
used to handling his own stump. Before the sutures are removed from
the healed stump a crêpe bandage is used, afterwards, the Elset 'S'
bandage or an elastic type bandage is applied.

Above-knee or through-knee stumps require a 4.5 metre (5yd),
15cm (6in) wide bandage; and the below-knee a 10cm (4in) one. Often
it is necessary to halve the length to a 2 metre bandage for the short or
thin below-knee stump. It is important to remember that the amount
of turns is directly proportional to the pressure build-up on the stump.
There are different methods of applying stump bandages (Figs. 18/12,
18/13, 18/14). The most important aspect is that there is more
pressure distally than proximally, and that all turns are diagonal. Most
methods require a fixing turn to hold the bandage in position, and
both patient and staff must be prepared to reapply the bandage several
times a day. It is also essential that the elasticity of the bandage is not
too stretched when applying it to the stump as it may act as a
tourniquet.

ABOVE-KNEE OR THROUGH-KNEE STUMP BANDAGING (Fig. 18/12)

1. With the patient in the half-lying position, place the end of the
bandage anteriorly at the inguinal fold, the patient or assistant holding
the two corners with his thumbs.
2. With the bandage at minimal stretch take it distally over the end of

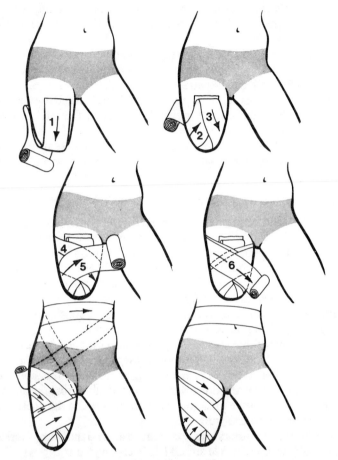

Fig. 18/12 Bandaging for an above-knee amputation

the stump and up the posterior aspect to the gluteal fold, the bandage is then held there by the patient's fingers. The next turn is taken again over the distal end of the stump slightly laterally and then returned anteriorly to the starting point, this turn again being held by the patient's thumbs.

3. Once more the third turn passes distally over the end of the stump, this time slightly medially. It is now passed proximally and laterally across the posterior aspect of the stump. It is held at this point and then brought diagonally downwards and medially across the anterior aspect (turn 4) and a turn is now taken firmly around the back of the stump at the distal end (turn 5).

4. Figure of eight turns are now continued around the stump working proximally until the whole of the stump has been covered and the turns taken well up into the groin.

5. A fixing turn is made by taking the bandage from the posterior aspect of the stump up over the buttock and then forward around the waist. It is best to have the patient turn on to the other side for this. As the turn is brought around the patient's back, he is asked to extend the stump. The bandage is then brought down again to the anterior aspect of the stump.

6. The rest of the bandage is used on one or two more turns on the stump, and fixed by two safety pins high up postero-laterally on the pelvis.

BELOW-KNEE STUMP BANDAGING (Fig. 18/13)

1. Place the end of the bandage anteriorly just below the tip of the patella, the patient or the assistant holding the two corners with his thumbs. With the bandage at minimal stretch take it distally over the end of the stump and up over the posterior aspect of the popliteal space. The bandage is held here by the patient's fingers.

2. The next turn is taken again over the distal end of the stump slightly laterally and then returns anteriorly to the starting point, this turn also now being held by the patient's thumbs.

3. Once more the third turn passes distally over the end of the stump, this time slightly medially. It is now passed proximally and laterally across the posterior aspect of the stump. It is held at this point and then brought diagonally downwards and medially across the anterior aspect (turn 4) and the turn now taken firmly around the back of the stump at the distal end (turn 5).

4. Figure of eight turns are now continued around the stump working proximally until the whole stump has been covered.

5. It is important not to put too much tension on the bandage or too many turns over the tibia as pressure sores can easily occur.

6. The bandage is finished by two or three turns above the knee. If the stump is short or the tibial shaft very superficial, the stump should be bandaged in extension and the knee joint included.

When the suture line of the below-knee amputation lies anteriorly, the turns of the bandage should be made in such a way that the bandage assists in approximation of the skin flaps and does not have the reverse effect.

Stump bandages should be reapplied at least three times a day or more frequently if necessary. The patient should be taught to apply the bandage himself; if this is not possible his wife or a close relative

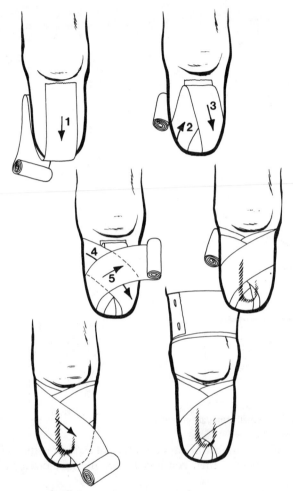

Fig. 18/13   Bandaging for a below-knee amputation

should be taught to do it for him. It will be essential for the stump to be bandaged until the patient is wearing his definitive prosthesis all day, at least three to four months.

Figure 18/14 shows another method of bandaging (Callen, 1981).

Plaster of Paris

Plaster of Paris rigid dressings also act as an early method of preventing oedema. In some cases patients have their rigid dressings

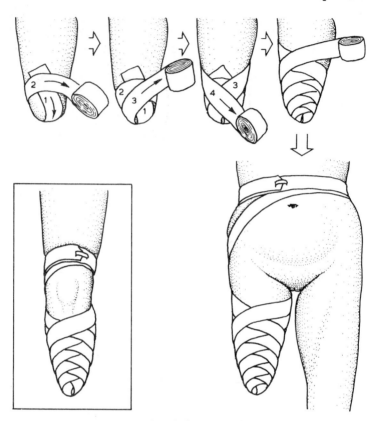

Fig. 18/14   Alternative method of bandaging

changed after a number of days for a second rigid dressing, while for
others bandaging is then continued after the first plaster of Paris
dressing.

Occasionally, instead of using the plaster of Paris just as a rigid
dressing, it can be used as an early weight-bearing method. A
prosthetic shin and foot, or length of tube, are put at the distal end of
the plaster and the patient learns to walk partially weight-bearing in
the parallel bars or using elbow crutches. At one time this was
commenced two or three days postoperatively but recently this system
is more likely to be used at a later stage of rehabilitation. Therefore
plaster of Paris dressings not only help to control oedema but
can help with early ambulation. It does, however, require a very
closely co-ordinated team of specialists, and the patient needs to be
in the care of a specialist unit. Any sign of the wasting of vastus

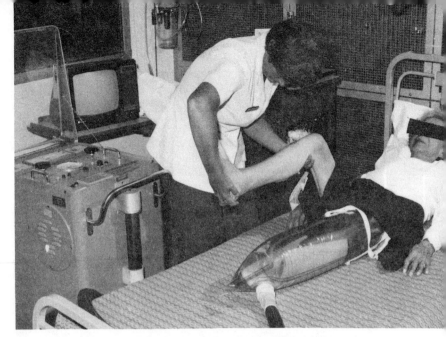

Fig. 18/15　Patient extending hip and knee while using the controlled environment treatment. The below-knee stump is totally visible in the Sterishield bag

medialis and vastus lateralis should be looked for, and these muscles may require extra strengthening after the removal of the plaster of Paris.

Controlled environment treatment (CET)

This method of postoperative management involves preventing and reducing oedema, and encouraging wound healing.

Originally it was used immediately postoperatively, the patient returning from theatre with his below-knee stump in a transparent plastic sleeve with a non-constricting seal proximally. Distally, the hose links the sleeve to the machine which delivers sterile warmed air under intermittent positive pressure. This gives an optimum environment for wound healing as well as aiding reduction and prevention of oedema. No dressings are necessary so healing and tissue reaction can be observed. The patient can exercise within the sleeve (Fig. 18/15); he can stand and hop in parallel bars or on crutches, and be reasonably mobile while attached to the machine.

Currently it is used more on stumps which are oedematous or slow healing. It can be used at any time postoperatively until the oedema is dispersed and the healing complete.

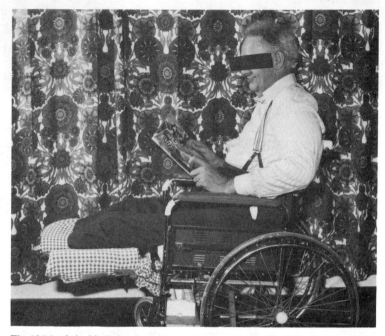

Fig. 18/16   A double, below-knee amputee using stump boards, sitting in a wheelchair that has been weighted behind the small front wheels for safety. (This is essential if the wheelchair does not have the large wheels set back 7.5 cm (3"))

Pressure environment treatment (PET)

This is a similar system, used in some departments, and is successful for reducing oedema quickly on below-knee stumps. The air is not sterile, but is filtered and there is no temperature control. Intermittent pressure can be controlled but only within a limited range. It should be used for a maximum of two hours per session.

Stump board

This is an essential piece of equipment for the control of oedema of the below-knee or through-knee amputee when sitting in a chair (Fig. 18/16). The board should extend beyond the distal end of the stump to protect it from being knocked. It gives support and the correct amount of elevation to prevent gravitational oedema. In the case of the below-knee amputee it prevents knee flexion contracture.

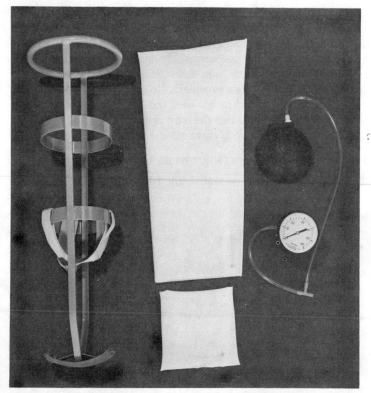

Fig. 18/17   The component parts of the pneumatic pylon (PPAM AID)

Pneumatic post-amputation mobility aid (PPAM AID)

This is an early walking aid. There is a certain amount of pumping effect in the inflatable bags as the patient walks, which helps to control and reduce oedema. The equipment consists of an outer plastic inflatable sleeve, a small inner plastic bag which is invaginated on itself, a metal frame with rocker base and a pump unit with gauge (Fig. 18/17).

The patient walks partial weight-bearing in parallel bars, and may progress to elbow crutches (Fig. 18/18). The PPAM AID is not worn outside the rehabilitation department. It does not have to be made and fitted for each individual amputee and can be put on the patient as early as five to seven days postoperatively, with the consent of the consultant.

It is important, particularly for the elderly, to encourage the patient to stand and walk as early as possible. In this way balance and postural reactions are maintained and improved, and the walking pattern retained. It can be used as an assessment to try and observe if the amputee will have the ability to balance and walk, before ordering a temporary pylon. This is particularly useful in the case of the hemiplegic patient. Bilateral amputees can also use the PPAM AID if they are able to walk on one prosthesis already. The PPAM AID can be used for above-knee, through-knee and below-knee amputations.

It must be remembered that the most important method of oedema control is daily and vigorous exercise.

RE-EDUCATION OF SENSATION OF THE HEALED STUMP

Once there is healing the patient should be encouraged to handle and

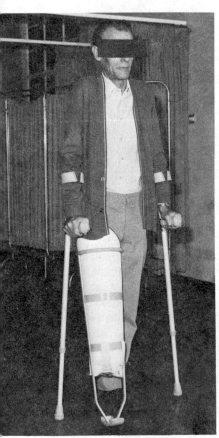

Fig. 18/18   Patient walking partial weight-bearing on PPAM AID

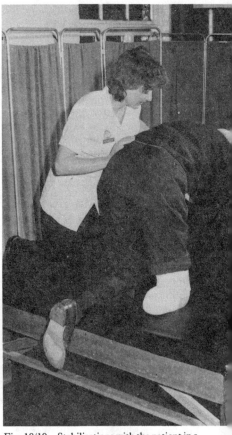

Fig. 18/19   Stabilisations with the patient in a kneeling position on a hard bed

percuss his stump. This helps to reduce the sensitivity of the stump and the patient becomes used to pressure. Exercises such as kneeling and weight-bearing through the stump also help (Fig. 18/19).

Referral to the Limb Fitting Centre

A few days postoperatively the surgeon and rehabilitation team will send the referral form, AOF3, to the regional limb fitting centre. The patient is examined by a medical officer and, if the stump is satisfactory, he will be measured for his first temporary prosthesis, the pylon. This will take two or three weeks to make and in the meantime the patient is usually discharged from hospital. It is important that his physical condition be maintained and improved; when practicable the patient should attend the physiotherapy department at the hospital nearest to his home. A young active patient will probably be able to carry out his own home programme so outpatient treatment will be unnecessary.

Prosthetic stage

As soon as the patient takes delivery of the temporary prosthesis arrangements are made to continue rehabilitation, either in the physiotherapy department of his original hospital or in the department at the limb fitting centre. The patient must learn not only to walk safely and well but also to be able to put on the pylon independently, to stand up from a chair, climb stairs, walk up and down a slope, on rough ground and possibly manage public transport.

It is advisable for the patient to attend daily, if possible, for a whole or half-day session. Elderly patients frequently experience difficulty in tolerating the prosthesis, and unless they wear this regularly for the greater part of the day their performance on an artificial limb is certain to remain limited. During all stages of treatment it should be remembered that many of these patients have undergone amputation for vascular conditions and therefore the other leg is likely also to be involved. It is important to observe the other leg, making sure that any lesions of the foot are dressed and sufficiently protected by adequate footwear when commencing gait re-education (Fig. 18/20). (See chapters on Peripheral Vascular Disease in *Cash's Textbook of Chest, Heart and Vascular Disorders for Physiotherapists*.)

When teaching a natural gait pattern to a patient wearing a temporary prosthesis, it is necessary to remember that if he is an above-knee amputee he will of necessity have to walk with a stiff knee. Hip up-drawing on the side of the prosthesis must be stressed and the

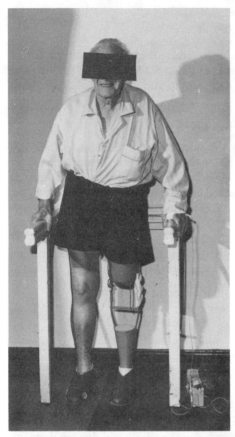

Fig. 18/20   Above-knee amputee wearing special Plastazote shoes to protect his remaining foot. Note the skin discolouration on the lower leg

Fig. 18/21   Patient learning how to lock her above-knee temporary prosthesis before standing

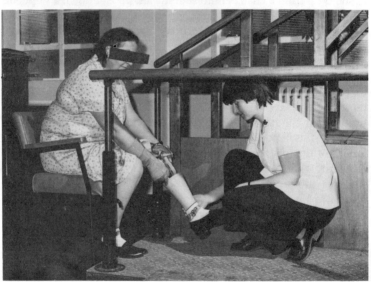

patient taught to bring the prosthesis forward without circumduction. All temporary prostheses have a type of knee mechanism which will only take the patient's weight if locked in extension. The knee lock can be released on sitting down. When the patient sits in a chair he puts his weight on the sound leg, releases the knee lock and sits down. On standing, he pushes on the arms of the chair and, with his weight on the sound leg and with the base of the prosthesis on the ground, he extends his stump as he stands, so locking the joint. Alternatively, the patient can be taught to lock the pylon before standing (Fig. 18/21) and to release the lock only after he has sat down. On climbing stairs, the patient puts the sound leg up first and brings the pylon on to the same step. To descend, the pylon is lowered first, the sound leg following.

The prosthesis is suspended on the patient by a pelvic band and shoulder strap. Occasionally there is a rocker base instead of a foot, which also facilitates weight transference and an even gait. It is, however, becoming more usual to have a foot on pylons (Fig. 18/22).

Although few allowances are made for cosmesis, the temporary

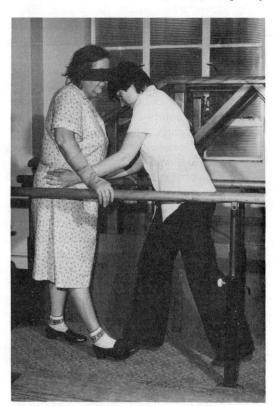

Fig. 18/22 Resisted walking in parallel bars

prosthesis is usually acceptable to the patient because it is functional and takes only two weeks to manufacture. It is lighter than a definitive prosthesis and it is relatively easy for the patient to walk well. Usually two walking sticks are the only aids required once the patient has learned the correct gait between parallel bars.

After one or two weeks the patient is normally discharged from outpatient treatment and he continues using his pylon at home, wearing it daily for the whole day. Some patients at this stage are able to return to work.

The below-knee amputee is more likely to be supplied with a patellar tendon weight-bearing prosthesis with a SACH foot (solid ankle cushioned heel), providing the wound has healed and the stump is suitable. If there is delayed primary healing then a rigid prosthesis would be supplied, and the stump must be bandaged. In this case the gait pattern would be similar to the above- or through-knee amputee.

Amputees wearing patellar tendon weight-bearing pylons will be able to walk using the knee joint normally thus giving a natural gait pattern.

The patient is reviewed by the medical officer in four to six weeks' time, and, if the stump has sufficiently reduced in size, a cast and measurements are taken for the definitive prosthesis. At present, this will take from six weeks to three months to manufacture, with at least one fitting. On completion of the prosthesis the patient returns to the limb fitting centre and, if all is satisfactory, takes delivery of the limb. He then attends at an outpatient department for final rehabilitation.

It will be necessary to teach the patient how to put on his new prosthesis and carry out all functional activities. His gait may be altered, for if he is an above- or through-knee amputee he may have been given a free-knee mechanism and he must learn to control the prosthesis accordingly. In this case, during the swing phase the prosthesis is brought forward by hip flexion to heel strike, the stump is then extended strongly against the posterior wall of the socket of the prosthesis which will ensure that the limb is fully extended and stable enough to take the patient's weight for the stance phase.

Stairs are negotiated in the same manner as with the pylon. A below-knee amputee, if previously supplied with the rigid pylon, will have to accustom himself to controlling his prosthesis with his normal knee joint and musculature which may have become weak.

It is advisable both with the temporary prosthesis and the definitive limb to start the patient in the parallel bars, teaching the basic fundamentals of gait with good weight transference, and then to progress to walking with two sticks. Occasionally two tetrapods will be necessary. The patient should be encouraged not to look down at his feet when walking, although this is inevitable in the early stages as it will compensate for the total loss of proprioception in the joints of the amputated part of the limb. As soon as possible he must learn to feel with the remaining joints the positioning of the prosthesis in the gait sequence.

A patient should never be allowed to walk with crutches while wearing his prosthesis as he will tend to bear weight on the crutches and not on the artificial limb. Very occasionally it may be necessary to teach the patient to walk with a frame, although this should only be done when he has proved unsuccessful with other walking aids. It is not possible to attain a good gait when using a frame and the patient will always be dependent on this rather bulky aid.

Elderly patients, particularly those living on their own, should be taught how to get up from the floor should they have a fall. This is best done by showing the patient how to pull himself across the floor to some stable piece of furniture, e.g. sofa, armchair, bed, and then to get himself from the floor on to this. Bilateral amputees are best advised to remove their prostheses first.

THE BILATERAL AMPUTEE

Occasionally as a result of trauma it will be necessary to amputate both lower limbs immediately. Unilateral amputees with vascular disease should be regarded as potential bilateral amputees within three years, depending upon the severity of the condition. It is not uncommon for the physiotherapist to be called upon to rehabilitate these severely disabled patients.

The pre- and postoperative treatment of the bilateral amputee follows that of the single amputee. Particular attention must be paid to strengthening and mobilising the upper limbs and trunk, and care taken to prevent flexion contractures of the hips developing while the patient waits for his pylons. All these patients will require a wheelchair which must be ordered for the patient while he is in hospital. All wheelchair activities, including transfers, will need to be taught, as well as balance.

The temporary pylons that the patient receives, i.e. rocker pylons with extension rockers, are very much shorter than the patient's normal legs, being 45–60cm (18–24in) high for the above-knee amputee and proportionately longer for the through-knee amputee. These short pylons lower the patient's centre of gravity and make balance easier (Figs. 18/23 and 18/24). In the case of the above-knee amputee, the patient takes weight on both ischial tuberosities and in effect is walking upon two stilts. He does not have a normal foot on the

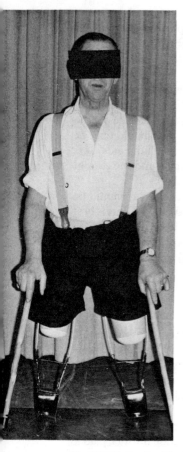 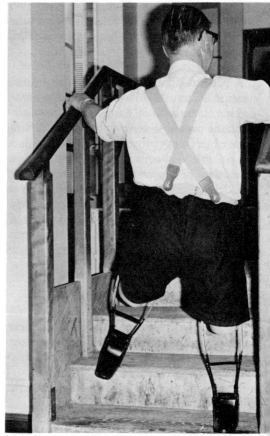

Fig. 18/23 (*left*)   Double above-knee amputee on short rocker pylons. Note the need for the wide base

Fig. 18/24 (*right*)   Climbing stairs – the rocker is placed on the edge of the step and the patient extends the hip on that side as he pulls with his hands on the rails

ground feeding in sensory information and helping with balance. It will be appreciated that these patients require a longer period of prosthetic rehabilitation, frequently four to five weeks of daily attendance. The bilateral below-knee amputee has the opportunity of using patellar tendon weight-bearing prostheses provided healing has occurred. These too will be reduced in height.

When the patient is mobile and competent on his pylons, he is reviewed by the medical officer when it will be decided whether the patient will be able to manage definitive prostheses. If he receives definitive prostheses, these will tend to be shorter than his normal legs, but nonetheless, cosmetically acceptable. A further period of rehabilitation will be necessary.

Sometimes a patient will not be fitted with prostheses, either as a single or a bilateral amputee. He may have multiple disabilities including hemiplegia, blindness or rheumatoid arthritis; his social conditions may make it unrealistic for him to be mobile on prostheses, or he may himself elect not to be fitted. These patients will need to be rehabilitated to a wheelchair life and adaptations in the home will have to be made where necessary.

The total care and management of the lower limb amputee is continuous. It is essential that at each stage of his rehabilitation he is reassessed so that his treatment is suitable to his needs. It is also important that the home conditions are known so that treatment, at all times, may be related to them. Before discharge all amputees should be allowed a trial visit home so that the return home will be successful.

UPPER LIMB AMPUTATIONS

Patients who undergo amputations of the upper limb do so most commonly as a result of trauma from accidents at work or road accidents. These patients tend to be in the younger age-groups, of employable age and are predominantly male.

The suddenness of the accident and the psychological shock of losing an arm cannot be underestimated. The physiotherapist can do much to help the patient in this respect as she will be treating the patient from the day following the operation, and much will need to be done to prepare the patient for wearing and using a prosthesis.

The aims of physiotherapy are as follows:

1. To strengthen the muscles controlling the stump and maintain full range of movement in the shoulder girdle.
2. To prevent contractures.
3. To control oedema of the stump.
4. To maintain a good posture.

On the day following amputation, exercises to the shoulder girdle and the unaffected arm are commenced. The patient will depend upon good mobility of this region for the control of his prosthesis, particularly flexion of the shoulder and protraction of the shoulder girdle.

The stump must remain in a good position and this must be supervised by both nurses and physiotherapists. The contracture most likely to develop in the above-elbow amputee is that of flexion, adduction and medial rotation at the shoulder, and frequently there is the danger of a frozen shoulder developing. The contracture most likely to occur in the below-elbow amputee is that of flexion at the elbow. When in bed the patient may rest the stump on a pillow provided it is in a contra-contracture position.

A few days following amputation, active exercises for the muscles controlling the stump can be started and gradually progressed to strong resisted exercises when the sutures are removed.

Once the sutures have been removed (usually on the 14th day) stump bandaging is commenced in the same way as for a lower limb amputee. Care must be taken to obtain more pressure distally, preventing a tourniquet effect, and the range of movement of the joints above the amputation must be retained.

A constant check on the posture of the patient is necessary to ensure a level shoulder girdle, and good position of the head and neck.

Four to five days postoperatively co-operation with the occupational therapist, who can fit a leather gauntlet which can be applied over the bandage, is useful. Into this gauntlet simple tools, such as cutlery for the below-elbow amputee, or a pencil or paint brush, can be fixed, and the patient encouraged to use his stump. Where possible early use of the stump for functional activities diminishes the risk of the patient becoming 'one-handed'. (Where there is no occupational therapy department, the physiotherapist will be responsible.)

Prosthetic stage

As soon as the stump is healed and the oedema controlled, the patient will be seen by the medical officer at the regional limb fitting centre, and measurements taken for a prosthesis.

Some centres fit the patient with a temporary prosthesis and commence arm training early, but this is not routine practice; normally the patient will wait six to eight weeks for the delivery of the definitive prosthesis.

Usually the arm training units in limb fitting centres are staffed by occupational therapists; the emphasis being placed upon training in functional skills towards personal independence, employment and leisure activities.

Upper limb prostheses are made in three weights – heavy working, light working and dress; the latter being cosmetic only. The choice of type of arm will be determined by the length of the stump, and the lifestyle of the patient. Working arms are controlled by the patient's body power through straps that pass posteriorly across his scapulae to the opposite axilla. The above-elbow amputee activates elbow flexion

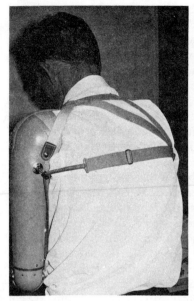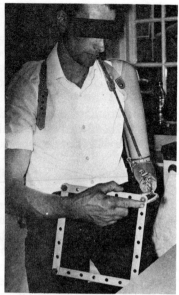

Fig. 18/25 (*left*) Posterior view of an above-elbow prosthesis showing leather operating cord (inferior) attached to the appendages. Protraction of the scapulae to operate terminal device

Fig. 18/26 (*right*) Anterior view showing the strap to operate elbow lock

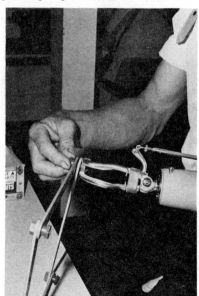

Fig. 18/27   Close-up of split hook

and the terminal device control by protraction of the scapulae and forward flexion of the shoulder joint (Fig. 18/25). The below-elbow amputee activates the terminal device by slight forward flexion of the shoulder and extension of the elbow. All arm prostheses are supplied with a cosmetic hand, but for practical activities numerous terminal devices are available, the most common being the split hook (Figs. 18/26, 18/27).

The occupational therapist will assess the patient to decide what devices will be needed to enable him to be independent and capable of work; these will then be supplied and suitable training in their use arranged.

Whatever prosthesis is prescribed in the working range, training should relate to employment potential. Most patients return to their former work, but for some retraining is required, and this should be considered early in the rehabilitation process. Most patients are well motivated to return to work and hold down jobs in any field of work.

Recent developments in upper limb prosthetics have produced a functional mechanical hand. Myo-electric and electronic controls are being tried but as yet are only experimental. These more sophisticated prostheses are appropriate for only a small number of patients, but research and development is continuing.

REFERENCE

Callen, S. (1981). A modern method of stump bandaging. *Physiotherapy*, **67**, 5, 137–8.

BIBLIOGRAPHY

Anderson, M. H., Bechtol, C. O. and Solars, R. E. (1959). *Clinical Prosthetics for Physicians and Therapists*. C. C. Thomas, Illinois.

Banerjee, S. N. (1982). *Rehabilitation Management of Amputees*. Williams and Wilkins, Baltimore.

Crosthwaite Eyre, N. (1979). Rehabilitation of the upper limb amputee. *Physiotherapy*, **65**, 1, 9–12.

Dickstein, R., Pillar, T. and Mannheim, M. (1982). The pneumatic post-amputation mobility aid in geriatric rehabilitation. *Scandinavian Journal of Rehabilitation Medicine*, **14**, 3, 149–50.

Humm, W. (1977). *Rehabilitation of the Lower Limb Amputee*, 3rd edition. Baillière Tindall, London.

Klopsteg, P. E. and Wilson, P. D. (1969). *Human Limbs and Their Substitutes*. Hafner Publishing Co, New York.

Kostuik, J. P. and Gillespie, R. (eds) (1981). *Amputation Surgery and Rehabilitation. The Toronto Experience*. Churchill Livingstone, Edinburgh.

Little, J. M. (1975). *Major Amputations for Vascular Disease*. Churchill Livingstone, Edinburgh.

Robertson, E. S. (1980). *Rehabilitation of Arm Amputees and Limb Deficient Children*. Baillière Tindall, London.

Symposium on Limb Ablation and Limb Replacement (1967). *Annals of the Royal College of Surgeons of England*, **40**, 4.

Troupe, I. M. and Wood, M. A. (1982). *Total Care of the Lower Limb Amputee*. Pitman Books Ltd, London.

Van de Ven, C. (1981). An investigation into the management of bilateral leg amputees. *British Medical Journal*, **283**, 707.

Vitali, M., Robinson, K. P., Andrews, B. G. and Harris, E. H. (1978). *Amputations and Prostheses*. Baillière Tindall, London.

ACKNOWLEDGEMENTS

This chapter is a revision of the one which appeared in *Cash's Textbook of Physiotherapy in Some Surgical Conditions*, 2nd edition, by Miss B. C. Davis MCSP. The present author and the book's editor are grateful to Bridget Davis for allowing this material to be used. They also thank Seton Ltd, Oldham for allowing the use of Figures 18/12 and 18/13 and the text of their leaflets on stump bandaging.

The author thanks the following for their help in the revision: Mr M. Vitali FRCS, past principal medical officer, Limb Fitting Centre, Roehampton, London; Mrs D. Dixey MCSP, senior physiotherapist, Limb Surgery Unit, Queen Mary's Hospital, Roehampton, London; Miss M. A. Mendez OBE, FCOT, district occupational therapist, Richmond, Twickenham and Roehampton Health Authority; Mr N. Babbage, consultant photographer, Bioengineering Centre, Roehampton, London; and Mrs G. Smith, secretary.

Chapter 19

Cranial Surgery

by M. LIGHTBODY, MCSP

Brain lesions may cause motor and sensory defects but may be accompanied by other severe disorders, for example of sight, hearing, intellect, speech and personality. Psychological disturbance, requiring full understanding and suitable management, may accompany both brain and spinal cord lesions. Early diagnosis of brain lesions and prompt admission to a neurosurgical unit is essential to ensure maximum benefit: delay may cause irreparable damage and permanent disability.

Although research continues to increase understanding of the central nervous system in terms of anatomy, physiology and function, much remains to be discovered. Increasing knowledge of brain areas, pathways, connections, spinal cord tracts and functions has opened up new fields in surgical neurology. Improved investigative and operative equipment and techniques, anaesthesia, antibiotics and other drugs continue to reduce operating time, and reduce to a minimum postoperative complications and morbidity.

Team work is essential for the fullest rehabilitation of patients. Apart from the doctors (surgeons and physicians) those involved include nursing staff, physiotherapists, occupational therapists, speech therapists, psychologists, social workers and chaplain, as well as the patient and his relatives who have an important contributory role. Interchange of knowledge between members of the team allows a full understanding of the particular problems of each patient. Encouragement, patience, and perseverance are of paramount importance during the rehabilitation period, which can be said to begin immediately the patient enters hospital. As rehabilitation proceeds, other support services may be required, e.g. the disablement resettlement officer (DRO), to arrange job retraining.

ANATOMY AND PHYSIOLOGY

For the purposes of description, the brain can be divided into the forebrain or prosencephalon, the midbrain or mesencephalon and the hindbrain or rhombencephalon. It must be remembered that the entire mechanism is extremely complex; no one part works as a separate entity, and the response of the brain is the result of the integrated action of its various systems. The anatomical units are not necessarily the functional units. For example, the extra-pyramidal system and the reticular formation appear to have specific functions and yet are comprised of widely spread grey and white matter; the distribution of the blood supply divides the brain into areas different from the anatomical lobes.

The effects of lesions at some strategic sites throughout the brain are given in the following brief guide.

Cerebrum (Figs. 19/1 and 19/2)

The cerebrum is the largest part of the brain, and consists of two hemispheres connected by bundles of nerve fibres, the corpus callosum. The surface of each hemisphere covered by layers of cells constitutes the cerebral cortex. This represents the highest centre of function and can be roughly mapped into areas, each concerned with a specific function. To facilitate reference each hemisphere is divided into four lobes, frontal, temporal, parietal and occipital. The right hemisphere controls the left side of the body, and the left hemisphere controls the right side of the body and usually speech function.

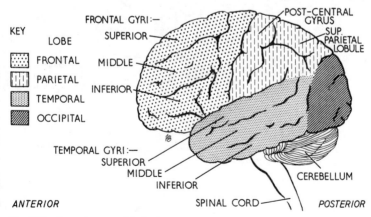

Fig. 19/1 Lateral aspect of the brain

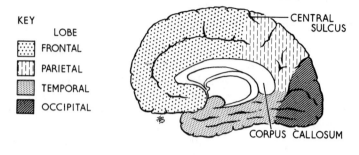

CENTRAL SULCUS

CORPUS CALLOSUM

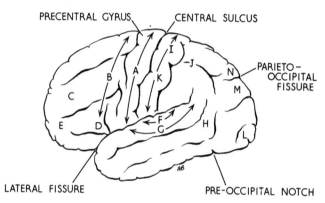

PRECENTRAL GYRUS   CENTRAL SULCUS

PARIETO-OCCIPITAL FISSURE

LATERAL FISSURE

PRE-OCCIPITAL NOTCH

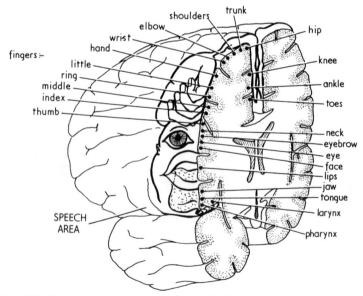

Fig. 19/4   The motor homunculus superimposed on the pre-central gyrus illustrates the proportions and positions of body representation in the motor cortex. For the post-central gyrus there is a similar representation for sensation

FRONTAL LOBE (Figs. 19/1 and 19/3)

Area	Function	Effect of a lesion
(A) Motor area (which gives rise to the cerebro-spinal tracts)	Controls voluntary movement of the opposite half of the body which is represented on the cortex in an upside down position (Fig. 19/4)	Flaccid paralysis. A lesion between the hemispheres produces paraplegia
(B) Pre-motor area	Localisation of motor function	*Spastic paralysis. Psychological changes
(C)	Controls movements of the eyes	The eyes turn to the side of the lesion and cannot be moved to the opposite side
(D)	Motor control of larynx, tongue, and lips to enable movements of articulation	Inability to articulate
(E) 'Silent area'	Believed to control abstract thinking, foresight, mature judgement, tactfulness	Lack of a sense of responsibility in personal affairs

*The effects of a lesion in the pre-motor area vary with the rate of onset; a lesion which occurs suddenly, such as a head injury or a haemorrhage, will result in a flaccid paralysis initially, spasm gradually developing over a variable period of time. A lesion which has a slow mode of onset, such as a slowly growing neoplasm, will produce spasm in the early stages.

TEMPORAL LOBE (Figs. 19/1 and 19/3)

Area	Function	Effect of a lesion
(F and G)	Hearing and association of sound	Inability to localise the direction of sound
(H) Auditory speech area	Understanding of the spoken word	Inability to understand what is said

Other areas on the medial aspect of the temporal lobe are associated with the sense of smell and taste. The optic radiations sweep through the temporal lobe to reach the occipital lobe and these may also be damaged by a lesion of the temporal lobe giving rise to a homonymous hemianopia (Fig. 19/5).

PARIETAL LOBE (Figs. 19/1 and 19/3)

Area	Function	Effect of a lesion
(I, J and K)	Sensory receptive areas for light touch, two-point discrimination, joint position sense and pressure	Corresponding sensory loss giving rise to a 'neglect phenomenon'. 'Body image' loss is associated with lesions of the non-dominant hemisphere

Visual defects arising from lesions in the parietal area may be highly complex and the patient unaware of them. Sensory loss gives a severe disability, which is out of proportion to any associated voluntary power loss.

OCCIPITAL LOBE (Figs. 19/1 and 19/3)

Area	Function	Effect of a lesion
(L)	Receptive area for visual impressions	Loss of vision in some areas of the visual fields (Fig. 19/5)
(M and N)	Recognition and interpretation of visual stimuli	Inability to recognise things visually

Brainstem

All nerve fibres to and from the cerebral cortex converge towards the brainstem forming the corona radiata, and on entering the diencephalon they become the internal capsule (Fig. 19/6). When the cerebral cortex is removed the remainder, or central core, is termed the brainstem. Its components from above downwards are: the diencephalon; the basal ganglia; the mesencephalon or midbrain; the pons; and the medulla oblongata.

The nuclei of the cranial nerves are scattered throughout this area.

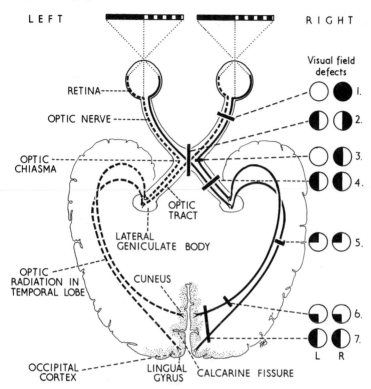

Fig. 19/5 The effects of injury in the visual pathway. (1) Complete blindness in one eye. (2) Bi-temporal hemianopia. (3) Complete nasal hemianopia right eye. (4) Left homonymous hemianopia. (5 and 6) Quadrantic defects. (7) Complete left homonymous hemianopia

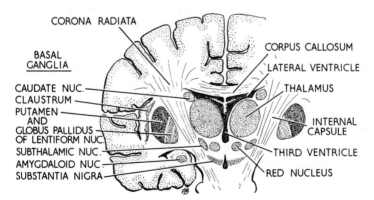

Fig. 19/6 Cross-section of the brain

Basal ganglia and extra-pyramidal system

Broadly speaking the basal ganglia include the corpus striatum, amygdala, claustrum, substantia nigra and subthalamic nuclei. The corpus striatum consists of the caudate nucleus and the lenticular nucleus, the latter being composed of the putamen and the globus pallidus.

The extra-pyramidal system includes parts of the cerebral cortex, thalamic nuclei connected with the striatum, corpus striatum, subthalamus, rubral and reticular systems and its functions are concerned with associated movements, postural adjustments and autonomic integration. Lesions may result in voluntary movement being obscured or abolished and replaced with involuntary movements.

Lesions of the extra-pyramidal system can produce either hyperkinetic or hypokinetic disorders.

Midbrain, pons and medulla oblongata

The midbrain, pons and medulla oblongata also act as a funnel for tracts passing from higher levels downwards to the spinal cord and for sensory tracts from the spinal cord passing upwards to higher centres. In view of it being a relatively small area, any lesion can give rise to widespread effects. Involvement of any of the following are likely.

Cerebellar function may be affected due to interference of the efferent and afferent pathways passing through the brainstem.

Sensation of all types may be affected as the fasciculi gracilis and cuneatus terminate in nuclei in the medulla oblongata. Nerve fibres then arise from these nuclei, cross the mid-line and continue upwards to the thalamus in the medial lemniscus. The spinothalamic tracts which cross in the spinal cord pass directly upwards through the brainstem.

Loss of motor function occurs if the cerebrospinal tracts are damaged. These pass downwards from the internal capsule to decussate at the lower end of the medulla oblongata.

The conscious level can be depressed if there is damage to the reticular formation which is scattered throughout the brainstem.

Vomiting and disturbed respiratory rate can occur with pressure on the vomiting and respiratory centres in the medulla oblongata.

Cranial nerve nuclear lesions may result with characteristic palsies.

CRANIAL NERVES (Fig. 19/7)

Cranial nerve	Function	Effect of a lesion
I. Olfactory	Sense of smell	Loss of sense of smell
II. Optic	Vision	Various visual field defects (Fig. 19/5). Visual acuity affected
III. Oculo-motor	Innervates medial, superior, inferior recti and inferior oblique muscle and voluntary fibres of levator palpebrae superioris. Carries autonomic fibres to pupil	Outward deviation of the eye, ptosis, dilation of the pupil
IV Trochlear	Motor supply to the superior oblique eye muscle	Inability to turn the eye downwards and outwards
V. Trigeminal	(a) Motor division to temporalis, masseter, internal and external pterygoid muscles (b) Sensory division: touch, pain and temperature sensation of the face including the cornea on the same side of the body	(a) Deviation of the chin towards the paralysed side when the mouth is open (b) Loss of touch, pain and temperature sensation and of the corneal reflex
VI. Abducent	Innervates the external rectus muscle	Internal squint and therefore diplopia
VII. Facial	Motor supply to facial muscles on the same side of the body	Paralysis of facial muscles
VIII. Acoustic	Sensory supply to semicircular canals. Hearing	Vertigo. Nystagmus. Deafness
IX. Glosso-pharyngeal	Motor to the pharynx. Taste: posterior one-third of the tongue	Loss of gag reflex. Loss of taste in the appropriate area

Cranial nerve	Function	Effect of a lesion
X. Vagus	Motor to pharynx. Sympathetic and parasympathetic to heart and viscera	Difficulty with swallowing. Regurgitation of food and fluids
XI. Accessory	The cranial part of the nerve joins the vagus nerve	
XII. Hypoglossal	Motor nerve of the tongue	Paralysis of the side of the tongue corresponding to the lesion, thus it deviates to the paralysed side when protruded

Cerebellum (Fig. 19/8)

The cerebellum lies in the posterior cranial fossa of the skull connected to the pons and medulla oblongata by the cerebellar peduncles. The surface is corrugated and consists of cells forming the cerebellar cortex. It is divided into two cerebellar hemispheres which join near the mid-line with a narrow middle portion called the vermis. Each hemisphere can be divided into the archicerebellum and the corpus cerebelli, of which the latter is composed of the paleocerebellum and the neocerebellum.

Although the whole of the cerebellum is highly integrated, and disease often results in diffuse damage, Lance and McLeod (1975) summarise the signs and symptoms of cerebellar syndromes as follows:

Archicerebellar syndrome: (a) ataxia of gait, (b) vertigo and (c) nystagmus.

Paleocerebellar syndrome (anterior or mid-line cerebellar syndrome): ataxia of gait and inco-ordination of the lower limb.

Neocerebellar syndrome: (a) hypotonia, (b) dyssynergia, (c) dysmetria, (d) static or postural tremor, (e) intention tremor, (f) ataxia of gait and falling to the side of the lesion, and (g) nystagmus.

Smoothly performed, accurate and skilled movements are the responsibility of the cerebellum, and the speed with which it can correlate the information it receives and effect controlled actions is phenomenal.

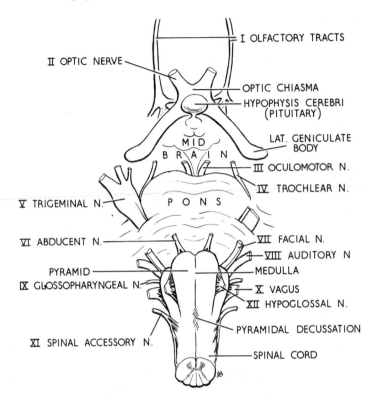

Fig. 19/7 The brainstem and cranial nerves (viewed from below)

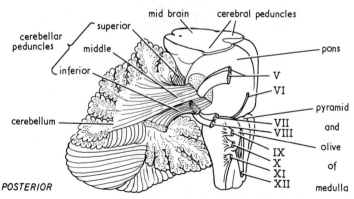

Fig. 19/8 Right antero-lateral view of the dissected cerebellar hemisphere and peduncles showing the lower cranial nerves

Circulation of the brain

The four major vessels which supply the brain, the right and left vertebral and internal carotid arteries, form an anastomosis at the base of the brain, called the Circle of Willis (see Fig. 19/13(c) p. 319). From this arterial complex many branches are given off, to be distributed to the brainstem, cerebellum and cerebrum. Interference with the circulation in any of these branches will cause characteristic deficits, depending on the parts of the brain deprived of blood supply.

The ventricular system

The ventricular system consists of four fluid-filled cavities within the brain. There is a right and left lateral ventricle, and a third and fourth ventricle in the mid-line. Cerebrospinal fluid (CSF) is produced in the choroid plexuses of the ventricles and circulates within the system to the fourth ventricle where it escapes through the foramina of Luschka and Magendie, into the subarachnoid space (Fig. 19/9). CSF flows all

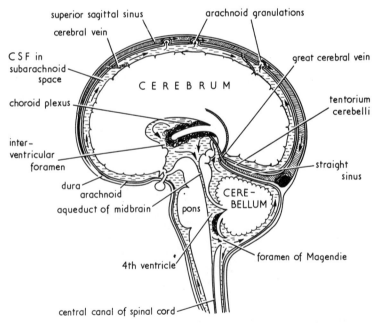

Fig. 19/9   Circulation of the cerebrospinal fluid

around the brain and spinal cord, bathing it and cushioning it against jarring forces.

Obstruction of the system leads to hydrocephalus, raised intra-cranial pressure and eventually neurological deficits as the underlying structures are compressed or distorted.

EXAMINATIONS AND INVESTIGATIONS

Before surgery can be considered, extensive examinations and investigations may need to be carried out to localise the lesion and decide upon its nature and likely prognosis.

Examinations

A history of the patient's present illness, previous illnesses and any relevant family illness is noted as are social circumstances, occupation, drinking and smoking habits. Whenever possible this information is obtained directly from the patient, but if the patient's level of consciousness or language function is disturbed it will have to be obtained from other sources such as spouse, parents or friends. If the patient has a history of unconscious episodes, such as epileptic attacks, a description of these attacks from an observer may provide useful information.

The patient undergoes a general examination but special attention is devoted to the central nervous system; each cranial nerve is tested, reflexes, motor power and all types of sensation are carefully checked. Full assessment of the central nervous system may be complicated by lack of co-operation, but adequate information is usually obtained to establish a diagnosis.

Assessment by the physiotherapist

Detailed and precise pre-operative assessment is ideal but this may be difficult if the patient requires immediate surgery, or if the conscious level affects co-operation.

The assessment will give a base line from which further improvement or deterioration can be measured. A postoperative deterioration may be the result of removal of brain tissue during the course of surgery, but more important it may be one of the signs of onset of postoperative complications, such as haemorrhage or thrombosis.

The assessment by the physiotherapist requires an accurate evaluation of:

1. Voluntary movement and muscle power, as this is useful both for diagnosis and future treatment. This should be recorded carefully, perhaps using a numerical scale, although this is not always appropriate in the presence of spasticity.
2. The range of movement which may be correlated with any incidental findings of importance, for example previous underlying orthopaedic pathology.
3. Muscle tone, which may be either hypo-, normo- or hyper-tonic. Changes in muscle tonus may be subtle but they are important indications of the patient's progress. Awareness of the state of muscle tone is an integral part of treatment. Muscle tone may be described as the resistance to stretch, and can be judged by palpation of the muscle belly, the resistance felt to velocity, sensitive passive movements, tendon responses, observation of active movements and posture.
4. Equilibrium and righting reactions.
5. The sensorium and mental status of the patient.
6. Sensory modalities particularly cutaneous, deep and proprioceptive responses.
7. The functional ability of the patient to determine the level and quality of his independence. (Chapter 5, *Cash's Textbook of Neurology for Physiotherapists*, describes the assessment of patients with a neurological disorder.)
8. The early assessment of the patient's respiratory function is desirable but will depend upon his physical state and the degree of urgency for operation.

Special investigations

These procedures may be carried out while the patient is having physiotherapy which may need to be modified.

LUMBAR PUNCTURE

A needle is inserted in the subarachnoid space between the third and fourth lumbar spinous processes; the pressure of the cerebrospinal fluid is determined and a sample of fluid taken for diagnostic purposes. Following lumbar puncture the patient is nursed lying flat in bed for eight hours, and active physiotherapy can be given in any of the lying positions. A severe headache may develop after a lumbar puncture. This can be relieved by elevating the foot of the bed for 24 hours.

RADIOGRAPHS

Plain films of the skull are usually necessary and can be supplemented by special views of various areas. A note is made of any intracranial calcification and possible displacement of a calcified pineal body. General radiographic examination may be indicated, and a chest radiograph is always taken.

COMPUTERISED AXIAL TOMOGRAPHY (CAT SCAN)

This technique has revolutionised the field of investigation. The patient's head is centred in a gantry containing an x-ray tube on one side, and banks of detectors on the opposite side. The gantry moves around the patient's head and the x-ray beam is measured by the detectors before entering, and on leaving, the head. The detectors are so arranged that tomographic cuts are obtained. All this information is processed by a computer and displayed on a TV screen as a cross-sectional picture of the head from which the operator can visualise the internal structure of the brain and identify certain abnormalities which may be present.

CEREBRAL ANGIOGRAPHY

This is an important procedure, which is often carried out under a general anaesthetic. Injections of radio-opaque solutions into the carotid or vertebral arteries are followed by taking films of the arterial, capillary and venous phases of the circulation. Displacement of the blood vessels shows the site of intracranial masses such as clots, tumours, abscesses or cysts. In a proportion of tumour cases, the circulation of the tumour itself may also be seen and may give an accurate assessment of its pathological type.

Angiography is of great value in cerebrovascular disease. The site of arterial stenosis or occlusion is easily seen. In spontaneous intracranial haemorrhage the site of an aneurysm or arteriovenous anomaly can only be determined by angiography. Postoperative angiography is a useful means of checking the efficiency of surgical treatment of aneurysms and anomalies.

Indirect methods of angiography are now more frequently used. A catheter is inserted into the femoral or axillary artery and its tip passed into the aortic arch. Large quantities of contrast medium injected under pressure allow the display of all major cerebral arteries.

Following angiography the patient is nursed flat for 24 hours, then allowed to sit up and get out of bed if no headache is present. Physiotherapy consists of breathing exercises and maintenance exercises. If the femoral or axillary artery has been used, care must be taken to ensure that the patient maintains full range of hip or shoulder joint movement.

LUMBAR AIR ENCEPHALOGRAPHY

This technique has been replaced by the CAT scan except in a few cases.

RADIO-ISOTOPE SCANNING

The use of radio-active isotopes in investigation of cerebral disorders may take the form of one of the following:

1. Intravenously in order to delineate masses such as tumours.
2. Introduced into the cerebral circulation to investigate the blood supply.
3. Introduced into the CSF for the study of obstruction to the circulation of the CSF. This helps to distinguish between atrophy and hydrocephalus with gross increase in intracranial pressure.

ELECTRO-ENCEPHALOGRAPHY

The electro-encephalograph (EEG) amplifies and records the electrical activity of the brain. It has been replaced by CAT scan, but is used as an aid to the diagnosis of epilepsy and location of a focus.

MONITORING INTRACRANIAL PRESSURE

A monitoring system can be used to measure intracranial pressure over a period of approximately 48 hours. The information gained allows fuller assessment of the patient's condition and his further management. (This means of measuring intracranial pressure over a period of time has been extremely useful in the management of certain head injury patients whose condition has remained static for no apparent reason. The monitoring can show up huge variations in pressure over a long period, which go undetected with random measurements, and can indicate the need for a 'shunt' to reduce intracranial pressure, with a resultant improvement in the patient's condition.)

Because the patient is connected to a delicate piece of apparatus, he is necessarily kept lying quietly in bed for the duration of the monitoring. Physiotherapy will probably need to continue, particularly chest care. It is important to note that moving or turning the patient, and coughing or straining, will dramatically alter the CSF pressure, and hence the recording needle may swing violently. It is necessary to note both type and time of physiotherapy so that when the results are analysed these changes in pressure are interpreted correctly.

GENERAL SIGNS AND SYMPTOMS OF CEREBRAL LESIONS

Raised intracranial pressure

Intracranial pressure depends on the volume of the skull contents. In a child under the age of 18 months, any slow abnormal increase in volume will result in a disproportionate increase in the size of the head. In individuals over the age of 18 months there is no increase in the size of the head, thus the effects of raised intracranial pressure will produce a disturbance of cerebral function more rapidly. Increased volume may be caused by a space-occupying lesion, such as a tumour or abscess, a blockage in the cerebrospinal fluid pathways or by haemorrhage from an aneurysm. With raised intracranial pressure the soft-walled veins become compressed, giving rise to oedema and subsequent lack of oxygen to the brain tissue, and although the symptoms vary in degree, the classical picture of raised pressure is a combination of the following features.

DROWSINESS

Drowsiness is the earliest and most important sign of raised intracranial pressure. The brain can adapt to very slowly increasing pressure and the patient may become gradually demented with little else to show. Rapidly increasing pressure will produce drowsiness and it becomes progressively more difficult to rouse the patient. Unconsciousness and death can follow in a short time.

HEADACHE

In the early stages of raised intracranial pressure, headache may be paroxysmal occurring during the night and early morning. With continued increase in pressure it becomes continuous and is intensified by exertion, coughing or stooping. The pressure headache is usually bilateral and becomes worse when the patient is lying down and is relieved when sitting up. Other causes of head pain are irritation of parts of the meninges, involvement of the Vth, IXth and Xth cranial nerve trunks, referred pain from disorders of the eyes, sinuses, teeth and upper cervical spine, and tension headaches due to muscle spasm.

PAPILLOEDEMA

This is oedema of the optic discs which can cause enlargement of the blind spot and subsequent deterioriation of visual acuity and complete blindness.

VOMITING

This occurs when the headache is most severe and tends to be projectile in nature.

PULSE AND BLOOD PRESSURE

Acute and subacute rises in pressure cause a slowing of the pulse rate, but if pressure continues to rise the pulse rate becomes very rapid. A rapid increase in intracranial pressure causes a rise in the blood pressure, but a chronic rise does not affect it, and in some lesions below the tentorium cerebelli the blood pressure is below normal.

RESPIRATORY RATE

This is not affected by a slow rise in pressure but a sufficiently rapid increase in pressure, which produces a loss of consciousness, usually results in slow deep respirations. This may change after a period and become irregular, of the Cheyne-Stokes type.

EPILEPTIC CONVULSIONS

Generalised fits may occur but it is not clear whether these are caused by the raised intracranial pressure or by the actual lesion itself.

Eye symptoms

It is essential to realise that eye symptoms are often present with a brain lesion and they can directly affect a patient's capabilities during his rehabilitation. Among those most commonly found are:

Damage to the optic nerve, optic chiasm or optic tracts will cause field defects (see Fig. 19/5).

Damage to the IIIrd cranial nerve can cause a ptosis, an inability to open the eye.

Nystagmus. This is frequently present in cerebellar or brainstem lesions and is an involuntary jerky movement of the eyes.

Diplopia or double vision. This is present if there is any imbalance of the eye muscles and may be overcome by covering alternate eyes on alternate days until the imbalance adjusts itself.

Ear symptoms

Deafness may be caused by tumours of the VIIIth cranial nerve such as acoustic neuromas; these tumours may give rise to vertigo.

Speech disorders

These have already been briefly mentioned and are mainly associated with lesions of the temporal lobe on the dominant side.

Level of consciousness

Numerous factors can be responsible for alteration in the level of consciousness:

1. Haemorrhage which can be either extradural, subdural, subarachnoid, or intracerebral;
2. Infection as in the case of meningitis and encephalitis;
3. Space-occupying masses causing increased intracranial pressure and compression of the brainstem;
4. Operational trauma;
5. Postoperative complications such as oedema or haemorrhage;
6. Certain types of trauma produce a craniocerebral injury.

Any known disturbance of hearing, vision or speech function must always be taken into account, and the patient given every opportunity to be able to respond.

General attitudes of the patient should be noted also:

1. A patient who lies curled up, turned away from the light, and does not like being interfered with, who is irritable to varying degrees and who may be confused or even delirious might be showing signs of cerebral irritation.
2. When the neck is held stiffly into extension, and the patient resists flexion sometimes accompanied by retraction of the head, it may be due to irritation from subarachnoid haemorrhage, meningitis or raised intracranial pressure.
3. Trunk and limb rigidity or stiffness may be signs of involvement of the base of the brain. The spine and lower limbs are held in total extension, the forearms pronated, elbows extended and the wrists and fingers flexed. This posture is usually described as decerebrate rigidity.

Other localising signs may include: ataxia; cranial nerve palsies; and reflex changes.

ASSESSMENT OF CONSCIOUSNESS

The conscious level is the most important observation made. Various ill-defined stages have been used to formulate different scales of consciousness in the past but these stages may mean different things to different people. An accurate scale where there can be little divergence is needed. One such scale is the Glasgow Coma Scale (Teasdale and Jennett, 1974). This assesses the patient's motor activity, verbal performance and eye-opening responses (Table I).

TABLE I NEUROLOGICAL OBSERVATION CHART FOR ASSESSMENT OF CONSCIOUSNESS (BASED ON THE GLASGOW COMA SCALE)

Time	0–24h	22.00 24.00 02.00 04.00 06.00
Eye opening	Spontaneous To speech To pain None	
Best verbal response	Orientated Confused Inappropriate Incomprehensible None	
Best motor response	Obeying Localising Flexing Extending None	

Motor activity, if not in response to commands, can be assessed by the response to painful stimuli. The response may be either 'localising', e.g. if the hand moves towards the stimuli, or 'flexor' or 'extensor' to indicate the direction of the movement. There may be no response. If one limb or one side is clearly worse than the other side, this is regarded as evidence of focal damage.

Verbal responses can indicate either full orientation and awareness of self and surroundings or confusion, inappropriate speech or incomprehensible speech.

Eye opening responses indicate whether the arousal mechanisms in the brainstem are active. The eyes may open in response to speech, to pain, or spontaneously.

CRANIAL SURGERY

Table II summarises the conditions for which surgery may be necessary. It is not proposed to describe in detail specific surgical procedures: the Bibliography on page 333 includes textbooks to which reference may be made for a description of the actual surgical techniques.

TABLE II   NEUROLOGICAL CONDITIONS FOR WHICH SURGERY MAY BE APPLIED

Condition	Adult	Paediatric and juvenile
Cerebral trauma	Head injuries	Head injuries
Neoplastic lesions	Cerebral – primary – metastatic Tumours from related structures, e.g. meninges; cranial nerves; pituitary fossa Cerebellar	Cerebral – primary Tumours from related structures, e.g. choroid plexus of ventricle Cerebellar
Cerebrovascular disease Haemorrhage Ischaemic lesions	Intracranial aneurysms Spontaneous subdural or extradural haemorrhage Angiomatous malformations Carotid stenosis	 Angiomatous malformations
Hydrocephalus	Secondary (e.g. with space-occupying lesions) Aqueduct stenosis	Congenital Secondary – tumours – spina bifida

Spina bifida		Spina bifida cystica
		   meningocele
		   myelomeningocele
		Encephalocele

Dyskinesia	Parkinsonism	Cerebral palsy
		   spastic hemiplegia
		   choreoathetosis

TABLE II (*continued*)

Condition	Adult	Paediatric and juvenile
Epilepsy	Intractable Primary focus	Primary focus, associated, for example, with Sturge-Weber syndrome
Cerebral infections	Abscess	Abscess
Repair of skull defects	Cranioplasty	Craniosynostosis
Psychiatric conditions	Psychosurgery, e.g. stereotactic amygdalotomy	
Miscellaneous	Intractable pain, e.g. trigeminal neuralgia	

GENERAL POINTS RELATING TO SURGICAL PROCEDURES

Most operations are performed under general anaesthesia and may take a considerable period of time to complete. During the course of surgery a bone flap may be turned back, but this is usually replaced at the end of the operation. Figures 19/10 and 19/11 illustrate some of the surgical approaches.

Postoperative treatment

On return from the operating theatre the patient will have a pressure bandage on the head to control swelling; this may be extended to include the eye on the side corresponding to the operational site, for the same purpose. Eyes are very vulnerable to swelling and do so as a result of operational trauma. The position of the patient on the operating table may also be a contributory factor, hence for the first two or three postoperative days the patient may be unable to open either eye.

Intravenous infusion begun during the operation may be continued for one or two days; then, if the ability to swallow is affected, the patient is artificially fed via a nasogastric or naso-oesophageal tube.

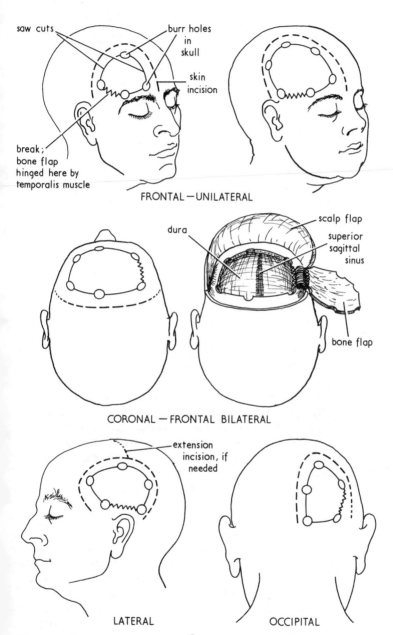

saw cuts

burr holes
in
skull

skin
incision

break;
bone flap
hinged here by
temporalis muscle

FRONTAL—UNILATERAL

dura

scalp flap

superior
sagittal
sinus

bone flap

CORONAL — FRONTAL BILATERAL

extension
incision, if
needed

LATERAL

OCCIPITAL

Fig. 19/10   Some supratentorial surgical approaches

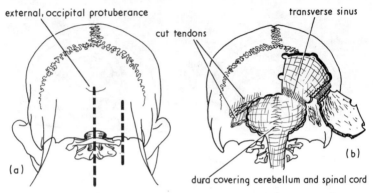

Fig. 19/11 Surgical approaches to the posterior fossa. (a) Mid-line or paramedian incision. (b) Craniectomy with an additional occipital bone flap when more exposure is necessary. The posterior arches of C1 and C2 have also been removed

Initially patients may be nursed without clothing, but well covered with bed linen, to ensure accurate observations of limb responses, and to facilitate skin care. A urinary catheter may be in situ.

Care must be taken to restrain a restless, confused patient, as he may attempt to remove head dressings, which will allow easy access of infection, and meningitis may result. Padding and bandages on the hands, which may need to be tied down, reduce this danger. Cot sides should be attached to the bed in the early postoperative phase. It is important to replace hand bandages and cot sides after any treatment.

During the first few postoperative days intensive nursing care is required, the patient's condition being carefully observed and charted. Deterioration can occur very rapidly due to postoperative complications, thus any change must be reported immediately as it can be a matter of life and death. Surgical resection of brain tissue may account for neurological deficits.

BONE FLAP

This may be removed if the brain is very swollen during operation, or if the skull is splintered as a result of a head injury. When bone has been removed the patient is not nursed on the affected side until he shows signs of recovery of his conscious level. Replacement of this flap is advisable once oedema has subsided, as the patient tends to suffer from headache, dizziness when stooping and is afraid of damage from a bump to the area. Following head injury, or invasion by tumour, the bone may be so badly damaged it has to be discarded, and the defect is then filled with plastic material.

The young active patient who is once more ambulant may be provided with a protective metal plate inside a cap, or a crash helmet to prevent further trauma, until the defect is repaired.

VENTRICULAR DRAINAGE

The patient may return from theatre with ventricular drainage if there are signs of inadequate cerebrospinal fluid circulation at operation. A catheter is introduced into a lateral ventricle by means of a burr hole in the skull and the cerebrospinal fluid drained into a bag; the height of the bag is dependent upon the pressure of the cerebrospinal fluid. Care should be taken when treating the patient to ensure that the level of the head is not altered in relation to the bag as this alters the drainage pressure.

If the doctor's permission has been given for postural drainage, the height of the bag must be adjusted as the bed is tipped and readjusted on its return to the horizontal, this being done under medical supervision.

LUMBAR DRAINAGE

This may be set up several days postoperatively if there are signs of continued raised intracranial pressure. The needle is placed as for a lumbar puncture and rubber tubing connects it to a drainage bag, the height of which is dependent upon the cerebrospinal fluid pressure. If the drainage is to be continuous the patient is nursed in side lying, well supported by pillows. Turning is done by lifting the patient from side to front, to his other side.

Complications

Apart from the complications arising from brain damage the following may also arise:

Cerebrospinal fluid may leak following the original operation, which may require further surgical repair.

Postoperative oedema, thrombosis or haemorrhage from cerebral blood vessels, or arterial spasm occurs in a small number of patients.

Thrombosis may occur elsewhere and pulmonary embolus.

Epilepsy may develop after a variable period of time.

Infection at the operation site is serious, particularly if the dura has been opened, as it can lead to meningitis and encephalitis.

Respiratory complications are fairly common.

PHYSIOTHERAPY

The general principles of physiotherapy in cranial surgery are virtually the same as for other surgical procedures.

1. Prevent respiratory complications.
2. Assess any problems and neurological deficits, and treat where appropriate.
3. Prevent the development of contractures and pressure sores.

Physiotherapy for specific conditions will be described as indicated.

General

Rather special anaesthetic conditions are required for neurosurgery (Greenbaum, 1976) and although techniques are continually improving, the operation may still take many hours and the patient be subjected to long periods of anaesthesia. Breathing exercises are taught and the patient is asked to practise them before operation and as soon as he is sufficiently awake afterwards. A check must be made that the patient can cough and he should demonstrate that he is able to cough effectively, as a shallow throat cough is quite ineffective in clearing secretions. Patients who are known smokers should be advised to stop before operation.

The patient should also be taught to move his legs frequently (particularly the feet and ankles) after the operation to prevent venous stasis and consequent deep vein thrombosis. Passive movements will be necessary when the patient is not able to actively move – in this instance the physiotherapist should show the nurses how to give them so that they may carry out passive movements every time they carry out nursing procedures.

Postoperative assessment of voluntary movement, power, muscle tone, sensation, degree of ataxia, balance and gait is carried out appropriately as the condition of the patient allows.

Respiratory complications

Postoperative complications such as cerebral oedema and haematoma formation may directly affect respiration. The cough reflex may be lost or diminished to an ineffective level, and the ability to swallow affected. The physiotherapist must be on the alert for those problems, as patients with coughing and swallowing difficulties are at risk from aspiration of food and fluids. Feeding by nasogastric tube is preferred until swallowing is established.

Treatment and prevention of chest complications may have to be carried out within limitations imposed by the patient's condition as follows:

1. Postural drainage may be contra-indicated immediately after operation as it may cause a raised intracranial pressure.
2. Blood pressure changes may govern the position in which the patient is nursed. It is imperative that the patient's charts are checked before treatment, and medical permission is obtained *before* using postural drainage.
3. If there is no bone flap in situ the patient may not be allowed to lie on one side.
4. The patient may have a diminished cough reflex or facial weakness and therefore have difficulty in expectoration.
5. A disturbed conscious level may make co-operation difficult. Deep breathing should be encouraged, and manual pressure on the chest wall as the patient breathes out is useful. Instruction to cough can be accompanied by pressure on the chest as this is attempted. Demonstration of coughing may help the dysphasic patient.

SUCTION

If there is a depressed conscious level or an ineffective cough suction may be necessary to clear secretions. It may be helpful if there are two people when treatment with suction is required: the nurse can use the suction while the physiotherapist assists the patient with breathing and attempts to cough. Suction is an aseptic technique and sterile gloves must be worn while handling the catheter.

Involvement of the lower cranial nerves (IX–XII) may increase the difficulties of maintaining an open airway. Patients who are unable to maintain their own airway for any reason will require intubation either orally or nasally. If clinical signs and blood gas analysis indicate poor oxygenation artificial mechanical ventilation may be necessary. If the patient is thought to require intubation for a lengthy period he may be given a tracheostomy.

FACILITATION TECHNIQUES

Some respiratory facilitation techniques suitable for the unconscious adult patient have been described by Bethune (1975). These include stimulating a co-contraction of the abdominal muscles, pressure on upper and lower thoracic vertebrae, stretch of isolated intercostal muscles, moderate manual pressure on the ribs, stretch of the anterior chest wall by lifting the posterior basal area of the supine patient, and peri-oral stimulation by firm pressure applied on the top lip.

INTRACRANIAL TUMOURS

Intracranial tumours may be primary or secondary. Secondary tumours are usually blood-borne metastases and derive from neoplasms of the bronchus, breast and kidney as well as from thyroid carcinomas, malignant melanomas and a variety of less common primary lesions. Primary intracranial neoplasms may be derived from the brain itself (cerebral hemispheres and the cerebellum), the meninges (meningiomas), cranial nerves, the pituitary gland, the pineal body and blood vessels.

Intrinsic tumours of the cerebral hemispheres (the glioma series) are locally invasive and thus considered malignant. The degree of malignancy depends on their rate of growth and histological character. Total removal of these tumours is seldom possible because of their infiltration of the brain tissue.

Meningiomas are generally benign and do not often invade the brain but present problems in view of their size and extreme vascularity. Total removal is often feasible.

The location of a tumour is the most important factor irrespective of its pathology because it may involve the vital centres, thus directly threatening life, or limiting surgical accessibility.

SIGNS AND SYMPTOMS

Some degree of raised intracranial pressure usually exists. Focal signs develop pointing to the site of the tumour.

INVESTIGATIONS

These include skull and chest radiographs, CAT scan and possibly angiography.

Surgical treatment

In order to attempt removal an operation (craniotomy) is necessary and, where possible, the tumour is removed totally, or as near totally as possible. If it is not possible to remove the tumour a biopsy will be taken to enable a diagnosis to be established. Tumours may recur following incomplete removal. Occasionally a bone flap may be removed to effect a decompression. Radio-sensitive tumours may be given a course of radiotherapy and cytotoxic (anti-tumour) drugs may also be given.

Surgical removal of intrinsic tumours of the dominant fronto-temporal or temporo-parietal areas is rarely attempted as this may lead to severe hemiplegia and dysphasia. Intrinsic brainstem tumours are rare and direct surgical intervention not possible.

PHYSIOTHERAPY

A patient without operative complications is encouraged to get up on the day following surgery. Hemiparesis or hemiplegia is treated accordingly. Where the prognosis is known to be poor, all steps must be taken to ensure maximum independence without recourse to sophisticated techniques (Downie, 1978).

Cerebellar tumours

The majority of cerebellar tumours arise in or near the mid-line and may extend into one or both cerebellar hemispheres. These tumours are most likely to be medulloblastomas or cystic astrocytomas in young children; haemangioblastomas in young adults or metastases in older age groups.

SIGNS AND SYMPTOMS

These differ considerably depending on the site of the tumour. The following occur in varying degrees: raised intracranial pressure, usually due to obstructive hydrocephalus; and focal signs: cerebellar, brainstem or cranial nerves, e.g. ataxia, probably most marked in walking, giddiness, nystagmus.

Surgical treatment

It may be necessary to treat hydrocephalus before approaching the lesion itself. This is achieved by 'shunting' (p. 324). To excise this type of tumour a different approach is necessary. A mid-line incision is made and the occipital bone covering the cerebellum is removed (craniectomy); the posterior arch of C1 is also removed because part of the cerebellum has often herniated through the foramen magnum by pressure from the tumour (see Fig. 19/11(b)).

PROGRESSION OF PHYSIOTHERAPY

A patient with a cerebellar lesion fatigues quickly. He will probably have a history of vomiting for a variable period of time before operation, leading to debility and dehydration. The treatment programme for physiotherapy and occupational therapy must be carefully graded to guard against exhaustion. As he improves progression will be made to:

Mat work: Resisted exercise is more accurately performed than free exercise, thus mat work begins with resisted activities such as rolling and bridging, stabilising in each new position. Activities are progressed to rolling and sitting up and moving about the mat. From prone lying the patient practises getting to four-point kneeling, sitting over from side to side and crawling in all directions. This is progressed to kneeling, half-kneeling and standing, again stabilising in each position attained.

Walking: Parallel bars and a mirror may be valuable in early mobilising. Stabilising in standing, resisted walking in all directions and walking to a constant rhythm (the therapist counting) with a moderate/fast pace helps the patient to combat unsteadiness and regain self-confidence. If a walking aid is necessary, elbow crutches or a reciprocal walking aid will be better for the more ataxic patient, a stick being suitable to support the less disabled person.

Tumours of the cerebello-pontine angle

A sub-section of posterior fossa tumours worthy of special mention are those occurring in the cerebello-pontine angle (Fig. 19/12). Surgery to these requires a more lateral approach. Several types of tumour occur in this confined and critical area, and any space-occupying lesion will gradually compress the nearby structures and result in deficits related to the appropriate cranial nerves, as well as producing a rise in intracranial pressure and long tract signs.

SIGNS AND SYMPTOMS

These may include: deafness, tinnitus and vertigo; facial weakness from compression of VIIth nerve; loss of corneal reflex, loss of pain and temperature sensations with compression of Vth nerve; ataxia of limbs on the side of tumour occurring with compression of the cerebellar hemisphere and cerebellar peduncles; and spasticity and dementia (with large lesions, the latter due to raised intracranial pressure).

The most common lesion to occur here is the acoustic Schwannoma (neuroma) which arises from the VIIIth nerve.

Surgical treatment

Some tumours in this area can be completely removed but large tumours, particularly those adherent to the brainstem may prove more difficult to excise and the lower cranial nerves may be damaged.

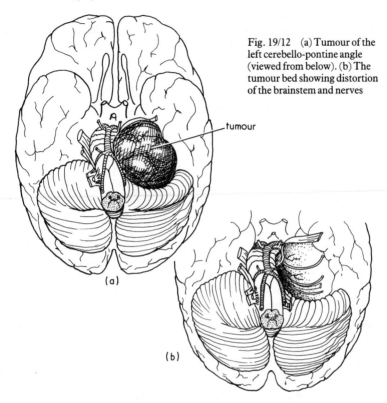

Fig. 19/12 (a) Tumour of the left cerebello-pontine angle (viewed from below). (b) The tumour bed showing distortion of the brainstem and nerves

tumour

(a)

(b)

POSTOPERATIVE TREATMENT

The patient may have swallowing difficulties and poor cough reflex; this requires the same care as for a cerebellar tumour. If there is a VIIth nerve palsy the patient will be unable to close his eye. The nurse devotes special care to the eye and a tarsorrhaphy (partial suturing together of the upper and lower lid) may be necessary to prevent damage to the cornea and infection.

PHYSIOTHERAPY

Physiotherapy is as for cerebellar tumours but special attention is frequently required to re-train oro-facial dysfunction. This is best done by a co-ordinated programme arranged between the speech therapist, physiotherapist and nursing staff. It can be a frustrating and humiliating experience for a patient to find he is unable to feed himself, to manipulate the food in his mouth and that he dribbles and drools. If he cannot control liquids adequately and coughs and splutters, he feels he is choking with every mouthful. Some of these difficulties can be overcome by ensuring correct head position, by facilitating a co-contraction of the tongue and cheeks and selecting food of appropriate consistency. Water is difficult as the patient is unable to control it with his slow and inaccurate movements. Lumpy or chunky foodstuffs are inappropriate initially and generally the most satisfactory consistency is that of ice-cream, purées and yoghurt. Slowly and carefully the patient progresses both to more-liquid and more-solid food as he learns to cope with the difficulty.

DAMAGE TO FACIAL NERVE

When the facial nerve cannot be preserved intact during surgery an attempt may be made to re-innervate the distal portion of the cut nerve. This can be achieved by an anastomosis with either the spinal accessory or hypoglossal nerves. Cross-facial nerve anastomosis to innervate both sides from one nerve is sometimes considered.

The spinal accessory nerve can be split to allow relative preservation of the shoulder girdle innervation, whereas using the hypoglossal nerve will cause some tongue paralysis. If facial-accessory anastomosis is used, particular attention is paid by the physiotherapist to shoulder girdle re-education. Facilitation techniques are very useful.

SUBARACHNOID HAEMORRHAGE

Intracranial aneurysms

Intracranial aneurysms are balloon-like dilatations occurring at the bifurcation of vessels of the Circle of Willis (Fig. 19/13). The precipitating cause is thought to be a congenital defect in the wall of the blood vessel. Aneurysms are also associated with arteriosclerosis and hypertension. Their size varies from a pea to a plum and multiple aneurysms may be present. Age-groups most affected are those between 30 and 50 years.

Rupture of an aneurysm is the most common cause of spontaneous subarachnoid haemorrhage.

SIGNS AND SYMPTOMS

These depend on the severity and site of bleeding. A minor leak from an aneurysm gives sudden severe (usually occipital) headache, which then radiates up over the head and settles in a generalised headache and neck stiffness. Severe haemorrhage will cause increased intracranial pressure and decreased level of consciousness with neurological deficits depending on degree of damage from haemorrhage.

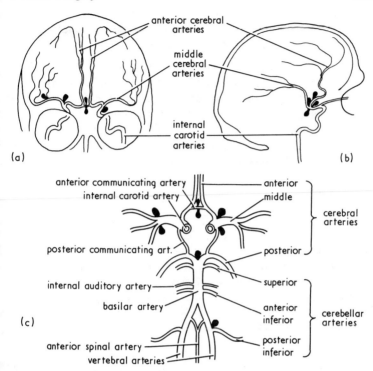

Fig. 19/13 Common sites for aneurysms. (a) Antero-posterior view. (b) Lateral view. (c) Vessels of the Circle of Willis

INVESTIGATIONS

These are: lumbar puncture to establish the presence of blood in the CSF, and to exclude bacterial meningitis; CAT scan to estimate position of haematoma formation; and angiography to determine the site of aneurysm.

Pre-operative treatment

As soon as subarachnoid haemorrhage is diagnosed precautionary measures are taken to prevent a fatal re-bleed before surgery.

There are two possible ways of reducing this risk:

1. Control of blood pressure if the patient is hypertensive. This is achieved by using beta blockers/diuretics, care being taken to avoid precipitous falls in blood pressure.
2. Use of antifibrinolytic agents to prevent clot lysis in and around the

aneurysm sac. There is doubt as to the efficacy of this form of treatment and there is, perhaps, increased risk of inducing a deep vein thrombosis and pulmonary embolus.

The patient is generally on strict bed rest and kept as flat as possible, but some neurosurgeons suggest that patients should be allowed to sit up and get out of bed for toilet purposes as this raises the intracranial pressure less than straining hard when lying down.

If headache remains severe an analgesic that does not depress respiration (e.g. codeine phosphate) is prescribed. Nausea and vomiting are controlled by anti-emetics.

Surgical treatment

Surgery is undertaken only if the patient is conscious and showing improvement from any neurological deficit arising from the initial bleed. This is usually 7–10 days post-bleed. Postoperative vasospasm of the vessels around the aneurysm site is a danger and there is less likelihood of this if surgery is delayed.

The aneurysm is usually occluded by placing a clip across the neck of the aneurysm, or by a clip and wrapping the aneurysm in cotton wool and glue or muscle.

COMPLICATIONS

Further bleeding may occur while the surgeon is attempting to obliterate the aneurysm. Traction upon blood vessels in the field of surgery can cause ischaemia of the area of brain which they supply. Oedema, thrombosis and vasospasm may follow surgery. These postoperative complications can be manifest within a few hours of surgery and can completely alter the neurological state and, therefore, outcome.

PHYSIOTHERAPY

This is similar to treatment following uncomplicated surgery for tumour. Once the aneurysm is clipped it is safe and will not re-bleed. Deficits are dealt with accordingly.

Ligation of common carotid artery

This is the procedure of choice when certain aneurysms are difficult to approach by a direct method, e.g. some of those arising directly from the internal carotid artery and those in the cavernous sinus. The patient's neurological state should be intact. If there is adequate cross-circulation in the brain, the vessel is ligated in the neck under local anaesthetic. If there is uncertainty regarding cross-circulation a clamp is put across the vessel and the vessel occluded over a period of 48 hours and, providing the neurological state remains the same, it is finally ligated.

POSTOPERATIVE TREATMENT

The patient is nursed in bed. Continuous nursing observations are required for blood pressure, pulse, conscious level, motor power and pupillary reaction to detect any deteriorioration.

Approximately 48 hours after occlusion of the artery the patient is gradually elevated in bed and allowed up on the seventh day. Prior to getting up he should be able to tolerate sitting upright in bed. The blood pressure is checked before getting out and any significant drop necessitates a return to bed.

PHYSIOTHERAPY

Treatment is fairly gentle. General bed exercises involving minimal disturbance are encouraged. Progression of treatment is slow and careful to allow the cross-circulation to compensate adequately. Sitting tolerance is gradually increased as the patient is mobilised, walking increasing distances, including stairs.

Rapid changes in position may cause dizziness, therefore, the patient is warned to move slowly and steadily when getting out of bed, standing up and turning around.

The stay in hospital is usually short, and on discharge home the patient is instructed to continue with the slow, gradual resumption of normal activities.

INTRACRANIAL ANGIOMATOUS MALFORMATIONS (ARTERIOVENOUS ANOMALIES)

These malformations are congenital abnormalities of vascular development; they occur on the surface of the brain or within brain tissue deriving a good blood supply from one or both hemispheres and are usually found in the younger age-groups including children.

The blood vessels of the malformation show degeneration of their walls, and direct communication between arteries and veins in some areas. If the malformation is small no diversion of blood from the capillary bed occurs, but a large one robs the brain of its blood supply.

SIGNS AND SYMPTOMS

These are variable but the following may occur: headaches of a migrainous character; focal epilepsy; subarachnoid haemorrhage; intracerebral haemorrhage which may produce focal signs such as mono- or hemiparesis together with a sensory or visual loss.

INVESTIGATIONS

Angiography and CAT scan will determine the site of the lesion. EEG may be used for investigating epilepsy.

Surgical treatment

A direct intracranial approach is made and the lesion excised if it lies superficially. A deep-seated hemisphere lesion is untreated by surgery. Sometimes complex lesions may be treated by the occlusion of the feeding vessels.

PHYSIOTHERAPY

This follows the same course as that for an aneurysm (p. 320).

CAROTID ARTERY STENOSIS

Discussion of occlusive cerebrovascular disease can be confusing because of the terminology used. Jennett (1977) has described it as follows: 'Stenosis implies narrowing only, occlusion a complete block, while thrombosis describes a pathological state which may sometimes be the cause of an occlusion but is more often a consequence of obstruction. Ischaemia refers to inadequate perfusion of an area of brain with functional failure; only if it is sufficiently severe and prolonged does infarction develop. Carotico-vertebral insufficiency is a useful term for symptomatic extra-cranial obstructive vascular disease.'

Atheroma is the most usual cause of stenosis of the common and internal carotid arteries, and thrombus formation may complete the occlusion. The site of the narrowing is most frequently at the origin of the internal carotid artery, and the severity is variable.

The deprived hemisphere is dependent upon the collateral circulation derived through the Circle of Willis for its blood supply.

If the major problem is caused by multiple emboli shooting off from the site of the thrombus, then anticoagulants may be used with great care.

SIGNS AND SYMPTOMS

A wide variety of symptoms and modes of onset can be produced by carotid artery occlusion.

Hemiplegia: This may be profound and occur suddenly, with loss of consciousness. There may be hemiparesis progressing to hemiplegia. There may be transient motor weakness ('stuttering') usually affecting one extremity.

Dysphasia, sensory loss, eye symptoms: These are associated in some degree with the loss of voluntary power.

Headache: Occasionally present behind the eye

INVESTIGATIONS

A CAT scan will differentiate between an infarct and haemorrhage. Angiography will reveal any stenosis or occlusion.

Surgical treatment

In carefully selected cases surgery is of value. Contra-indications are gross arteriosclerotic involvement of other cerebral vessels, and loss of consciousness with the onset of symptoms, which carries a poor prognosis.

Surgical measures aim to restore the normal blood flow and prevent further emboli to the blood vessels of the brain causing ischaemia and infarction.

Endarterectomy: The atheromatous portion of the artery and any thrombus is removed, by opening the artery and then resuturing it.

PHYSIOTHERAPY

A patient with stable neurological signs after uncomplicated surgery may be mobilised early.

Immediate measures are required for the re-education of hemiplegic limbs. Bearing in mind the likely sensory loss and visual field defects the patient must be reminded constantly of the affected limbs. Patients with deficits remain on bed rest longer and are mobilised at a slower pace.

HYDROCEPHALUS

Hydrocephalus in adults may be secondary to a mass lesion particularly in the posterior fossa, third ventricle or midbrain where a tumour may block the flow of CSF through the ventricular system (obstructive hydrocephalus); or following a subarachnoid haemorrhage or meningitis when adhesions occur in the subarachnoid space and prevent CSF circulating over the brain (communicating hydrocephalus).

Aqueduct stenosis may produce a slowly developing hydrocephalus in which an acute episode may be precipitated by a mild head injury.

The commonest underlying causes of hydrocephalus in the neonatal period are birth trauma and meningitis. Congenital malformations such as spina bifida are found in about one-quarter of cases (Jennett, 1977).

Surgical treatment

Treatment is often by 'shunting'. CSF is drained from the lateral ventricle via a tube and valve system into the internal jugular vein, thence to the right atrium (ventriculo-atrial) or to the peritoneum via subcutaneous neck and trunk tubing (ventriculo-peritoneal).

PHYSIOTHERAPY

Patients are nursed flat in bed for two to three days and are gradually sat up over the next two days. More severe cases are nursed head down for one to two days and may take five to six days to be upright. There is danger of a subdural haematoma forming as the result of traction on the veins in the subdural space if the patient is sat up too rapidly. Once up, the patient can be steadily mobilised. Further operative procedures may be necessary where tumour is involved.

CEREBRAL ABSCESS

A brain abscess develops either in the cerebral hemispheres or cerebellum according to how pus enters the brain. Approximately half of them arise from local spread (usually ear, mastoid and otitis media and air sinuses) and half by bloodstream spread. The inflammation around the pus causes considerable oedema so patients are drowsy and have headache but rather less obvious focal signs. Cerebral abscess still carries high mortality due to speed of development, and epileptic fits are common sequelae.

Surgical treatment

Treatment is vigorous. Pus is aspirated through burr holes, and large doses of antibiotics are administered intravenously. If repeated aspiration does not clear the pus then it will be necessary to turn a bone flap to effect this.

PHYSIOTHERAPY

Treatment is as for craniotomy for tumour. In cases where there is markedly raised ICP, the conscious level will be decreased and careful attention is paid to the chest, limbs and positioning. Any neurological deficit is treated accordingly.

PARKINSONIAN SYNDROME

Parkinsonism is described in *Cash's Textbook of Neurology for Physiotherapists*, and only points relating to the surgical management of the condition will be discussed. Stereotaxic surgery is used mainly for the treatment of tremor, and careful selection of patients is essential, particularly as many of these patients are elderly and frail.

INVESTIGATIONS AND ASSESSMENT

Plain skull radiographs, EEG and neurophysiological measurements of the tremor may be carried out. The patient is fully assessed by the physiotherapist, speech therapist and occupational therapist.

Surgical treatment: Stereotaxy

This surgical technique is used in the treatment of certain movement disorders, epilepsy, intractable pain and some psychiatric conditions. The procedure involves making destructive lesions, or stimulating small, accurately located targets within the brain. The general procedure requires fixing to the skull a special frame capable of holding the apparatus used to make the lesion. Contrast medium is introduced into the ventricles via a burr hole and radiographs taken. Measurements on the radiographs are taken relating the outlined structures to the target area. The target point is then related to the stereotactic frame, and an electrode introduced to the target point. The trajectory of the electrode is checked by recording from the nervous tissue during advancement of the electrode. For destructive lesions a radio-frequency current is passed and the lesion made at the electrode tip. The size of the lesion is adjusted by the electrode size or by moving it slightly. Usually the lesion is only about 5mm×3mm (Hitchcock, 1978).

Specific lesions may be made in the thalamic or dentate nuclei of the brain, and are sometimes indicated for the abolition or reduction of involuntary movements such as dystonias, dyskinesias and spasticity. The classic example is in the treatment of Parkinsonian tremor. Some psychiatric conditions benefit from discrete surgical lesions and occasionally leucotomy, amygdalotomy, cingulectomy and partial fronto-thalamic lesions are made.

In operation for Parkinsonian tremor, after affixing the frame, contrast ventriculography is performed to outline the anterior and

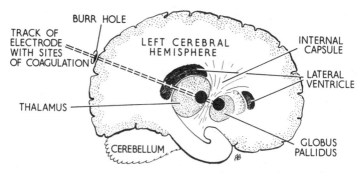

Fig. 19/14   Position of a burr hole and electrode track in stereotaxic surgery for parkinsonism

posterior commissures. An electrode is passed through a frontal burr hole to the thalamus (Fig. 19/14). Coagulation is carried out in the ventro-lateral nucleus of the thalamus to reduce tremor and in the globus pallidus to reduce rigidity.

While stereotaxy is used mainly for the relief of tremor, rigidity is treated largely by drug therapy, L-dopa being widely used.

PHYSIOTHERAPY

Chest care is important. Coughing may be difficult for the patient whose main symptom is rigidity. If bilateral lesions are made there may be speech and swallowing problems so chest physiotherapy is particularly important. Functional re-education may be required. After loss of severe tremor, stabilising exercise helps the patient regain functional use of his limbs particularly the upper limbs. Full range joint mobility is rapidly regained when symptoms have been relieved.

The patient is encouraged to get up the day after surgery. Balance re-education is important where rigidity is the main symptom. A patient with mainly tremor has little or no problem in regaining balance. Re-education of standing up and sitting down, walking, walking with arm swinging and turning round require patience and perseverance. Moving from standing to sitting and vice versa is difficult for a Parkinsonian patient. He must be taught to tuck his feet well underneath him, then use his hands on the edge of the chair to push his weight forward over his feet, then straighten up. When sitting down he should feel for the chair and lower himself down gently.

To re-educate walking it must be impressed upon the patient to lift his feet and take a big step. Lifting the feet is over-emphasised at the onset; marking time on the spot prior to walking can be a useful preliminary followed by stepping over lines on the floor. Poles are useful to re-educate arm swinging while walking. The patient holds one end of the pole in each hand, the physiotherapist walking behind holding the other. Arm swinging is done at first by the physiotherapist pushing the appropriate pole with the patient gradually taking over. When turning, the great tendency is to jerk round suddenly. The patient should be taught to turn round slowly, lifting his feet up. There is usually no difficulty with stairs but the patient's balance may be unsteady initially.

Progress is rapid and work is increased to include class participation, mat work and mobility.

EPILEPSY

Epilepsy can be described as a paroxysmal transitory disturbance of the functions of the brain which develops suddenly, ceases spontaneously, with a strong tendency to recurrence. Many varieties of epileptic attack exist depending upon the site of origin, extent of spread and the nature of the disturbance of function.

CAUSES

Epilepsy may be caused by: a local lesion in the brain, such as tumour or abscess; complications of a head injury; hereditary predisposition; and unknown causes.

INVESTIGATIONS

EEG recordings of the electrical activity of the brain can help to pinpoint the cause of epilepsy. If a focus can be determined, its nature can be investigated by other means. Other appropriate procedures will be selected according to the particular history and clinical features of the patient.

Surgical treatment

Surgery is of value to a patient who has epilepsy as the presenting feature of a brain lesion, or a definite focus which gives rise to his epileptic attack. Surgical procedures vary with the type of lesion to be excised. Temporal lobe epilepsy may be treated by lobectomy. Stereotaxic procedures are occasionally employed to treat certain forms of epilepsy particularly that of diffuse origin which cannot be treated by drugs or cortical excision.

PHYSIOTHERAPY

Rehabilitation follows general principles with deficits being treated accordingly.

INTRACTABLE PAIN

There have been considerable advances in the treatment of intractable pain over the past decade due largely to the establishment of several regional centres for pain relief which are able to combine the services of physicians, surgeons, anaesthetists and radiotherapists to provide comprehensive treatment.

Intractable pain describes chronic severe pain which may persist after the primary lesion has been treated and cannot always be totally relieved even by constant narcotic therapy. This becomes progressively less effective and there is a danger of addiction to the drugs used. Figure 19/15 shows some pain pathways.

Pain is difficult to quantify and has different characteristics depending on its origin. Innumerable factors can influence it; some of the most important being the patient's personality, intelligence and emotional maturity. Careful clinical and psychological assessments are thus essential before surgical measures are undertaken to relieve pain. Figure 19/16 shows some of the surgical procedures used in pain alleviation.

Pain is of malignant or benign aetiology. Carcinomas outside the nervous system are frequently the cause of malignant intractable pain. Among the benign causes are herpes zoster, scar tissue, amputation stump neuromas, phantom limb pain and some cord lesions.

A general principle of surgical treatment is to start with the smallest effective procedure working up to large ones if necessary,

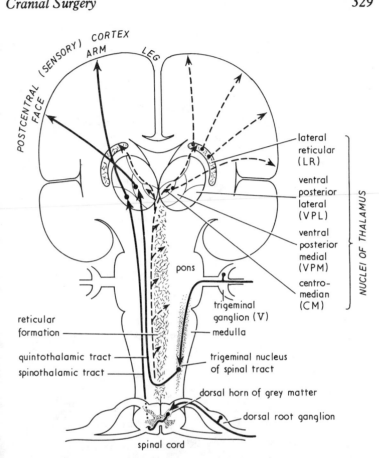

Fig. 19/15   Projections of some pain pathways. The centromedian nucleus (CM) and the ventro-postero-medial nucleus (VPM) of the thalamus are sites for stereotaxic interruption of central pain pathways. Interruption of the trigeminal nerve tract at spinal or pontine levels or at the trigeminal ganglion are possible sites for treating facial pain

and wherever possible to start peripherally in the nervous system and work centrally. Surgery can be directed at peripheral nerves and nerve roots, spinal cord and the brain, and may involve open operations or percutaneous procedures. Many such operations involve making small electrical lesions at various points within the nervous system or local administration of drugs using catheters placed in the epidural space.

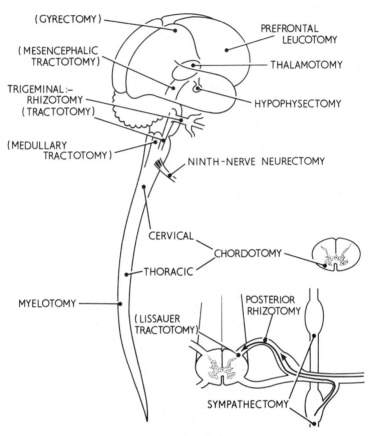

Fig. 19/16   Some surgical procedures used to alleviate pain

Surgical treatment

LOCAL SURGERY

A local procedure to excise a neuroma or a form of percutaneous or transcutaneous electrical stimulation may be all that is necessary to effect relief.

POSTERIOR RHIZOTOMY

The appropriate posterior spinal nerve roots are sectioned between the spinal cord and the posterior spinal ganglion on the same side of the body that the intractable pain is felt. Due to the overlap of the sensory supply from one dermatome to another, it is necessary to section at least two sensory roots above and below the area in which pain is localised by the patient. This operation has been used for post-herpetic pain and painful scars, but after a period of time the intractable pain has a tendency to recur. It is of no use for limb pain, as it destroys muscle and joint sensation which would give rise to a severe disability.

DORSAL ROOT ENTRY ZONE

This procedure involves operations on the root entry zone of the spinal cord (see Further Advances, p. 332).

CORDOTOMY

Fibres of the lateral spinothalamic tract are divided on the opposite side of the body to that on which the pain is experienced. To achieve a permanent result the procedure must be done at least several segments higher than the localisation of pain to allow for the fact that fibres carrying pain and temperature sensations enter the spinal cord and ascend for several segments before crossing the mid-line to join the lateral spinothalamic tract, and that no matter how deep the incision made at operation the level of sensory loss always descends during the first postoperative week.

Spinothalamic cordotomy is used to relieve pain for malignant disease especially affecting the pelvic region. It has poor results for upper limb pain and de-afferentation pain (i.e. pain in an already numb area).

Bilateral cordotomy may be necessary for bilateral symptoms but this can produce weakness below the level of the surgical lesion. Bladder and bowel function may be disturbed. High cervical cordotomy can damage the innervation to the diaphragm and intercostal muscles producing ipsilateral paralysis.

Stereotaxic cordotomy can bring greater accuracy in making a lesion in open cord surgery. Percutaneous cordotomy is an alternative to open procedures: it only requires local anaesthesia and there is no painful wound. However, precise localisation of the lesion can be more difficult.

MYELOTOMY

This is essentially a mid-line lesion in the cord involving the pain fibres that cross in the mid-line. It is used for bilateral leg pain but runs the risk of producing sphincter dysfunction.

THALAMOTOMY

Thalamotomy is used for de-afferentation pains and for other types of pain where cordotomy is inappropriate or has failed. Destructive lesions are made stereotactically without causing significant sensory loss.

PHYSIOTHERAPY

The patient is encouraged to get up on the second day post-surgery. Chest care is important if there is diaphragm and intercostal muscle paralysis. Static muscle contractions start two or three days after surgery progressing to active extension exercises after a week. Following high cervical cordotomy gentle neck mobilisation can start five or so days post-surgery.

It is important to teach the patient to look after any area of pain and temperature loss and he should be reminded to test the temperature of water with the sound side before immersing the affected side.

Further advances

Cordotomy and many peripheral procedures are of little value in treating de-afferentation pain (e.g. phantom limb pain) or pain occurring in the upper limbs. Some recent advances are stereotactic methods of stimulation of the peri-aqueductal grey matter (for general mid-line and bilateral limb pains) and chronic thalamic stimulation for certain forms of de-afferentation pain. Lesions can be made at the dorsal root entry zone (DREZ) of the spinal cord for pain in limbs. This procedure involves making small electrical lesions at open operation at the point of entry of the pain fibres from the sensory roots into the spinal cord, thereby avoiding loss of touch and proprioception which would render the limbs useless.

REFERENCES

Bethune, D. D. (1975). Neurophysiological facilitation of respiration in the unconscious adult patient. *Physiotherapy* (Canada), **27**(5), 241.

Downie, P. A. (1978). *Cancer Rehabilitation: An Introduction for Physiotherapists and the Allied Professions*. Faber and Faber, London.

Greenbaum, R. (1976). General anaesthesia for neurosurgery. *British Journal of Anaesthesia*, **48**, 773.

Hitchcock, E. R. (1978). Stereotactic surgery for cerebral palsy. *Nursing Times*, **74**, 50, 2064.

Jennett, B. (1977). *An Introduction to Neurosurgery*, 3rd edition. William Heinemann Medical Books Limited, London.

Lance, J. W. and McLeod, J. G. (1975). *A Physiological Approach to Clinical Neurology*, 2nd edition. Butterworths, London.

Teasdale, G. and Jennett, B. (1974). An assessment of coma and impaired consciousness. A practical scale. *Lancet* (July 13).

BIBLIOGRAPHY

Bickerstaff, E. R. (1978). *Neurology for Nurses*, 3rd edition. Hodder and Stoughton, London.

Bobath, B. (1971). *Abnormal Postural Reflex Activity caused by Brain Lesions*, 2nd edition. William Heinemann Medical Books Limited, London.

Bobath, B. (1978). *Adult Hemiplegia: Evaluation and Treatment*, 2nd edition. William Heinemann Medical Books Limited, London.

Carr, J. H. and Shepherd, R. B. (1980). *Physiotherapy in Disorders of the Brain*. William Heinemann Medical Books Limited, London.

Downie, P. A. (ed) 1982). *Cash's Textbook of Neurology for Physiotherapists*, 3rd edition, Faber and Faber, London.

Downie, P. A. (ed) (1983). *Cash's Textbook of Chest, Heart and Vascular Disorders for Physiotherapists*, 3rd edition. Chapters 8 and 9. Faber and Faber, London.

Dunkin, E. N. (1981). *Psychology for Physiotherapists*. The British Psychological Society in association with Macmillan Press Limited, London.

Matthews, W. B. and Miller, H. (1979). *Diseases of the Nervous System*, 3rd edition. Blackwell Scientific Publications Limited, Oxford.

Mitchell, G. A. G. and Mayor, D. (1977). *The Essentials of Neuroanatomy*, 3rd edition. Churchill Livingstone, Edinburgh.

Northfield, D. W. C. (1973). *The Surgery of the Central Nervous System – A Textbook for Postgraduate Students*. Blackwell Scientific Publications Limited, Oxford.

Purchese, G. (1977). *Neuromedical and Neurosurgical Nursing*, Baillière Tindall, London.

Walsh, K. W. (1978). *Neuropsychology – A Clinical Approach*. Churchill Livingstone, Edinburgh.

Walton, J. N. (ed)(1977). *Brain's Diseases of the Nervous System*, 8th edition. Oxford University Press, Oxford.

Williams, M. (1970). *Brain Damage and the Mind*. Penguin Books Limited, Harmondsworth.

van Zwanenberg, D. and Adams C. B. T. (1979). *Neurosurgical Nursing Care*. Faber and Faber, London.

ACKNOWLEDGEMENTS

This revised chapter is based partly on the chapter which appeared in the second edition and the author and the book's editor are grateful to Miss P. A. Dawe MAPA for allowing the continued use of it. The present author thanks Mr C. B. T. Adams MA, MChir, FRCS and Mr Peter Teddy DPhil, FRCS, consultant neurosurgeons at the Radcliffe Infirmary, Oxford, for their help and advice in the revision of this chapter.

Chapter 20

Acute Head Injuries

by M. LIGHTBODY, MCSP

The role of the physiotherapist in the treatment of patients with severe head injury is vital in the acute stage of management and in their rehabilitation.

HEAD INJURIES

The injuries may be either open or closed.

Open

These injuries mean that the skin and skull have been penetrated by a missile or sharp object possibly causing penetration through the dura into the brain, i.e. a compound (through the skin), penetrating (through the dura) depressed fracture of the skull.

Closed

These are the most common form of head injury and may cause only a linear skull fracture, but of more importance is the effect on the brain. The real damage results from the brain being suddenly shaken within the skull by a sudden *acceleration* (such as a blow to the back of the head) or *deceleration* (the moving head comes in contact with a fixed object). This causes, at its mildest, concussion, but more severe damage causes serious brain injury or even death.

HISTORY

When the patient first arrives in the casualty department the admitting doctor must take an accurate history, from witnesses if the patient is unable to communicate. This should include: type of accident; an assessment of level of consciousness at the time of injury and any deterioration or improvement; any respiratory or bleeding problems; any evidence of fitting; and, if possible, any relevant past medical history should be obtained as this may influence the management of the head injury.

Assessment

The immediate assessment concerns the respiratory state, the conscious level and the cardiovascular state. The result of this assessment will dictate priorities of treatment. It will be followed by a thorough neurological and general examination.

RESPIRATORY STATE

Respiratory distress and, therefore, inadequate ventilation may be caused by:

1. *Obstruction of the airway*: The airway may be partially or completely blocked by inhalation of vomit or blood; the tongue flopping against the back of the throat; jaw fractures; false teeth or other foreign bodies inhaled at the time of the accident.
2. *Depression of the respiratory centre*: The brain injury may damage the respiratory centre in the brainstem affecting control of rate and rhythm of respiration.
3. *Associated injuries*: Primary damage to the chest wall and lung tissue can lead to further respiratory disturbance requiring immediate attention.

CONSCIOUS LEVEL

This is the most important observation. It is best described in terms of speech or movement with or without stimulation, and a scale of response measured in these terms is used. This gives an overall impression and an accurate picture can be made over time by different observers without wide variation in meaning (e.g. Glasgow Coma Scale, p. 306).

Any alteration in response can be seen easily if the observations are plotted on a graph.

CARDIOVASCULAR STATE

Hypotension will lead to reduced cerebral perfusion and neurological deterioration.

NEUROLOGICAL EXAMINATION

Neurological examination will include: level of consciousness; pupil reaction; pulse, BP, respiratory state; and movement of limbs (lateralising and focal signs).

From the examination an assessment of severity of the injury can be made. The Glasgow Coma Scale is a method of putting a numerical figure on the severity of the injury.

A retrospective assessment of the severity of damage can be made by the length of post-traumatic amnesia (PTA) which can be described as 'the period of time from the moment of injury to the time when continuous awareness and memory return' (Potter, 1974). Some attempt at prognosis can be made using the Glasgow Outcome Scale (Jennett and Bond, 1975).

INVESTIGATIONS

Skull and chest radiographs are mandatory. A CAT scan and cervical spine radiographs may be indicated in more severe injuries. Blood chemistry relevant to surgery, and investigations relevant to other suspected injuries are also necessary.

ASSOCIATED INJURIES

Many patients with a head injury have additional injuries. These injuries may be relatively minor and can await attention, or they may demand as urgent attention as the head injury itself. For example, chest injuries causing hypoxia and hypercapnia may further aggravate cerebral oedema. Abdominal bleeding from damaged viscera may cause hypotension reducing cerebral perfusion. Fracture-dislocation of the cervical spine may be caused by hyperextension movement when damage is to the front of the skull and face. Fractures of the face, ribs, pelvis and long bones may be present.

Priorities of treatment have to be decided upon.

Treatment and early complications

The primary brain damage sustained in a head injury is not in itself treatable, but subsequent deterioration due to secondary damage may be prevented and reversed in some cases. Treatment is aimed at preventing and minimising these secondary effects.

Raised intracranial pressure

Damage secondary to the primary brain injury is caused by the development of raised intracranial pressure (ICP). This raised ICP is caused by: haematoma formation (extradural, subdural or intracerebral); cerebral oedema; or hydrocephalus.

The skull is essentially a closed box lined by dura containing CSF (10 per cent) brain (80 per cent) and blood (10 per cent). If any of these increases in volume then the pressure will increase. The brain, given time, can adapt to very slowly increasing pressure, and produces signs and symptoms at a later stage. However, rapidly increasing pressure will produce unconsciousness and death in a short time.

HAEMATOMA FORMATION

Extradural haematoma (EDH): An EDH usually develops within 12 hours of the injury. A skull fracture is almost always present in adults. This causes tearing of blood vessels in the dura, particularly the middle meningeal artery.

Subdural haematoma (SDH): Acute SDH is generally associated with severe head injury and profound underlying brain damage. It is thus only part of the total brain injury and not always the most important component. The size may not relate to the severity of brain damage.

Intracerebral haematoma (ICH): This may be present and, like an acute SDH, is only part of the total brain injury.

Prompt removal of an extradural haematoma by craniotomy can produce complete recovery. An acute subdural haematoma may be evacuated through burr holes or craniotomy but tends to carry poor prognosis.

CEREBRAL OEDEMA

Just as any other damaged tissue swells when injured so cerebral oedema may occur and will produce a rise in ICP. It may have a delayed onset and give rise to problems some days later. Hypoxia and hypercarbia which may result from raised ICP will further aggravate damage and thus a vicious circle is set up.

Attempts are made to reduce the swelling. These include the use of mannitol (and other diuretic drugs), and intermittent positive pressure ventilation (IPPV) to reduce carbon dioxide levels if spontaneous ventilation is inadequate.

HYDROCEPHALUS (See p. 323)

Fat embolism

Fat embolism is associated with severe trauma especially extensive long bone fractures. The mechanism of production of 'fat embolism' is not clear. It may be due to fat globules from the fracture site entering the bloodstream and when lodged in the lung reduce gas exchange leading to hypoxia and confusion. The main treatment is the appropriate management of the respiratory problem.

Skull fractures

LINEAR

Most skull fractures are linear and undisplaced. They may radiate to the base of the skull and through foramina damaging blood vessels and cranial nerves.

DEPRESSED

An area of bone is displaced on to underlying dura and brain with the possibility of damage to these structures. They may require surgical elevation.

COMPOUND DEPRESSED

These fractures invariably require exploration and elevation.

Infection

If the scalp overlying a depressed fracture is torn a route of infection is created. Meningitis and cerebral abscess may result. Thorough surgical exploration is, therefore, mandatory.

CSF rhinorrhoea and otorrhoea

Fractures involving the base of the skull may create a fistula between the subarachnoid space and nasal cavity or middle ear. This is a further route for infection and may require surgical intervention to close the communication, especially if it involves the nasal cavity.

Epilepsy

Epilepsy may follow a head injury and it may occur at any time. It reflects brain bruising or occasionally a developing haematoma (see later complications).

PATIENT CARE

Management of the unconscious patient

The unconscious patient is best nursed in an intensive therapy unit (ITU) as these units maintain the high levels of care required by these patients.

Patients who are managing to maintain their own airways and adequate oxygenation are unlikely to require intubation and mechanical ventilation. They are nursed in side lying to prevent inhalation of secretions and turned at regular intervals, usually every two hours, to prevent chest complications such as consolidation and collapse, and pressure sores. Problems may arise with positioning and turning if there are associated injuries which require splints, such as plaster casts or traction, although these can usually be minimised. A nasogastric tube is passed to allow appropriate nutrition to be given.

Neurological observations are carried out frequently so that immediate action may be taken if any deterioration is noted.

CHEST CARE

This is best carried out to coincide with turns and before a feed.

The chest is vibrated on the expiratory phase of breathing and facilitation methods to produce reflex, involuntary respiratory movement reactions may be used (Bethune, 1975). Postural drainage can be used *only* if there are no contra-indications, and the medical staff have been consulted. Suction is required to remove secretions. Suction procedures via the nose are contra-indicated if CSF rhinorrhoea is present: this indicates a CSF leakage through a skull fracture with a risk, therefore, of ascending infection. The frequency of treatment depends on the individual patient, but even if there are no obvious lung problems treatment is given to prevent any unnecessary extra complications. Modification of techniques will be required with associated chest injuries.

Patients with known, or suspected, raised ICP need careful handling and may be attached to ICP monitoring equipment (see p. 302).

GENERAL CARE

Unconscious patients must be treated as a whole person and not as a series of joints and muscles. As consciousness returns the clinical features resulting from the head injury are evident but the predominant problem, spasticity, will be evident early on. Handling these patients is often made more difficult from spasticity with the release of primitive neuromuscular activity such as reflex patterns. Techniques to preserve mobility and inhibit primitive responses are employed as far as possible. These, combined with careful positioning after treatment sessions and every turn, should help to reduce the problems to which hypertonicity leads at a later stage. *Never* assume that these patients are unaware of what is happening around them. Talking to them, telling them what you are doing and why, asking them to try and help, provide important stimuli from other sensory pathways alongside the stimuli from movement and handling.

Management of the severely head injured patient

Hypoxia causing further brain damage is an important cause of neurological deterioration. Cerebral hypoxia may be produced by: airway obstruction from inhalation of blood or vomit or head position; depression of the respiratory drive; associated chest injury, infection or pulmonary oedema; and fits.

If the patient is unable to maintain his own airway a cuffed endotracheal (ET) tube is passed. This may be sufficient to obtain adequate oxygenation and remove any retained secretions to stop any further deterioration. When it is evident that the respiratory effort is inadequate, artificial ventilation (IPPV) is required.

CHEST CARE

Techniques of shaking and vibration are best used while the patient is being ventilated by bag squeezing, i.e. off the ventilator. Careful suction via the ET tube should stimulate adequate coughing and clearance of secretions. Postural drainage should be used only with permission from medical staff.

CHEST CARE OF PATIENTS WITH RISING/RAISED ICP

This deserves special mention.

The brain is able to compensate to some degree while its structures are being distorted and displaced. The compensatory mechanisms will eventually reach a level where a small rise in intracranial volume may cause a dramatic rise in ICP (Fig. 20/1). This rise may well be

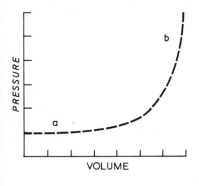

Fig. 20/1   The relationship between a small *volume* rise and the resultant dramatic pressure rise: a=stage of compensation; b=stage of decompensation

precipitated by various procedures such as postural drainage, shaking, bag squeezing, prolonged suction and coughing.

It is important to keep the chest clear of secretions as patchy collapse with sub-clinical hypoxia and hypercarbia is probably more damaging to the brain than any other factor. Therefore, it is important that if the stage of decompensation is being reached the patient must be protected during chest physiotherapy; effective treatment can be carried out without provoking large increases in ICP. This can be achieved by sedation, analgesia and muscle paralysis.

Patients having controlled IPPV usually need continuous sedation using anaesthetic agents and analgesics. A bolus dose of sedation is given prior to physiotherapy and, once stable conditions have been established, the techniques mentioned previously are employed and the ICP recording observed for significant changes.

There are other indications for the use of IPPV including repeated fitting, spontaneous hyperventilation, cyanosis and underventilation and associated pathology, e.g. chest injury. An acute head injury requiring significant intracranial operative procedures may need to be ventilated after surgery.

The duration of controlled IPPV is 12–24 hours in patients ventilated purely because of intracranial operative procedures and in those who show signs of rapid improvement. For the majority, two to three days of controlled IPPV is indicated, while in those with signs of advanced intracranial compression a much longer period of ventilation may be implemented.

LATER MANAGEMENT AND COMPLICATIONS

The variety of physical problems evident after head injury may present in combination with sensory and emotional features.

Physical and motor problems include spasticity and rigidity, and ataxia.

Sensory disturbance will involve perceptual problems including vision and hearing, apraxia and agnosia.

Emotional and intellectual disturbance will involve memory and behavioural disorders.

Vigorous management of patients in the acute stage will be of little value if proper and adequate rehabilitation is not undertaken following the initial recovery. Rehabilitation at this later stage is a team effort, and co-operation among all the disciplines can only lead to improved care and the best possible outcome for the patient.

REFERENCES

Bethune, D. D. (1975). Neurophysiological facilitation of respiration in the unconscious adult patient. *Physiotherapy* (Canada), **27**(5), 241.

Jennett, B. and Bond, M. (1975). Assessment of outcome after severe brain damage. *Lancet*, **1**, 480.

Potter, J. M. (1974). *The Practical Management of Head Injuries*, 3rd edition. Lloyd-Luke Ltd, London.

BIBLIOGRAPHY

Campkin, T. V. and Turner, J. M. (1980). *Neurosurgical Anaesthesia and Intensive Care*. Butterworths, London.

Evans, C. D. (1981). *Rehabilitation after Severe Head Injury*. Churchill Livingstone, Edinburgh.

Field, J. H. (1976). *Epidemiology of Head Injuries in England and Wales*. HMSO, London.

Jennett, B. (1976). Resource allocation to the severely brain damaged. *Archives of Neurology*, **33**, 595.

Jennett, B., Snoek, J., Bond, M. and Brooks, N. (1981). Disability after severe head injury: observations on the use of the Glasgow Outcome Scale. *Journal of Neurology, Neurosurgery and Psychiatry*, **44**, 285.

Jennett, B. and Teasdale, G. (1981). *Management of Head Injury*. Contemporary Neurology Series. F. A. Davis Co, Philadelphia.

Chapter 21

Paediatrics – 1

by B. KENNEDY, MCSP

In working with children the physiotherapist can expect a wide and varied case-load. The range includes neurological, respiratory, orthopaedic and rheumatic conditions as well as mental subnormality and multiple handicaps. That paediatrics has become a specialty of physiotherapy is due more to the differences between children and adults than to the actual conditions, some of which are specific to childhood, while others closely resemble the adult forms. It is the study of normal patterns of development, learning, behaviour and basic needs of childhood which provide the necessary framework on which to build up physical treatment for any particular condition. Observation of normal children of all ages will reveal a wealth of information which can be utilised when dealing with those less fortunate.

One natural advantage which the physiotherapist can put to good use is the child's enjoyment of movement. This is apparent from the earliest days when the baby learns to move his arms and legs, to play with his hands, and to kick off his blankets. It is seen in the toddler who is never still, and quite tireless in practising his new-found skill of walking. In the playground children can be seen running and jumping and twirling for no other purpose than the pleasure it gives them.

EARLY DEVELOPMENT

As the greatest changes in growth and development of the central nervous system, and therefore in the general activity of the child, take place in its first year of life, the study of this period is of the utmost importance. Probably for parents the major milestones are smiling, sitting, standing, walking and talking. Between and around these achievements there are a host of others – less spectacular but of equal or even greater importance in providing the total framework from which all activity springs. Physical and mental activity develop side by side, and up to a point are interdependent.

In early life all movements are reflex. Later these reflexes are modified by 'higher', more complex ones, e.g. righting reflexes, balance reactions, and by willed movements. It is important to bear in mind the fact that the later willed or voluntary movements depend on the variety and quality of the earlier ones. Even the simplest voluntary movement depends on: (a) an adequate stimulus; (b) the integration of the stimulus at conscious or unconscious levels and (c) the resulting motor response.

Interference for whatever reason with any of these functions will result not only in limiting the immediate response; because the pathways are not working to their full capacity the sensory feedback will also be inaccurate, and there will be a deficiency of stored experience which, in its turn, will affect any future response. In this way, learning is affected.

Thus a baby who is backward in development may be so for a number of reasons.

LACK OF ADEQUATE STIMULATION

From their earliest days all babies need the comfort and stimulation of human contact. They need to be cuddled and to be fed in mother's arms, where they feel content and secure. They enjoy 'baby play' and quickly begin to learn about their immediate surroundings. Unfortunately, babies may be left alone for long periods, deprived of auditory or visual stimulus. These babies have no incentive to move and no opportunity to learn. Frequently the mothers of such children are depressed or may, from choice or necessity, leave their offspring with unsuitable daily minders. Sometimes, physically handicapped children, those who have prolonged hospitalisation or immobilisation, are also in danger of being deprived, unless special care is taken to ensure that they have the opportunity to see and hear and touch those things which they would experience in normal circumstances.

LOSS OF SPECIAL SENSES

Blind or deaf babies will obviously be behind in activities requiring sight or hearing – though later they may partially compensate for this. There may be sensory loss in children with neuromotor defects, either because they cannot move, and therefore cannot appreciate movement, or because sensation itself is deficient.

BRAIN DAMAGE

Depending on the area affected, brain damage may result in

impairment of the appreciation of sensation, of integration, or of the motor response.

MILESTONES OF DEVELOPMENT

It is more satisfactory to regard these rather as a related sequence than as isolated events which must be achieved in a certain number of weeks or months. Babies vary greatly and there is a wide age-span covering the rate at which a normal child develops. The following plan should be read only as a guide to the sequence of normal development:

1. Head control
2. Hands
3. Rolling
4. Sitting
5. Creeping, crawling and bottom shuffling
6. Standing and walking
7. Gait

These headings have been arranged to show the sequence in which the beginnings of control are acquired, but it is stressed that all these activities overlap and are related to one another.

Head control

At birth the baby's head lolls when unsupported. If placed on his tummy he will turn his head to the side. In supine it is also generally turned to one side.

At six to eight weeks, when his eyes begin to focus, he starts to turn his head to look and will survey things in mid-line in the supine position. In the prone position he is beginning to lift his head off the bed.

At about three months he has full control of head rotation in supine, is getting good extension in prone, and is less wobbly when sitting on mother's knee. Quite soon he can lift his head in prone to look round from side to side.

By six to seven months he holds his head high in prone, and is beginning to raise it in supine. Although unable to maintain a sitting position, he can control his head if his trunk is supported.

With practice, head control and sitting balance improve. Head raising in supine develops together with increasing trunk and arm movements. Independent sitting and the ability to sit up from supine are both achieved by nine to ten months.

THE PULL TO SITTING TEST (Fig. 21/1)

This test is often used to demonstrate the degree of head control. The examiner takes hold of the baby's hands and pulls him into a sitting position. At birth and for a few weeks after, the head falls back with no attempt to right itself. By three months there is less head lag and by five or six months it will compensate throughout the movement, and it may even actively flex as the child tries to sit up as soon as he grasps the examiner's fingers.

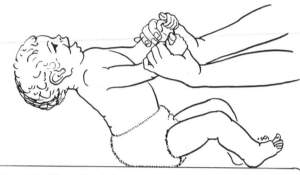

Fig. 21/1   The pull to sitting test – note the moderate head lag

Hands

Hands are used for manipulation and support. At birth the baby shows predominant flexor tone throughout the body, and his hands are mainly fisted with the thumb held across the palm, though there is occasional extension of the fingers. By stretching the flexors of the fingers anything pressed into the palm elicits the grasp reflex, which in the first month or two is strong enough to lift the baby up by holding on to the examiner's fingers. The grasp reflex gradually fades in three to four months, and is replaced by voluntary grasping.

MANIPULATION

At four months, when eyes and head have gained some control, he is able to grab and hold a rattle and take it to his mouth for further investigation. Later he learns that it is fun to hold and release, to grab and throw. Also at about four months, he begins to play with his own hands, watching them move in front of his face. He also holds toys in his two hands, and transfers from one hand to the other at six to seven months. Early grasp is a simple flexion of the hand and fingers, the little and ring fingers playing the major part. This is known as palmar grasp.

By about nine months, the action of the hand has changed, the index finger has become the dominant feature, and is used for poking, and, with the thumb in a pincer grasp, to pick up quite tiny objects. This is the beginning of fine manipulation which will continue to develop over many more months as all the fingers become independent and fine skills are acquired by practice.

SUPPORT

Hands are used for support:

1. In prone, from about six months when the child pushes up on straight arms.
2. In sitting (see below and Fig. 21/3).
3. In saving reactions which begin to develop concurrently with the use of hand support (Figs. 21/2 and 21/3).

PARACHUTE REACTION (Fig. 21/2)

This test is often performed when screening children for cerebral palsy or other conditions where there is brain damage. The child is

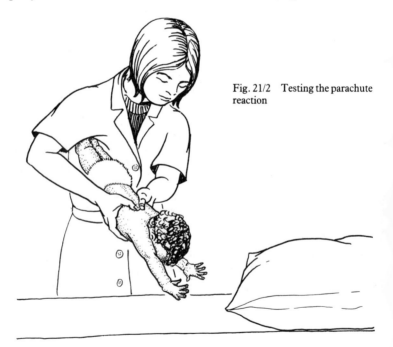

Fig. 21/2   Testing the parachute reaction

held under his chest, and moved rapidly forwards and downwards towards the bed – from six months onwards he should extend his arms and open his fingers as if to save himself – flexion or retraction of one or both arms indicate some neurological abnormality.

Later still the child uses his hands to pull himself to standing and to hold on as he learns to walk.

Rolling

This is an important part of development requiring co-ordination of most parts of the body. The earliest rolling is from side to supine or side to prone, depending on which position the baby prefers. This in its turn may well depend on how the baby was nursed in his early days. Rolling from prone to supine occurs at about five months, i.e. when he can lift and rotate his head and upper trunk while the lower trunk and legs flex. Here is the beginning of trunk control and rotation. Rolling from supine to prone generally follows about one month later (head flexion in supine occurring later than head extension in prone), and about the same time as progress is being made in sitting.

Sitting (Fig. 21/3)

Before six months the baby can be placed in a sitting position but needs support. At about five months it is not uncommon for him to reject the position and throw himself backwards when his mother wants him to sit up. Active sitting starts at about six months, when he is able to lean forward on his hands (Fig. 21/3(1)), but has no balance and is liable to fall. By seven months he can sit unsupported for one minute; by eight months he has acquired sufficient balance to sit steadily and to save himself with his hand if falling sideways. Between eight and ten months he is able to save himself if tipped backwards, extending his hands behind him (Fig. 21/3(4)). About this time he also learns to pivot on his bottom and to get from sitting to all fours. During this time, head and trunk control have improved in all positions and he is able to sit up from supine, rolling over on his elbow to do so, and at first pulling himself up with the other hand on the side of the cot. This pattern of sitting up, using trunk rotation, continues until the age of four or five years, when the child is able to sit up symmetrically.

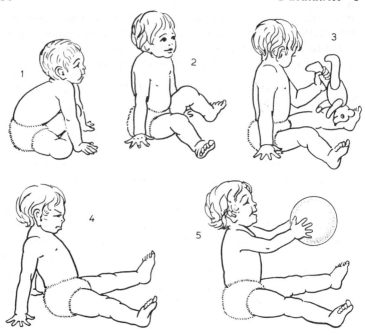

Fig. 21/3   This series shows the inter-related development of hand support and
balance in sitting:
(1) Leaning forward on his hands at 6 months
(2) Supporting himself in sitting   ⎫
(3) Support with one hand while picking up a toy ⎬ 7–8 months
(4) Saving himself from falling backwards ⎫
(5) Balance and play!   ⎬ 8–10 months

Creeping, crawling and shuffling

These are all valid modes of progression of which a child may use each
in turn, one only, or none at all. Unfortunately, there is great
confusion about the terms *creeping* and *crawling* and in any discussion
one must be quite sure that all concerned are using the same terms for
the same actions. In this Section, *creeping* refers to progress in prone
with tummy on the floor; *crawling* refers to progression on hands and
knees, moving one arm and one leg alternately.

CREEPING

This may start with pivoting in a circle at about six months. Some
babies push up on their extended arms and move backwards, others
kick their legs and wriggle forwards. There are many variations and
the preference for one is of little significance unless combined with

other signs of abnormality, e.g. if a child consistently uses only his arms to creep and has difficulty in sitting one might suspect some neurological abnormality of the legs.

CRAWLING

This occurs at about the same time as sitting balance is acquired, and the child is generally already beginning to pull up to stand. Quite a large number of normal children never crawl, but go straight to standing and walking. Some crawl for only a few days, others for many weeks, but this seems to have little bearing on their general development.

BOTTOM SHUFFLING

This is a self-descriptive method of progress and is sometimes an alternative to crawling. Obviously, the pre-requirement is the ability to sit and balance while moving either one arm and leg, or both legs. Normal and abnormal children may be seen to bottom shuffle, so it is not a diagnostic sign unless associated with similar and consistent patterns in other activities, e.g. the refusal to use the other arm and leg and inability to sit symmetrically would lead one to suspect infantile hemiplegia. It is of interest to note that normal children who bottom shuffle are often late in walking.

Standing and walking

Although the stepping reflex can be demonstrated in the newborn infant, this is only a transitory state which disappears in a week or so. However, at a few weeks he starts alternate kicking, and soon enjoys 'feeling his feet' when held upright with his feet on mother's knee.

By the time he is five months old he sustains most of his weight, and starts to bounce. Most children start to pull themselves to standing soon after they have learnt to sit. They then enjoy standing at the cot rail; often their first steps are taken moving sideways along it. The actual age at which children stand and walk varies greatly. Some will stand at eight months and walk at 10, others not until 18 or 20 months. The average is reckoned to be 10 months for standing and 13 months for walking unaided.

Gait

At first the child walks on a wide base in a rather square-set fashion. He has little balance and no movement of the pelvis. Gradually, with practice, his balance improves and his feet get closer together, and he learns to run. However, not until the age of three or four years does walking resemble adult gait, i.e. with pelvic rotation. Given the opportunity most children start climbing as soon as they get on their feet, but walking up- and downstairs using alternate legs is not achieved until two or three years, neither is the ability to stand on one leg, or jump on two. Hopping on one leg takes another year.

Conclusion

To summarise briefly, it may be seen that there is a definite link between the development of different motor skills. Rolling and sitting both require some head control; sitting also needs the support of the hands and arms; sitting up uses and consolidates the same pattern of movement as rolling and so on. It becomes evident that one must understand this progression of acquired skills in the normal child in order to appreciate and treat effectively the abnormal.

THE IMPORTANCE OF PLAY (Figs. 21/4, 21/5, 21/6)

The value of play to a child cannot be over-emphasised because this is how he learns. When a mother plays with her baby, he learns to watch her face, listen to her voice, to follow with his eyes, reach with his

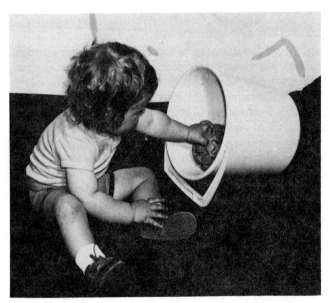

Fig. 21/4   Playing with a plastic bucket!

hand, to localise sound, later to imitate both sound and expression. He touches his mother's face and hair and finds it soft, holds his bottle or rattle, and discovers it is hard. So he learns about texture and temperature, shape and weight. Then he can learn about the purpose of things, rattles to shake, or punch, or roll, some noisy, some cuddly. He learns to select what is appropriate for his purpose – a soft toy to sleep with, a rattle to bang when he wakes.

Although good toys tend to be expensive, they are a good investment provided they are carefully selected. They may be supplemented by improvisations, using everyday household materials, such as a wooden spoon and saucepan which can be used for a variety of activities, cardboard boxes, particularly large ones, are great fun for climbing in and out and under, and later provide much imaginative play. A plastic bucket also has many uses, as container, seat, table, or just something to carry about (Fig. 21/4).

Although a large selection of toys are available in the shops, the choice of suitable ones is important if both the donor and the recipient are not to be disappointed. A great deal of money is wasted on toys which are either too complicated or too delicate for the child's ability; something which has been chosen more thoughtfully might provide enjoyment as well as practice in acquired skills. This is particularly true in the case of handicapped children whose intellectual, physical and emotional needs are not always at the same developmental level. Parents and friends of such children often seek advice for Christmas and birthday presents. Guidance along these lines may be a means of introducing a much wider concept of treatment, demonstrating how play and daily activities can become an important part of therapy. It is useful to be able to lend out the catalogues of firms who supply well made or educational toys, so that the rest of the family can see what has been suggested. Toy libraries are another means of finding suitable toys; some toys may be of interest for only a short time and it is better to borrow these than to buy them. In addition there are often ideas for making satisfying and original toys cheaply.

The physiotherapist will also want to give advice on the use and suitability of large toys, such as bouncers, swings, walkers and tricycles. It is, however, much more difficult to give advice once the article in question has been purchased; so it is essential to raise the question of these things at the earliest opportunity. In fact, this makes a good starting point to introduce ideas of management to parents when they first bring their child for treatment. It can be explained to them that baby may well be helped by one or other of these things, but that it would be better to delay buying any of them until his problems have been fully assessed. It is helpful to be able to try out the different types of equipment on the market, and see which is beneficial, and which harmful to each individual. Equipment should never be recommended for home use unless the physiotherapist has seen the child use it, and is certain that it will continue to be used to advantage.

Of this group of equipment, the baby bouncer is perhaps the most controversial problem, as everyone has a friend whose baby loves it, and for whom it works wonders! One must be rather wary of recommending these for handicapped children, particularly until one has made a careful assessment, e.g. it is tempting to 'bounce' the lethargic, floppy baby, but one must be sure that it is not in the process of developing extensor spasticity of the legs – which might be increased by the bouncing.

Care must also be taken when treating mentally handicapped children, though they may well benefit from using the bouncer to stimulate activity and build up their muscle tone which is often low. One of their characteristic problems is that of perseveration of movement, so strict limits should be imposed on the length of time spent in the bouncer. It is also important that other activities, e.g. rolling, creeping and crawling which may be more useful developmentally, even if less convenient for the mothers, should not be neglected. The bouncer should be discarded when it has served its purpose, and the child is able to progress to a new activity.

Provided they are used with discretion and the contra-indications are recognised, bouncers can provide useful and enjoyable activity to meet specific needs. Occasionally the bouncer may have a more static use as an aid to standing or even sitting by giving trunk support to the very hypotonic child, to whom it is difficult to give the experience of an upright posture in any other way. It gives the physiotherapist a chance to position the child's legs and to encourage it to take some of its weight.

Baby walkers can be useful, but must also be used with discretion. There is a variety of these on the market, and each child must be assessed individually for his particular needs. This includes safety. If he is too tall for the model chosen, or too floppy, the child may cause the walker to overbalance. Care should also be taken where the floor is uneven. The older child may use the Cell Barnes walker, but should be supervised in case he tries to climb out and becomes stuck or falls. Other types of walkers should be selected with equal care.

Baby chairs and swings must be similarly considered for fit, safety and function. More will be said about these later.

It is important to remember that much early play takes place at floor level. Young children suffering from spina bifida or other conditions which make mobility a problem can use a crawler or tummy trolley to

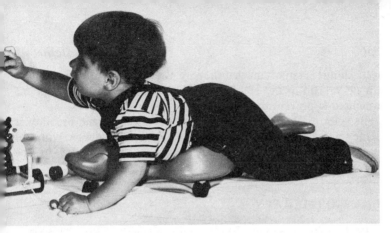

Fig. 21/5 Floor play using a crawler for mobility gives enjoyment while strengthening arm and back muscles

keep pace with their peers (Fig. 21/5). At the same time they strengthen arms and shoulders in preparation for more advanced activities later. Ride astride toys are also popular and have many uses. A great number are available and one should look for the more stable ones that will not easily tip over, and also consider the variations of height and width. Pushing toys can help young children learning to

Fig. 21/6 Pushing trucks may be a stage in learning to walk. Trucks must be the correct height for the child

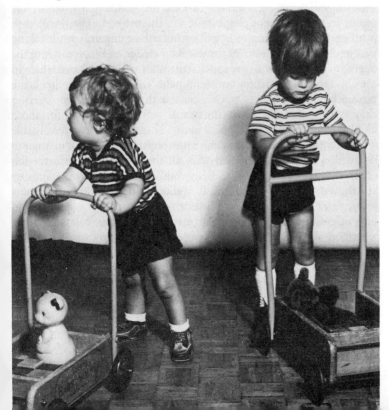

walk, but it is important that they are of a suitable height and do not tip up or run away. Handles can be raised and trucks or prams weighted to prevent this (Fig. 21/6).

Bicycles, tricycles and Go-karts provide exercise and mobility at some stages of treatment. If necessary, they can be adapted with seat backs and foot straps, and can sometimes be provided by the Department of Health and Social Security.

PHYSIOTHERAPY

With an increasing number of paediatric physiotherapists working in the community, children may receive treatment in different places including day or boarding schools, nurseries, play groups, at home as well as in hospital. It is important to choose the place that is most appropriate to the current needs of the child and his family. Thus treatment at home may be suitable for young babies or for assessment, but the isolating effect on the family, and difficulties of giving adequate treatment in a restricted space must be weighed against problems of transport to a centre which can provide a more supportive environment as well as better treatment facilities.

When working in schools it is essential that teachers should understand the need and purpose of treatment, and the difficulties which a child may encounter in class or in the playground; for example, the mild hemiplegic child in a mainstream school will have problems with two-handed activities and will be ungainly while taking part in physical education or games. Knowledge and acceptance of the degree of disability will save much frustration on all sides and will help the child to achieve maximum attainment. In some special schools the physiotherapist is able to work alongside the teacher so that together they may devise the most functional working position for those children with particular physical needs. Nursery staff can be valuable allies in continuing and complementing physiotherapy; but in order to do so they must be provided with all the appropriate information about the child's problems. A daily routine should be worked out by all who are involved in the child's welfare. The same applies in play groups and in residential establishments. In hospital it is desirable to have a children's room or department so that they can have their treatment separately from adult patients: their needs are different in every way. Parents and children become more relaxed and confident when they do not have to worry about making too much noise or getting in the way; they can see that other children feel at home and are able to enjoy themselves. Many parents find it helpful to meet other parents who have similar problems to their own.

It is important to get off to a good start and the first visit should be carefully planned, allowing time for the child to settle down without any feeling of haste. Parents should be given adequate explanation of the importance of observation and assessment. Many children are shy and respond badly to a direct approach. Playing on the floor or on mother's knee may give them the chance to make their own adjustment to new people and new surroundings. This is a good opportunity to watch their patterns of movement and behaviour, and to talk to the parents, thus gathering information which will influence the planning of treatment. All families are different in their commitments, priorities and expectations. Some may have unrealistic hopes of treatment while others need encouragement to accept treatment. A clear explanation of the aims of treatment will help parents to understand what is being planned and how they can become involved. For a successful result parents, child and therapist must work together.

Play and movement are normal parts of life, so physiotherapy is often presented in the form of play. It must be organised so that set goals are achieved, at the same time remembering that play is only an incentive for as long as it is fun. Free play is also important for the child to develop skills, initiative and personality. It is sometimes necessary to ensure that time for play *is* included in the child's daily routine. Physiotherapy assessment should include observation of free play as this will indicate deficits, needs and progress. Very severely handicapped children may be unable to engage in any form of play without help; this does not mean they do not need play, and ways of providing them with the opportunity to do so should be sought constantly.

Babies need to be handled in a quiet, calm manner as they are easily upset by sudden noises or movements. In spite of this they can move very quickly, wriggling and rolling into dangerous places unless precautions are taken to protect them. A baby must never be left unattended in any place from which he can fall. In the ward, cot sides must be left raised and locked. Fires and radiators are another hazard to be considered, particularly with children who have defective sensation.

Powers of concentration vary, not only between one child and another, but in the same child from day to day. It is necessary to recognise the 'off' days and adjust the treatment accordingly, thus avoiding frustration and preserving a good working relationship for next time.

A few children in the under-five group will respond to a direct approach and can be taught straightforward exercises. Others need the incentive provided by toys and games for longer. At all stages it is important to maintain the child's interest and to change the activity before he becomes bored. Encouragement is the greatest spur; even a dull child will work for praise, whereas threats or bribes provide only another distraction. Praise, of course, must not be given indiscriminately, but it is usually possible to find some simple achievement to provide a starting point.

Games and toys must be chosen to provide the activity which is required and not merely for their own sake, otherwise valuable time will be wasted. Similarly, older children may enjoy the interest and companionship of classwork but it must be remembered that the aim is treatment of the individual and that each has his own specific needs.

In selecting a child for a class, various aspects must be considered; these include the age, personality and physical needs of the child, as well as the size and nature of the class and the experience of the physiotherapist. Most children begin to enjoy working together at about the age of four or five, but at this stage will need considerable individual help, either during or in addition to a group session. Classwork in its generally accepted sense is better delayed until the age of seven or eight.

Schoolchildren attending for specific exercises, e.g. breathing, posture, re-education after injuries, are generally more satisfactorily treated if their parents are not present. Once he has learnt them, the child is pleased to demonstrate the exercises to his parents and feels that he is responsible for his own treatment when it is continued at home.

Younger children, and severely handicapped older ones, are normally treated with mother present, so that she can learn what to encourage in the daily routine, and what to include in her home treatment sessions if these are recommended. Sometimes it is desirable to work entirely through the mother, so that it is she who handles the child throughout the treatment, the physiotherapist giving the instructions and explaining why they are necessary. This is particularly useful in the case of young children in hospital who need tipping, and can be persuaded to do so over mother's knee, possibly while the physiotherapist gives the same treatment to dolly or teddy.

Home treatment

This must be kept as simple as possible, and within the limits of medical necessity, as short as possible. Parents and child should understand the importance of regular treatment, and over-enthusiastic parents restrained from insisting on prolonged sessions in the early stages which can result in exhaustion and frustration for all concerned. Notes should be kept of treatment given. Home programmes should be revised regularly so that they continue to be effective and the child does not become bored. It is also wise to ascertain that the treatment prescribed is practicable at home, e.g. that there is enough space to perform the exercises and that any apparatus required is available. Further reference to home treatment and management of the handicapped child is made in Chapter 23.

BIBLIOGRAPHY

Andre-Thomas and Autgaerden, S. *Locomotion from Pre- to Post-natal Life.* Clinics In Developmental Medicine, No 24. Spastics International Medical Publications in association with William Heinemann Medical Books Limited, London.

Bobath, B. and Bobath, K. (1975). *Motor Development in the Different Types of Cerebral Palsy.* William Heinemann Medical Books Limited, London.

Gesell, A. (1971). *The First Five Years of Life: A Guide to the Study of the Pre-School Child.* Methuen, London.

Griffiths, R. (1964). *The Abilities of Babies.* Hodder and Stoughton Educational, London.

Leach, P. (1980). *Baby and Child.* Penguin Books, Harmondsworth.

Lear, R. (1977). *Play Helps: Toys and Activities for Handicapped Children.* William Heinemann Medical Books Limited, London.

Levitt, S. (1981). *Treatment of Cerebral Palsy and Motor Delay*, 2nd edition. Blackwell Scientific Publications Limited, Oxford.

Matterson, E. M. (1970). *Play with a Purpose for Under-Sevens.* Penguin Books, Harmondsworth.

Sheridan, M. (1975). *Children's Developmental Progress from Birth to Five Years: The Stycar Sequences*, 2nd edition. NFER Publishing Company, Windsor.

Sheridan, M. (1977). *Spontaneous Play in Early Childhood – Birth to Six Years.* NFER Publishing Company, Windsor.

Toy Library Association (1982). *The Good Toy Guide.* Inter-Action Inprint, London.

Chapter 22

Paediatrics – 2

by B. KENNEDY, MCSP

CONGENITAL ABNORMALITIES

A congenital abnormality may be defined as a defect already present in the infant at the time of birth. Sometimes more than one abnormality may be present, for instance a congenital heart condition may be associated with talipes or congenital dislocation of the hip.

The three main causes of congenital abnormalities are: genetic factors; intra-uterine pressure; intra-uterine infection.

The conditions described here are some of those most commonly seen in the physiotherapy department.

TALIPES EQUINOVARUS (Fig. 22/1)

As the name suggests, the foot is twisted downwards and inwards. The head of the talus is prominent on the dorsum of the foot, the medial border of which is concave. In severe cases the sole of the foot may face upwards and if untreated, the child walks on the dorsum of the foot. The majority of cases are bilateral.

Aetiology

The cause is uncertain, but there is often a genetic element. It has been suggested that the development of the foot is arrested before birth as a result of some unidentified infection of the mother, and that the initial abnormality may be in the bones with secondary changes in soft tissue. Alternatively, it is possible that moulding of the foot occurs when the fetus lies awkwardly in the uterus, and that the primary change is in soft tissue, the bones only becoming misshapen later, if the deformity is not corrected.

There are three components of the deformity:

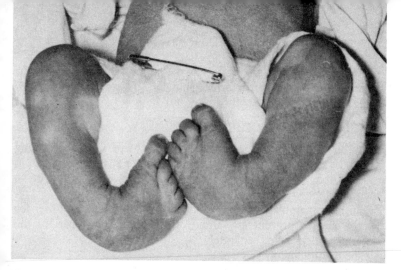

Fig. 22/1   Congenital talipes equinovarus showing severe bilateral deformity

1. Plantar flexion at the ankle (equinus). The talus may lie almost vertically instead of in the horizontal position.
2. Inversion at the sub-taloid and mid-tarsal joints. The calcaneus faces inwards (varus).
3. Adduction of the forefoot at the tarsometatarsal joint. Some cases also have internal rotation of the tibia.

There is shortening of tibialis anterior and posterior, and the long and short flexors of the toes. The calf muscles are wasted and the tendo-calcaneus drawn over to the medial side of the heel.

Similarly, the ligaments and joint capsules on the medial side of the ankle and foot are tight and the plantar fascia forms a tight thickened band on the medial side of the sole. On the lateral side of the leg, the peronei and lateral ligaments and capsules are overstretched and weak.

Treatment

Treatment should be commenced early, on the first day of life if possible, and continued until the child walks. It consists of over-correction of the deformity by manipulation, and maintenance by splinting and active use of all the leg muscles, particularly the peronei. In severe cases open reduction of the deformity may be performed within a few weeks of birth if conservative methods appear inadequate. Full over-correction of the deformity within two or three weeks is desirable for a good prognosis. If this is not achieved, either because of very severe deformity, muscle imbalance or delay in starting treatment, there is increased likelihood of relapse; operations to release or lengthen soft tissues on the postero-medial aspect of the ankle and foot may be performed initially, followed if necessary by bony procedures as the child gets older.

MANIPULATION (Figs. 22/2, 22/3)

Manipulation to obtain over-correction may be performed on young babies by the doctor or physiotherapist without anaesthesia. In mild cases where no splinting is necessary, the mother is taught to manipulate the feet each time she changes the nappy.

During manipulation, the baby's knee is flexed and the lower leg firmly held to prevent any strain on the knee. Each part of the deformity is stretched separately.

The manipulations are:

1. To correct the heel: the heel is pulled down and out, stretching the tendo-calcaneus and structures on the medial side. For a good

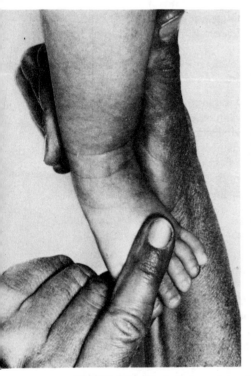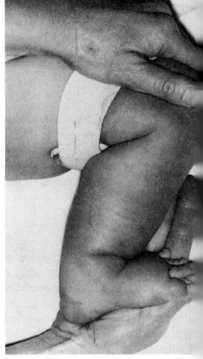

Fig. 22/2 (*left*)   Manipulation to abduct forefoot

Fig. 22/3 (*right*)   Manipulation to gain combined eversion and dorsiflexion

result the heel must be fully corrected in the first two or three weeks of life. After this time an inverted heel is unlikely to respond to manipulative measures.

2. To abduct the forefoot: the baby's left heel rests in the palm of the physiotherapist's right hand so that her thumb supports the outer side of his leg, and her index and middle fingers hold his heel. The ball of the thumb acts as a fulcrum as the foot is bent sideways over it, the physiotherapist using her left thumb and index finger to grasp along the base of the toes (Fig. 22/2).

3. To combine eversion and dorsiflexion: the fully corrected foot can be pushed up and out so that the dorsum touches the outer side of the leg (Fig. 22/3). Care must be taken to ensure that dorsiflexion occurs in the ankle joint and not in the sole of the foot. This depends on adequate correction of the tightness of the tendo-calcaneus; sometimes a tenotomy is needed to achieve this.

SPLINTING

Splinting may be by strapping, Denis Browne splints or plaster of Paris. The splints or plaster will be applied by the doctor and will maintain the feet in eversion and dorsiflexion. Strapping may be applied by the doctor or by the physiotherapist under his direction.

It is important that treatment should not be interrupted, so every effort must be made to maintain the skin in good condition. Three points are worth noting:

1. Care of the skin by painting it with Tinct. Benz. Co. before the strapping is applied. If, in spite of this, the skin becomes wet and soggy, gentian violet may be liberally applied and strapping continued. Occasionally it may be necessary to leave the skin exposed for 24 to 48 hours. Very rarely a baby may be allergic to zinc oxide strapping but may tolerate Dermicel or a similar preparation.

2. Reinforcement of the corrective straps so as to prevent these from dragging on the skin.

3. Padding pressure points with adhesive felt.

STRAPPING (Figs. 22/4, 22/5)

This method of strapping to be described has been used by the author for many years and has proved satisfactory. Minor adaptations can be made to suit the individual case. The lateral malleolus is protected by a small piece of adhesive felt. Another piece 1–2.5cm (½–1in) wide depending on the size of the foot, is wrapped round the medial side of the big toe and under the base of the toes.

Three strips of 2.5cm (1in) wide zinc oxide strapping are used; one

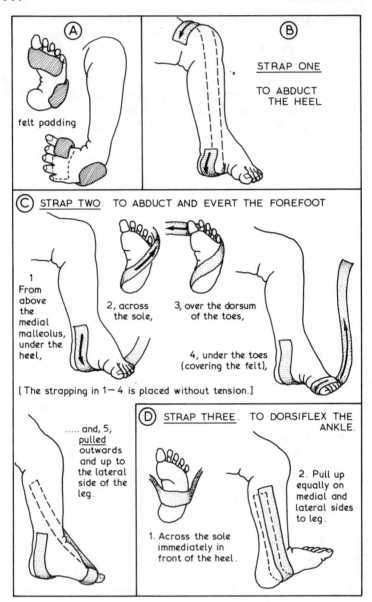

Fig. 22/4   Strapping for talipes equinovarus

to correct each part of the deformity. In very tiny babies the strapping width will need to be reduced to 1.9cm (¾in).

1. The first starts below the medial malleolus, passes under the heel, up the outer side of the leg and over the bent knee (Fig. 22/4 A & B).

2. The second starts above the medial malleolus and passes across the sole of the foot, around the forefoot (covering the felt). N.B. It is important that no tension is applied up to this point. The strap is then pulled upwards and outwards to the lateral side of the leg (Fig. 22/4C, 1–5).

3. The third strap maintains dorsiflexion and passes under the sole of the foot and up both sides of the lower leg (Fig. 22/4D, 1–2).

Reinforcement by strips of zinc oxide 5–7.5cm (2–3in) in length applied diagonally across the strapping on the lateral side helps to prevent these from dragging on the skin. A cotton bandage secured with more strapping is useful protection and can be reapplied if it becomes soiled.

Initially, strapping is renewed or reinforced daily progressing to every two or three days until full over-correction can be maintained without undue circulatory disturbance, generally in two or three weeks if treatment is started early. It is then reapplied weekly or fortnightly. Some form of splinting must be retained until the child is standing when its own body weight acts as a corrective force. Before this time there is a strong tendency for the condition to relapse. In the later stages some form of removable splinting may be used such as Denis Browne night boots (Fig. 22/6) or a plastic splint moulded to

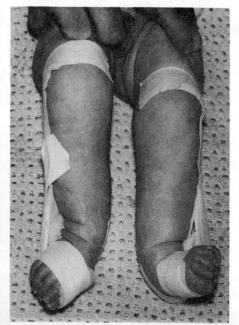

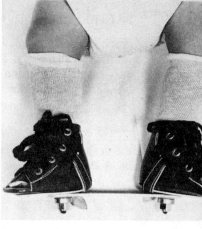

Fig. 22/5 (*left*)   Strapping for bilateral talipes equinovarus

Fig. 22/6 (*above*)   Denis Browne night boots

maintain the over-corrected position. Whatever appliance is used it must be well-fitting, and reviewed frequently as the child grows. Parents must understand the function of splints and be competent and conscientious in their use.

EXERCISE

Whatever form of splinting is used, the baby is encouraged to kick at first against his mother's hands, the end of the pram or, when he is old enough, against the floor. This strengthens his muscles and reinforces the correction of the deformity. Each time the strapping is removed, the peronei can be stimulated by stroking over the muscles, or along the outer border of the foot. When intermittent splinting is introduced the infant should be encouraged to exercise without splints during his waking hours. Parents should be taught to move the foot through its full range, to stimulate the peronei and encourage the child to stand.

Advice to parents

Parents must understand:

1. The importance of continuous treatment.
2. The danger of the feet relapsing if treatment is stopped too soon.
3. The necessity of keeping splints or strapping dry. This should not be too difficult if the baby wears plastic pants.
4. The importance of inspecting the toes to check the circulation, particularly after splinting has been renewed. The baby should return immediately to hospital if the toes become blue or swollen.

TALIPES CALCANEO-VALGUS

This is much less serious than the equinovarus deformity. It tends to recover spontaneously. The baby is born with the feet in a position of eversion and dorsiflexion. All the anterior tibial muscles are shortened together with the ligaments over the front of the ankle.

Causes

It is probable that the deformity develops shortly before birth due to the awkward position in which the fetus lies.

Treatment

Treatment consists of gentle stretching of the foot into plantar flexion and inversion, and encouraging active movements in the same direction. The mother is taught to do this several times a day. If the condition is severe or persists, a small splint may be made to keep the foot in plantar flexion and inversion.

TORTICOLLIS

Wry neck or torticollis is occasionally seen by the physiotherapist. The child holds his head tilted to one side so that the ear is drawn towards the shoulder on the tight side. At the same time, the face is turned to the opposite side.

Structural torticollis

A cervical hemivertebra may be the cause of torticollis but this is very rare and there is no treatment.

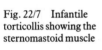
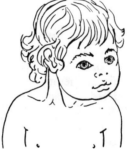

Fig. 22/7   Infantile torticollis showing the sternomastoid muscle

Infantile torticollis (Fig. 22/7)

This is the type most commonly seen. It is often associated with sternomastoid tumour. A small hard lump consisting of fibrous scar tissue can be felt in the muscle belly at birth or shortly afterwards. The scar tissue contracts, so shortening the muscle. The clavicular head of the muscle may stand out in a tight band and the head is pulled over into the typical position.

CAUSE

The cause is unknown. A fibrous tumour may be present before birth or a haematoma may result from a traction injury during birth. Facial asymmetry and moulding of the head is often a factor, but this slowly improves if the muscle can be stretched and the head held straight. In untreated cases facial asymmetry may persist and after some years it becomes irreversible.

Fetal torticollis

The appearances are similar to the infantile type described above but there is no tumour and little or no limitation of passive movement.

Asymmetric moulding of the head, probably from the position in utero, results in it being held consistently on one side. Active rotation to the other side is made difficult by the shape of the head. The infant frequently prefers to lie on one side only.

The condition often improves spontaneously as the baby grows and gets more active. The moulding of the head disappears more slowly in about a year.

Physiotherapy is sometimes given if the infant is slow to start moving. It follows the pattern given below.

Treatment

Physiotherapy, consisting of stretching, active exercises and general management, should be started early, usually at about four weeks, and is generally successful up to the age of six months. After this time the muscle is more difficult to stretch, and although it is worth while continuing with physiotherapy, tenotomy of the sternomastoid may have to be considered at a later date.

STRETCHING

The movements performed in stretching the sternomastoid are:

1. Side flexion of the head and neck away from the tight side
2. Rotation of the head so that the face is turned towards the tight side
3. Both movements combined, side flexion followed by rotation.

If the baby is small the mother can do the stretching while he lies on her lap (Fig. 22/8). In order to make him feel secure, she must sit on a chair low enough for both feet to rest firmly on the floor. The baby lies across the mother's knee, in the case of a right torticollis his head rests on her right knee. She places her left hand over the point of his right shoulder to hold it down; her left forearm keeps his arms and trunk tucked close in to her own body. She places her right hand on the right side of the baby's head, avoiding his ear, and brings his chin to the

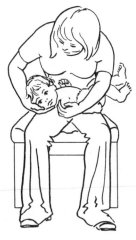

Fig. 22/8   Mother
manipulating her child's
torticollis

mid-line before performing side flexion (bringing the head towards
her) and rotation (turning the face away from her).

   If the child is too big, a second person must be enlisted to help. The
child lies supine on a flat firm surface – a thin sponge bath mat on a
table is ideal as it will not slip. The assistant holds the baby's shoulder
down, while the mother takes his head between her hands and
performs the movements as before.

   Each movement should be through the fullest range possible,
performed five or six times at each session and repeated two or three
times each day. Although the mother must be taught to stretch the
neck as soon as possible, the physiotherapist must realise that she is
bound to be frightened of doing so, especially as the baby is likely to
cry. She should be reassured and gain confidence, by being allowed to
practise getting her hands into the correct position without actually
stretching. When she is able to do this easily she starts stretching the
neck under supervision before doing so at home.

ACTIVE EXERCISE

From about 10 weeks old the baby can be encouraged to turn his head
through the full range of rotation by attracting his attention with a
coloured toy or rattle. At first this is done in supine, later in prone,
later still in sitting. It is important to move the rattle slowly, giving the
infant time to fix his eyes on it and accommodate to the movement. By
changing his position, by holding down one shoulder the movements
of flexion, extension and side flexion may be encouraged in a similar
fashion.

GENERAL MANAGEMENT

The baby should be encouraged to lie on alternate sides; frequently one side is less used than the other.

The cot or pram should be placed so that the baby is encouraged to look towards the tight side; toys should be hung on this side.

The baby should not be sat up too early or for too long; his head will drop to the tight side if his muscles are weak or tired.

Ocular torticollis

Occasionally children of three or four are sent for treatment because they hold their head on one side. There is a full range of passive movement and the child is able to correct the head position actively with help, but resumes the torticollis position as soon as left alone.

The cause lies in weakness of one eye and physiotherapy should be delayed until this has received attention. Usually the head is held straight as soon as the eyes are treated.

BRACHIAL PALSIES

These are not very common but sometimes follow a difficult birth. They may be caused by pressure between neck and shoulder or by traction on the arm or head. There is damage to the nerves or nerve roots, resulting in paralysis of the muscles in the arm supplied by them. The prognosis will depend on the degree of damage. This can vary from mild bruising followed by recovery in a few weeks, to severe tearing of the nerves resulting in permanent paralysis and the danger of deformity. Fortunately the latter cases are rare.

Erb's palsy (Fig. 22/9)

The fifth and sixth cervical nerve roots are damaged resulting in paralysis of deltoid, supraspinatus, infraspinatus, teres major, biceps and supinator.

SIGNS AND SYMPTOMS

The arm may be completely flaccid at birth but soon assumes the typical position of adduction and internal rotation at the shoulder, with pronation of the forearm and flexion of the wrist and fingers.

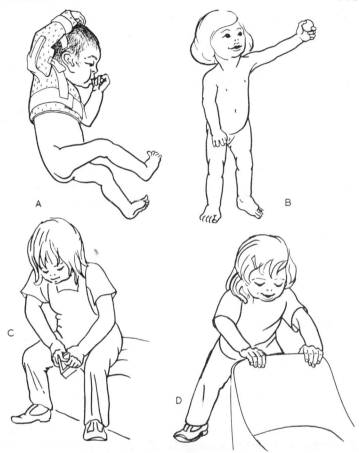

Fig. 22/9   Erb's palsy. A. The shoulder in a splint. B. The typical deformity (right): arm turned in and fingers flexed; drooping shoulder line and a disproportionately short upper arm. C. Using toys so that the fingers of both hands are used. D. Using both hands to push a chair.

TREATMENT

This should be started as soon as possible with the aims of protecting the shoulder joint and preventing deformities.

A splint may be used to support the shoulder in abduction and lateral rotation, with the elbow in 90 degrees of flexion and the fore-arm supinated. Light splints made of Plastazote or Orthoplast are comfortable, and can be altered as the baby grows (Fig. 22/9(A)). Pinning the sleeve of the nightdress to the pillow is not recommended because of the danger of straining the shoulder joint if the baby moves.

Passive movements and the encouragement of whatever active movements are possible are started immediately and taught to the mother so that she can continue at home.

In severe cases where splinting must be continued for several months it is important to see that the infant has opportunities for the activities normal for his age, e.g. in the prone position, rolling over, and sitting himself up, and it is essential to give the help necessary to achieve this.

The greatest recovery takes place in the first few months, after which time only slight improvement can be expected. Functional activities assume greater importance and the child should be given opportunities to develop the use of his arm and hand as fully as possible (Fig. 22/9 (C and D)).

Klumpke's paralysis

The seventh and eighth cervical and first thoracic nerve roots are affected.

SIGNS AND SYMPTOMS

Paralysis of the extensors of the wrist and fingers results in the wrist being held in the flexed position. The small hand muscles are also affected.

TREATMENT

Small cock-up splints for the wrist can be made from plaster of Paris, Plastazote or Orthoplast.

Passive movements are started early and active use of the hand encouraged as recovery takes place. Play involving the use of two hands together, clap hands, finger play, holding a ball or toy, should be assisted if necessary, as soon as the child would normally be expected to do so (about six months), so that normal sensory development should not be lost.

RESPIRATORY CONDITIONS

These form a large part of the physiotherapist's work with children. Although the structure and function of the respiratory tract are similar to those of the adult, the fact that the lungs are so small increases the danger of the infant quickly developing severe respiratory distress. Consideration of the size and age of the patient also suggests variations of treatment in presentation and technique, even though basic principles remain the same.

NEONATAL RESPIRATORY PROBLEMS

Premature, low birth-weight and other very sick infants may be cared for in special units in regional centres or large hospitals. Many of these babies have respiratory problems which will at some stage require physiotherapy. Work in such a unit is highly specialised, and it is necessary to be acquainted with local procedures and to work closely with the medical and nursing staff.

It is possible for infants to survive from the age of 26 weeks' gestation and with birth weights below 1000 grams. Their special requirements are:

1. *Minimum handling*: Small, premature and very sick infants respond badly to handling, and will show signs of apnoea, bradycardia and cyanosis.
2. *Warmth*: Babies lose heat very rapidly because of their relatively large surface area.
3. *Oxygen*: Immature or damaged lungs may require an increased supply of oxygen. It is important that this should be adequate but *not* in excess of requirements. High levels of oxygen for long periods can damage the baby's eyes.
4. *Ventilation*: The premature baby may be physiologically unable to maintain respiration without mechanical assistance. Low birth-weight and other sick babies may also need to be ventilated.
5. *Feeding*: By intravenous catheter or by nasojejunal or nasogastric tube. In the latter case physiotherapy should be given before feeds; continuous tube feeds should be discontinued and the stomach aspirated before treatment, with the contents being returned to the stomach afterwards.
6. *Constant observation and monitoring*: It is essential that any change in condition is noted so that deterioration or improvement may be acted upon immediately.

Equipment

There is a large amount of equipment which must be confusing for anyone entering the unit for the first time.

1. *Incubators* enable infants to be nursed and observed in a constant warm and humid atmosphere with minimum disturbance.
2. *Ventilators* are required by many of the babies. Intermittent positive pressure ventilation (IPPV) may be used initially progressing to continuous positive airways pressure (CPAP) as the infant begins to initiate his own respirations.

3. *Oxygen* may be administered via the incubator, sometimes into a headbox if it is necessary to maintain a high concentration. Oxygen can also be given directly into the endotracheal tube through the ventilator or via nasal prongs when using CPAP.

4. *Suction apparatus and catheters* must always be ready for use. The size of catheters used in these infants is usually number 6, 8, or 10.

5. *Monitors* come in many shapes and sizes and are used to record ECG, heart rate, blood pressure, respiratory rate, temperature, oxygen concentration in the incubator and levels of oxygen in the blood. When the machinery is available the latter is measured using a transcutaneous electrode which gives a continuous reading of tP_{CO_2}.

Apnoea alarms may be in use either in the form of a highly sensitive pad on which baby lies or a disc electrode attached to his chest. In either case the alarm sounds if the baby ceases to breathe for more than the pre-set number of seconds.

It is important to note the readings on monitors before, during and after treatment. For this age-group normal heart rate is about 150 per minute. Normal respiratory rate is 50–60 per minute, but may rise to over 80.

Physiotherapy

In spite of the difficulties it is possible for physiotherapy to make an effective contribution in suitable cases. The most common of these are:

1. Chest infection with increased secretions.
2. Increased secretions following prolonged intubation.
3. Collapse of lung due to mucus plug or aspiration of feed.
4. Meconium aspiration.

Before commencing treatment it is important to check that all necessary equipment, e.g. gloves, catheters, suction apparatus, is to hand and in working order.

Techniques must be adapted to each baby's condition. *Postural drainage* may not be tolerated if the baby is very sick. In any case it is rarely possible to treat more than two areas at any one treatment. *Tipping* can be accomplished by winding the tray of the incubator up or down. *Percussion* is possible using three fingers of one hand and supporting the chest with the other. As an alternative a small Bennett mask may be used for percussion, which must be given firmly enough to influence underlying tissues. *Vibrations* using two or three fingers with pressure on expiration can be effective in clearing secretions. It is quite easy to do this in time with the ventilator. If not ventilated the baby's respiratory rate may be high – the vibrations can then be given on every second or third expiration. In some units the padded head of an electric toothbrush may be used to give vibrations by nursing or physiotherapy staff.

SUCTION

The removal of secretions is an important part of treatment and may be required before, during and after physiotherapy, as well as at other times. It is most important to acquire a good technique in order to minimise the almost inevitable damage caused by introducing a catheter into the delicately lined airways. There is need to be aware of the dangers of both inadequate and over-enthusiastic use.

Secretions may be removed from the nasopharynx via the nostril, or from the oropharynx via the mouth. Before suction 0.5ml of normal saline may be instilled into the endotracheal tube. Suction should only be applied during withdrawal of the catheter, which should be the largest size that can be introduced with ease. When suctioning through the endotracheal tube it must be borne in mind that the catheter will, in effect, fill the airway, and speed is essential so that the child can breathe. Suction pressure should be no higher than 50cm H_2O (5kPa).

Instructions for positioning and turning babies between physiotherapy sessions should be worked out with the nursing staff, together with the times of treatment.

BRONCHIOLITIS

Bronchiolitis is an acute viral infection occurring in infants, especially in their first year.

It is characterised by bronchiolar obstruction due to oedema and mucus accumulation. This results in coughing, wheezing and dyspnoea. The respiratory rate is greatly increased, often to more than twice normal, which for a sleeping baby is 30 per minute. In severe cases the baby is limp and pale and may be cyanosed. Immediate complications include cardiac or respiratory failure and broncho-pneumonia.

Treatment

Nursing care and observation are of the utmost importance. The baby frequently requires oxygen and sometimes humidity. The upper airways must be kept clear by the careful use of suction. In the acute stage any disturbance causes further coughing, increased oedema and obstruction, so handling of the baby is kept to a minimum.

Physiotherapy is not indicated. It may be useful at a later stage if the condition does not resolve, e.g. if there is collapse of part of the lungs.

PNEUMONIA

Pneumonia is fairly common in childhood.

Bronchopneumonia

Bronchopneumonia is often preceded by an upper respiratory tract infection and may be a complication of infectious diseases such as measles and whooping cough.

Aspiration pneumonia follows inhalation of food or vomit.

SIGNS AND SYMPTOMS

Cough, fever and a raised respiratory rate are usually found.

Crepitations may be heard on listening to the chest.

A plug of mucus may block one of the smaller bronchi, resulting in collapse of the lung tissue beyond. This area of collapse can be seen on the radiograph.

Lobar pneumonia

This is a more acute condition and results from bacterial infection by the *Pneumococcus*.

SIGNS AND SYMPTOMS

There is a sharp rise in temperature accompanied by coughing, rapid shallow breathing and often pain in the chest. The chest pain is sometimes referred to the abdomen, simulating appendicitis. Consolidation of the whole or part of the lobe may follow the inflammatory reaction to infection. The consolidated area may be easily recognised on the chest radiograph.

Treatment

In the acute stage the treatment is by drugs and, if necessary, the administration of oxygen.

In the subacute and chronic stages, where there is obstruction of the bronchi, collapse or consolidation, postural drainage with vibrations, percussion or breathing exercises as appropriate are given to assist expectoration and so clear the bronchial passages and to increase air entry.

It may be necessary to give physiotherapy to babies in their incubators. When their condition permits, more effective treatment can be given if they are able to lie on a pillow on the physiotherapist's lap.

As already mentioned, mechanical suction should be available for use if necessary. The technique requires experience, skill and great care in order to avoid damaging the delicate membranes lining the respiratory passages.

In older children postural and mobility exercises may help to improve their general condition where this is poor following prolonged illness.

INHALATION OF A FOREIGN BODY

Inhalation of a foreign body is a common cause of collapse of lung tissue in children. One commonly inhaled object is a peanut, which because of its oily texture is not only difficult to shift, but causes irritation of the lung tissue. Other items include small beads, bits of plastic toys, as well as teeth or fragments of tonsil following operation for their removal.

SIGNS AND SYMPTOMS

These may follow a specific incident when the child was seen to choke and cough. Alternatively, there may be no known history and the symptoms are noticed over a period. The child may appear quite well, but has a persistent cough and is often breathless on exertion. There may be obvious diminution of movement on one side of the chest, and a dull note on percussion indicating diminished air entry.

Radiographs are always a necessary part of diagnosis in chest conditions. In this case they will demonstrate the area of collapse and/or indicate the position of the foreign body.

Treatment

Foreign bodies must be removed by bronchoscopy. Often no further treatment is necessary. If the affected area does not re-expand spontaneously, physiotherapy may be given as for lobe collapse.

BRONCHIECTASIS

CAUSES

This chronic condition of dilatation of the smaller bronchi may follow any prolonged or repeated chest infection, particularly if there has been blocking of one of the larger bronchi by a plug of mucus or a foreign body. A congenital weakness of the walls of the bronchi may be a predisposing factor. The small bronchi become over-stretched by the accumulation of secretions, which become thicker and more infected. The elasticity of their walls is lost as well as the sensitivity of the tissues lining them. Eventually the walls of the bronchi collapse, forming cavities filled with thick sticky purulent material.

SIGNS AND SYMPTOMS

Bouts of coughing occur, often, but not always, producing purulent sputum, greenish in colour and foul-smelling. These may be precipitated by a change of posture which causes the secretions in the lungs to move into contact with healthy tissue and stimulate the cough reflex. This is often apparent when the child goes to bed or when he wakes in the morning.

In the long-standing cases there may be clubbing of the fingers and even of the toes.

The child is often thin and small for his age.

Diagnosis is confirmed by a bronchogram which demonstrates the dilation of the bronchi. With improved child health care and treatment of the causative conditions by modern drugs, bronchiectasis is now uncommon in the United Kingdom.

Treatment

MEDICAL TREATMENT

This includes the control of infection by antibiotic drugs and investigation into the cause of the condition, e.g. the exclusion of cystic fibrosis.

SURGICAL TREATMENT

If the condition is limited to a well-defined area, lobectomy or partial lobectomy offers a good prognosis. The healthy remainder of the lung quickly expands to fill the space created by removal of the infected part and normal function is restored.

PHYSIOTHERAPY

The principal aim of treatment is drainage of the affected area. Therefore the physiotherapist must know the exact site of the lesion and the appropriate drainage positions (Fig. 22/10).

Postural drainage, percussion, shaking and vibrations, and breathing exercises are used to facilitate coughing and expectoration. Sputum should be collected and measured each day. If there has been little or no sputum prior to treatment the amount may increase in the first day or two, but should then gradually decrease in quantity, becoming thinner, clearer and less purulent.

Some adaptations of treatment for babies are given on pages 383–4.

CYSTIC FIBROSIS

Cystic fibrosis is a disorder of the exocrine glands. The mucous secretions are abnormally viscid and tend to block the ducts of the glands, thus preventing the proper function of the organ as a whole. Lungs and pancreas are affected as well as the sweat glands, which secrete an excessive amount of salt.

CAUSE

The condition is inherited by an autosomal recessive gene, which if carried by both parents gives a one in four chance of a child being affected.

SIGNS AND SYMPTOMS

In its early months the baby may suffer from malabsorption, due to the lack of pancreatic secretions, and fail to thrive.

He is underweight and may pass a large number of pale, bulky and unpleasant smelling stools.

He is particularly prone to chest infections which do not resolve and frequently progress to a condition similar to bronchiectasis. Formerly these chest infections would prove fatal before the child reached his teens.

DIAGNOSIS

Diagnosis is made from analysis of sweat which contains an abnormally high proportion of chloride and sodium.

Treatment

Early diagnosis and treatment with the administration of pancreatin and other drugs, and attention to diet now makes the prognosis less gloomy. Particular care is needed to avoid respiratory infections and to provide immediate treatment when they do occur.

Chest physiotherapy plays a vital part and should be started in infancy. All areas of the lungs should be drained and coughing encouraged in order to clear the respiratory passages. This should become a daily routine at home, and increased to three or four times a day when there are signs of developing chest infection. It is therefore important to teach the parents to carry out the technique, and for older children to learn to perform their own postural drainage and breathing exercises.

ASTHMA

Asthma is a common condition characterised by spasmodic episodes of wheezing and breathlessness. Severe attacks may be prolonged and are known as 'status asthmaticus'.

CAUSE

Allergy is the most common cause. There may be sensitivity to the house dust mite, feathers, pollens, some foods and dust in the coats of animals. The house dust mite is a minute organism found in most normal situations but particularly in woollen blankets, carpets, etc.

In many cases there is a family history of asthma or hay fever. Acute attacks of asthma may be provoked by respiratory infection. A psychological factor is sometimes present; the degree of this varies in different individuals.

Irritation of the mucous membrane lining the smaller bronchi results in it becoming oedematous and therefore narrows the lumen of the bronchi. Further narrowing occurs from spasm of muscle in the walls of the bronchi. Air and secretions become trapped in the areas beyond the obstruction.

SIGNS AND SYMPTOMS

Some children appear normal between acute attacks, others have an almost permanent mild wheeze. Most asthmatics quickly become wheezy or breathless on exercise.

Acute attacks often occur at night or in the early morning. They may commence suddenly or build up slowly, with wheezing and a hard dry cough. The child feels unable to breathe and uses his accessory muscles of respiration to try to get more air into his lungs, but has difficulty in breathing out. The chest is held stiffly in the position of inspiration. Initially no permanent changes occur, the chest returning to normal between attacks. In time the lungs tend to remain hyperinflated, the chest and shoulder girdle rigid.

Asthma and eczema are often found in the same patient, one deteriorating as the other improves. In severe cases appetite and general health are often poor. The child looks pale, small and underweight but may be of high intelligence.

The degree of airway obstruction can be measured with a Wright's peak flow meter. Regular recording of the peak expiratory flow rate, (PEFR) may be used to assess the severity of the condition.

Treatment

Medical treatment can be divided into (1) that which is given during an acute attack and (2) long-term prophylaxis.

IN THE ACUTE PHASE

In an acute attack bronchodilators may be administered orally, intravenously or by inhalation. Salbutamol and aminophylline are the most commonly used. The easiest way to inhale salbutamol (Ventolin) is from a nebuliser. This treatment takes about 20 minutes and is repeated four-hourly until the attack subsides. The effectiveness is measured by peak flow readings taken before and 20 minutes after the inhalation. Nebulisers are sometimes prescribed for use at home under parental supervision, thus reducing the need for hospital admissions. Salbutamol can also be inhaled from an aerosol spray (Medihaler), but as accurate timing is necessary to release the spray and inhale at the same time, this method is only suitable for older children who can co-ordinate this. If the attack is severe or prolonged, steroids may be given.

PROPHYLAXIS

Prophylactic treatment with sodium cromoglycate (Intal) in a spinhaler is often successful in reducing the number of asthmatic attacks. Intal acts by reducing the sensitivity of the lungs, so it is important that it is used regularly, (usually three or four times a day) even though the child is well. Becotide, a locally acting steroid, from an aerosol may be used in a similar manner. Both aerosol and spinhaler require considerable skill and co-operation from the child and are therefore unsuitable for the very young.

OTHER ASPECTS OF MANAGEMENT

As many children are allergic to dust and feathers, bedding, pillows and furnishings should be of synthetic materials; these should be washed, shaken or vacuumed frequently. The child should not be in the room while bedmaking or dusting take place.

The child should be treated as normally as possible, attending school and partaking in whatever activities he can. Occasionally it may be necessary to impose restrictions on competitive sports or those requiring sustained physical effort.

Physiotherapy

1. In the acute phase, active treatment is not indicated. The child should be comfortably supported with pillows under his head and shoulders either in a half-lying or side-sitting position. If those around him are calm and confident, this will be communicated to the child and will help him to relax. If he has been taught diaphragmatic breathing, it may be helpful to practise this after nebulisation or other medication.

2. In the subacute phase of an attack, postural drainage and breathing exercises may assist in removing secretions from the lungs and encourage effective coughing. This is of particular importance when the attack has been exacerbated by respiratory infection.

3. Where complete control by medication is not being achieved, some children can be helped by learning relaxation, diaphragmatic breathing and general mobility exercises. This can help to minimise the development of the typical posture and barrel chest deformity. Mild wheezes can sometimes be controlled by positioning and relaxation; parents are more confident if they can help their children in this way and are able to institute postural drainage for those children prone to chest infections.

4. Instruction and supervision of the use of Intal or other inhalers may be undertaken by the physiotherapist. Before using the Intal spincap which contains a fine powder, the child should first learn to take a deep breath in while maintaining a good lip seal round the mouthpiece; he should remember to remove the spinhaler from the mouth before breathing out. When the spincap is introduced the child may complain of some discomfort as the powder strikes the back of the throat, and he will need encouragement to continue. A whistling device can be attached to the spinhaler which is popular with some children. With practice it is possible to empty the spincap in two or three attempts. Manufacturer's instructions are provided with each spinhaler, and are a useful reminder to parents of its correct preparation, use and maintenance.

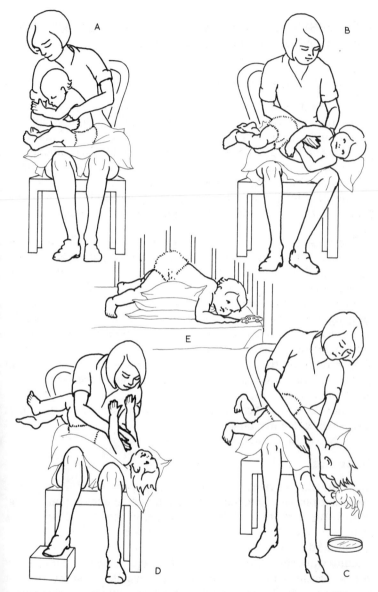

Fig. 22/10   Postural drainage for babies. A. Apical segments of the upper lobes.
B. Right middle lobe. C. Posterior segment of the lower lobes. D. Anterior segments of
the lower lobes. E. Draining the posterior segments of the lower lobes by lying over
pillows in the cot

SUGGESTIONS FOR CHEST PHYSIOTHERAPY FOR BABIES AND YOUNG CHILDREN

Postural drainage (Fig. 22/10)

This is most easily done with the baby lying on a pillow on the physiotherapist's lap (Fig. 22/10A,B). The baby feels comfortable and secure and can lie in the prone, supine, side- or half-side-lying positions with additional support provided by the physiotherapist's hands on his chest. The physiotherapist should sit on a low chair so that she can regulate the degree of tip by moving her knees. In Figure 22/10D) she achieves this by having her right foot on a low platform; in (C) she produces the same effect by extending her left knee.

Thus, all areas of the lung can be drained with minimum disturbance. If possible, the baby should be positioned so that his face can be seen, so that his colour can be checked frequently. A toy unbreakable mirror can be useful if arranged so that the physiotherapist, and the baby, can see his reflection, particularly when draining the posterior segments of lower lobes. Other toys, mobiles, or musical boxes may also be arranged to hold the attention of toddlers who are often happier treated on the lap, but still tend to get restless. They can, of course, also be tipped over pillows and are often found afterwards administering the treatment they have received to their favourite doll or teddy.

Details of the correct drainage positions for each area of the lungs are shown in the diagrams.

'Exercises'

It is quite easy to give vibrations and shaking in time with the baby's natural expiration. Toddlers will often imitate sounds and may 'sing' Ah-Ah-Ah while their chests are clapped or vibrated. Laughing is good exercise and if not too ill, most babies enjoy being tickled and encouraged to use their arms, by grasping the physiotherapist's thumbs while she performs 'circles' or 'hugging and stretching'. They quickly learn to participate; and so help to maintain mobility of chest and shoulder girdle, which can become quite stiff even in very young children.

All children love bubbles and blowing them is often a good introduction to the very young as well as helping to overcome the fears of many slightly older children, who may be away from home for the first time and view any new face or treatment with apprehension. Bubble-blowing requires little effort and therefore does not cause tension in the muscles of the throat or chest – even if the child does not blow them he enjoys watching and will reach out to catch them and a great deal of activity can be stimulated in this way.

Fat, lethargic babies are sometimes 'chesty' and may benefit from a spell in the baby bouncer. The activity improves their general musculature as well as increasing the rate and depth of respiration.

Simple direct breathing exercises should be commenced as soon as it is possible to get the child's co-operation. This varies from about the age of two years to four or even five years. The easiest starting positions are side lying or supine with knees bent. The child's hands rest over his diaphragm and he feels his 'tummy get smaller as the air goes away' and larger as he fills up again with air. This can then be repeated with hands on the lower ribs.

BIBLIOGRAPHY

Batten, J. (1975). Cystic fibrosis in adolescents and adults. *Physiotherapy*, **61**, 8.

Carter, C. O. (1975). Genetics and incidence of cystic fibrosis. *Physiotherapy*, **61**, 8.

Collins, J. V. (1983). *Clinical Aspects of Medical Chest Disease*, 1 and 2. Chapters in *Cash's Chest, Heart and Vascular Disorders for Physiotherapists*, 3rd edition, (ed Downie, P. A.). Faber and Faber, London.

Davis, A. J. (1983). *Medical Chest Physiotherapy*, 1 and 2. Chapters in *Cash's Chest, Heart and Vascular Disorders for Physiotherapists*, 3rd edition, (ed Downie, P. A.). Faber and Faber, London.

Ellis, R. W. B. and Mitchell, R. G. (1973). *Disease in Infancy and Childhood*, 7th edition. Churchill Livingstone, Edinburgh.

Gaskell, D. (1977). Physiotherapy for adolescents and adults with cystic fibrosis. *Physiotherapy*, **61**, 8.

Gaskell, D. V. and Webber, B. A. (1980). *The Brompton Hospital Guide to Chest Physiotherapy*, 4th edition. Blackwell Scientific Publications Limited, Oxford.

Hodge, G. J. (1975). Physiotherapy for children with cystic fibrosis. *Physiotherapy*, **61**, 8.

Holzel, A. (1975). The quest for the basic defect in cystic fibrosis. *Physiotherapy*, **61**, 8.

Jones, R. S. (1976). *Asthma in Children*. Edward Arnold (Publishers) Limited, London.

McCrae, W. M. (1975). Emotional problems in cystic fibrosis. *Physiotherapy*, **61**, 8.

Mearns, M. B. (1975). Inhalation therapy in cystic fibrosis. *Physiotherapy*, **61**, 8.

Norman, A. P. (1975). Medical management of cystic fibrosis. *Physiotherapy*, **61**, 8.

Robertson, N. R. C. (1981). *A Manual of Neonatal Intensive Care*. Edward Arnold (Publishers) Limited, London.

Scrutton, D. and Gilbertson, M. P. (1975). *Physiotherapy in Paediatric Practice*. Butterworths, London.

Shepherd, R. (1980). *Physiotherapy in Paediatrics*, 2nd edition. William Heinemann Medical Books Limited, London.

Chapter 23

Childhood Handicap

by B. KENNEDY, MCSP

WHAT IS A HANDICAP?

A handicap has been described as 'a disability which for a substantial period or permanently, retards, distorts or otherwise adversely affects normal growth, development or adjustment to life' (Younghusband et al, 1970).

Blindness, deafness, mental handicap, cerebral palsy, spina bifida and progressive diseases of the muscular and nervous systems are among the most obvious handicapping conditions, but other disabilities such as cystic fibrosis, Still's disease, pathological clumsiness and perceptual difficulties may also handicap a child in competition with his non-affected peers.

Although the first part of this chapter is concerned with conditions resulting in handicap it must always be remembered that it is the *child* that has the handicap not the reverse. The second part deals with the child, his family, care and management.

TYPES OF HANDICAP

Although the terms mental handicap and physical handicap are in common use the diagnosis may not always be clear cut. Particularly in the young infant continued observation and assessment may be necessary to discover where the greatest needs lie. Children with gross motor and intellectual disability are often referred to as multiply handicapped. At the other end of the scale less severe disabilities may present major obstacles in a family with high expectations in a particular direction, for example the child with mild diplegia will appear more handicapped in a family of keen athletes than in one whose interests lie in more academic pursuits.

Mental handicap

In recent years attitudes to mental handicap have changed, and are still changing. As the general public becomes better informed and as services for mentally handicapped people improve, their integration into society becomes more accepted.

A child whose intellectual ability is below normal for his age and is likely to remain so as he gets older can be described as mentally handicapped. This may be due to inadequate or abnormal development of brain cells in the area affecting intelligence, or to damage incurred in the course of development. The 1981 Education Act recognises the special needs of all children with learning difficulties. Implementation of the Act in 1983 introduces a new classification of special educational provision. Assessment for education is now based on the child's special needs rather than on categories of handicap. Special education and training which meet their needs may enable many children to live full and interesting lives and to acquire some degree of independence. The profoundly handicapped will continue to need full support services.

Although damage to brain or nerve cells cannot be repaired some improvement can be anticipated in the majority of cases if suitable help can be provided, preferably early in life. Intelligence is only one aspect to be considered, and personality and behaviour are equally important factors in the making of a happy, well-adjusted child who is able to take his place among his family and friends. It is therefore always necessary to consider the whole child and not just those parts of him considered to be in need of treatment. Patience, loving care and consistent, but firm, handling are of even greater importance in the management of the handicapped than in the 'normal' child.

CAUSES

Even after thorough investigation it is not always possible to find the cause of mental handicap. Environmental factors may play a contributory role in some cases of mild handicap, e.g. poor home conditions, dull parents, lack of stimulation. Such cases may show considerable improvement given help and encouragement for their material and intellectual needs.

In severe mental handicap there is little evidence of any environmental or class distinction – all being equally vulnerable.

Where specific causes can be identified they may be considered under antenatal, perinatal and postnatal.

1. *Antenatal causes*: The abnormality occurs before birth but is not

always immediately apparent. The cause may be genetic or may relate to maternal conditions in pregnancy. Some genetically determined conditions are recognisable at birth, one of these is the chromosome abnormality of Down's syndrome. This is the most common cause of severe mental handicap in children. The defect is due to an extra chromosome which increases the normal number of 46 to 47. The child is often the youngest of several and there are seldom more than one in the same family. Such children are easily recognised at birth by their typical facial appearance, broad and flattened with small nose and slanting eyes; the tongue may appear too large for the rather small mouth. Hands and feet are broad and short; frequently the terminal phalanx of the little finger is in-curved and a single deep crease runs right across the palm (simian crease).

There is generalised hypotonia with hypermobility of the joints. Milestones are always delayed and speech may remain infantile and difficult to understand. A large number suffer from congenital heart defects and a high proportion of these do not survive early childhood; usually they succumb to repeated respiratory infections. In general they are happy, sociable children, fond of music and anxious to join in all that goes on. The range of intelligence varies greatly among this group. The more intelligent children become independent in self-care and can learn simple repetitive work. Others remain severely subnormal.

Causes not associated with genetic factors include:
1. Maternal infections during pregnancy, e.g. rubella, cytomegalovirus, toxoplasmosis.
2. Certain drugs taken by the mother.
3. Alcohol taken in excess during pregnancy.
4. Exposure to x-ray irradiation.

2. *Perinatal causes*: Brain damage may occur due to lack of oxygen during a difficult birth. In the period immediately after birth pre-term or low birth-weight babies may have respiratory problems or suffer from other conditions which reduce the supply of oxygen to the brain, causing permanent damage to brain cells.

3. *Postnatal causes*: Postnatal brain damage can result from injury or disease. Serious head injuries from falls, road traffic accidents or from non-accidental injury may result in permanent brain damage. Meningitis, encephalitis, metallic poisoning and severe dehydration in infants, may be also responsible for mental handicap in previously normal children.

EARLY SIGNS AND SYMPTOMS

Many babies appear normal until they start to fall behind in their physical development. Smiling is frequently delayed. These children are often poor feeders, making little effort to suck, and in due course resisting the introduction of solid foods. The general muscle tone is often low and they lie passively in their cots, taking little notice of their surroundings. Alternatively some are irritable and restless with a high-pitched cry which is difficult to calm.

Infants are slow to make eye contact and fail to smile and respond to stimulation at the expected time. They are disinterested in people and do not attempt to grab toys or to hold on to toys placed in their hands. At a later stage some children may show a superficial brightness which may initially be interpreted as intelligence until it becomes evident that the smile is too fixed and automatic to be meaningful and there is little constructive play at an age-appropriate level.

Most subnormal children lag behind because they lack the drive and inquisitiveness to investigate and try out new channels of activity; thus they never experience those things normal to a child of their age and so they fall even further behind. As they get older they have a strong tendency to repeat the same action, or sound, or word, over and over again (perseveration). They dislike change and easily develop set patterns of behaviour which are hard to break, like sitting and rocking, or various mannerisms of the hands. Drooling is also common even when there appears to be no physical reason for it.

Initially it may be difficult to distinguish between mental and physical handicaps (cerebral palsy, deafness, defects of vision). An accurate diagnosis may only be possible after prolonged observation. Delay in social responses and motor behaviour and the exclusion of other handicaps indicates the likelihood of mental subnormality.

PHYSICAL HANDICAP

Cerebral palsy

Cerebral palsy is a common but very complex condition, treatment of which is a specialty in its own right and is fully described in *Cash's Textbook of Neurology for Physiotherapists* (1982). It is due to damage or maldevelopment of the brain before, during, or soon after, birth. There can be many reasons for this, including intra-uterine anoxia, birth asphyxia and prematurity; the initial cause is not always known.

SIGNS AND SYMPTOMS

It should be remembered that the lesion is irreversible and non-progressive; the manifestations of damage may change as the brain and nervous system mature. Quality and variety of movement are always affected. Balance may be poor and position sense is often defective. Young babies may have difficulty in sucking. Usually they are floppy (hypotonic) in infancy but very severe cases may be stiff (spastic or hypertonic) from the beginning. Later, floppy babies may develop either spasticity or athetosis (involuntary movements). Ataxia, a disturbance of co-ordination, is occasionally seen, and is sometimes found in conjunction with hypotonia or with spasticity.

Deformities may result from unequal pull of spastic muscles; the most common deformities are equinus of the ankle, adduction/flexion of the hip, and flexion of the knee. In the upper limb flexion of elbow, wrist and fingers with pronation of the forearm may become a fixed deformity.

Associated problems may include those of hearing, speech, vision, perception, intellectual impairment and fits.

The severity of the symptoms can vary from mild disability with little interference of normal activities to major handicap, where virtually no useful movement is possible.

TREATMENT

It is generally accepted that some advice or treatment should be given early and that parents should quickly become involved (see p. 398). The selection and extent of specialised treatment will depend on the age and condition of the child, resources of the family, and of the services available.

In brief the following points about the different methods of treatment are important:

(a) The student is advised to acquire some practical experience and understanding of the condition before seeking deeper theoretical knowledge.

(b) Many workers may be involved in the management of the cerebral palsied child, e.g. doctors, speech therapists, occupational therapists, teachers, nurses, and social workers as well as the physiotherapist and of course the parents. It is vital that there should be close liaison and frequent discussion between them.

(c) It is characteristic of cerebral palsy that signs and symptoms can vary in different situations. Where spasticity or involuntary movements are present they are likely to be more marked when the child is excited, tired or self-conscious. Treatment must be adapted to the child as he is at the moment, not the child to the treatment.

(d) It follows that keen observation and continual assessment are an essential basis for treatment.

(d) With experience the physiotherapist may learn to foresee and sometimes forestall future problems.

Spina bifida

A more detailed account of this condition is given in *Cash's Textbook of Neurology for Physiotherapists* (1982). As it is one of the commonest physical handicaps at present found in children of school age, some of the basic points are also included here.

Maldevelopment of the vertebrae and spinal cord may occur at any level but is most frequent in the lower dorsal or lumbar region. The cause is unknown but there may be a genetic element.

SIGNS AND SYMPTOMS

Involvement of the spinal cord in the swelling (myelocele or meningomyelocele) which protrudes through the open arch of the vertebrae produces a mainly flaccid paralysis below the level of the lesion, though some spasticity may also be present. In addition there is severe sensory loss, the implications of which must be continually borne in mind. The greatest care must be taken when moving on rough surfaces or near heaters (radiators) as well as seeing that clothing, calipers or toys do not cause friction or undue pressure.

The degree of involvement of the lower trunk and legs depends on the level and severity of the lesion. In high lesions the whole trunk and upper limbs may be affected to some degree.

COMPLICATIONS

1. Hydrocephalus is frequently present and it appears soon after birth. If a valve has been inserted there is the possibility of it becoming blocked. Physiotherapists and parents should be aware of this and report signs of drowsiness or vomiting to the doctor or surgeon at once.

2. Deformities may be present at birth or may occur later if muscle tension is not balanced. Unopposed flexors and adductors of the hip joint quite often cause subluxation or dislocation of this joint.

3. Urinary incontinence predisposes to skin inflammation and chronic urinary infection; absence of bowel control is a major problem – (but the danger of infection is absent).

4. Fractures are liable to occur particularly following immobilisa-

tion in plaster. Where possible weight-bearing and full activity should be encouraged so as to maintain, as far as possible, the circulation and stimulation of bone growth.

TREATMENT

Early management is again important and is directed towards giving maximum normal experience, developing what muscle potential is available and obtaining independent mobility as soon as possible. If the child's condition permits, calipers for walking may be fitted between the ages of one and two years. The motivation to get about unaided is strong at this age. Unfortunately this is not always possible and in any case achievement comes slowly, so it may be desirable to keep alive the spark of independence, by using some other means of mobility, e.g. the Shasbah trolley or a junior wheelchair. Various aids are available for walking. When possible walking exercises should be objective, i.e. the child should learn to walk as a means of getting from place to place, not merely as an exercise performed only in the physiotherapy department.

The clumsy child

At first sight the clumsy child may appear to be minimally handicapped, but a more discerning examination may reveal very real difficulties in gross and/or fine motor activities, together with perceptual sensory and proprioceptive deficiencies. It is a fact that the absence of an obvious disability often deprives the child of any understanding and sympathy with his problems from parents, teachers and play fellows.

SIGNS AND SYMPTOMS

Diagnosis is unlikely before school age because of the wide variation of normal in the pre-school child.

Neurological signs may not be present although a few children with minor degrees of cerebral palsy may in addition have the same type of perceptual problems.

Children may be referred to the physiotherapist because of the following:

Poor balance
Frequent falls
Poor posture and general 'weakness'
Difficulties going up/down stairs
Clumsy hands and fingers.

These children may find it difficult or be unable to:

Kick or catch a ball
Dress themselves, especially putting on pants or trousers
Manage buttons and laces
Manipulate a pencil, etc.

In school, problems may arise in copying shapes or designs (therefore in learning to write), recognising shapes (learning to read), copying positions or movements (in PE) or distinguishing left from right.

The child may be labelled lazy, inattentive, easily distracted or stupid. In fact, the child may try hard to please and become frustrated by repeated failure and if not recognised this may lead to behaviour problems.

Further investigations may show that body image and body awareness are poor and this may include:

Difficulties in finger recognition
Difficulties in co-ordinating both sides of the body
Difficulties of balance reactions, particularly if sight is excluded
Difficulty in judging distance and direction.

TREATMENT

The treatment programme combines sensory stimulation, body awareness, balance and perceptual training. In some units this is planned by the physiotherapists and occupational therapists working closely together; the occupational therapists undertake perceptual training, the physiotherapists the motor development.

The child's difficulties should be discussed with him so that he can understand the reasons for treatment. If the parents are present during the initial investigations, they too will be able to see where the problems lie. Careful explanation as to how help may be given may relieve tension and pressure on the child both from school and home routine. Allowing a little extra time may enable the child to become more independent and less frustrated. Dressing can be made easier by using Velcro fastening, until the child becomes more skilful in managing buttons and laces; elastic at the waist of shorts or skirt, or slip-on shoes. Games can be adapted so that the child is able to participate at his own level, or to help to develop or practise new skills.

Hypotonia in infants and young children

DIFFERENTIAL DIAGNOSIS

Some babies and young children are referred to physiotherapy for assessment of hypotonia or delayed development. Some possible reasons have already been discussed (social deprivation, mental handicap, cerebral palsy). Two other main groups of conditions which should also be kept in mind are the myopathies and muscular dystrophies (see Bibliography).

Spinal muscular atrophy (Werdnig Hoffman disease) may be present at birth or may only become apparent some weeks or months later. In the severe form all muscles are extremely weak, particularly the respiratory muscles. Less severe cases may be floppy but capable of some movement, although respiratory problems are still likely.

Signs and symptoms of muscular dystrophy do not usually cause problems before the age of three or four years, though parents may remark that the child has always been slow or floppy. The two main physical diagnostic signs are the child's inability to rise from the floor to standing without using his hands to 'walk up his legs' (Gowers' sign), and his firm, apparently overdeveloped, calf muscles. This is due to muscle being replaced by fibrous tissue which tends to contract causing the child to walk on tip toe.

ADDITIONAL HANDICAPS

Other disabilities which have an increased incidence in association with physical and mental handicap include epilepsy; sensory defects; communication problems and behaviour disorders.

Epilepsy

Epilepsy is not a disease: it is a transitory disturbance of brain function giving rise to seizures. Attacks are due to a sudden neuronal discharge, the duration of which may vary, which usually ceases spontaneously. Epilepsy is found at all levels of intelligence but the incidence is higher in the severely mentally handicapped.

There are many types of seizures ranging from those where there is loss of consciousness, incontinence, tongue biting and stiffness followed by jerky movements of the whole body (tonic clonic attacks (grand mal)) to akinetic drop attacks lasting only a few seconds. In the latter there is sudden momentary loss of tone and the child drops to the floor but recovers instantly and continues as if nothing had happened. Protective helmets may be supplied to children who have frequent attacks. Infantile spasms or 'salaam' attacks may appear in infants known to be brain damaged, and sometimes in those with no previous history. In either case the prognosis for future mental development is poor. The attacks are brief but often frequent, and present as a sudden total flexion of the body; when they first occur they may be confused with colic pain.

Absence attacks may last only seconds and do not cause the child to fall. They may be mistaken for inattention unless accurately observed. Physiotherapists should be alert to the possibility of these attacks when working with children who have problems with learning and concentration. Careful observation and accurate reporting of the details of attacks can assist the paediatrician in their management. Although not a cause of brain damage in the first instance, continuing, uncontrolled seizures can result in further cerebral deterioration.

It is known that seizures can be precipitated by infections, emotional upsets and flashing lights (e.g. the television screen), therefore management may include avoidance of the latter and early treatment of infections with antibiotics. The anticonvulsant drugs most commonly used are phenytoin, sodium valproate and clonazepam. Good control of seizures is sometimes difficult to achieve, but when it is, regular administration of the prescribed dose is essential for the control to be maintained.

Sensory defects

It is not surprising that children who have brain damage causing severe mental and/or physical handicap may also suffer other disabilities as a result of damage extending to other parts of the brain. Sight and hearing may be affected singly or in combination.

The child whose only disability is visual or auditory will develop more slowly than the normal child, but will be able to make up for his sight or hearing loss by the use of the senses that remain (hearing, sight, touch, taste, smell). The child whose sight and/or hearing problems are additional to his mental handicap will need very special help and training. Physiotherapists can help parents of young infants by advising on positioning and handling, and choosing suitable toys which will help develop remaining abilities.

Communication problems

Many mentally and physically handicapped children have difficulty in communicating with other people. This places even greater restrictions on their lives and is often the cause of frustration and temper tantrums. Therefore, the establishment of some form of basic communication is necessary for the success of any plan of treatment or management. It should be noted that communication is a two-way process involving the person sending the message and the person receiving it. Breakdown can occur at any level depending on the extent and location of brain damage; one area may be damaged leaving others intact, for example the mentally handicapped child may hear perfectly but not understand speech (though he may understand the tone of voice), while the child with cerebral palsy may be unable to speak or use gesture effectively because of his motor problem, but have good understanding.

Communication is not restricted to speech but can include gesture, signing or the use of symbols. These children benefit from assessment and treatment by a speech therapist who can institute the use of the system most appropriate to the child's abilities and needs. Makaton sign language is used successfully by many mentally and some physically handicapped children before they learn to speak. The signs are reinforced by the spoken word so that both are learnt. In time the child may start to say the word also, confident that the sign, at least, will be understood.

Blissymbolics have been developed for use by the physically disabled who cannot use speech or signing but are able to point to symbols on a chart or electronic board. The system is built up from a core of picture-type symbols and can be expanded to give a wide vocabulary. The symbol has the word written beneath it so that the system can be understood by people with no previous knowledge.

Not all children will learn to talk; some will only be able to use very simple gestures or signs. Others will learn to express complicated and abstract ideas – all will become more friendly, happier and less isolated.

Behaviour disorders

Behaviour disorders are not uncommonly associated with mental handicap, brain damage and epilepsy. The primary cause of behaviour disorders lies in the specific site of brain damage. As an example some cases of infantile or traumatic hemiplegia may be hyperactive, aggressive and have temper tantrums and epileptic seizures. Secondary factors are frequent causes of behaviour disorders: they include rejection by parents and peers, inability to keep up with educational expectations, poor self-image and problems of communication, all of which are likely to cause frustration and difficult behaviour. The absence of a stable environment will tend to exacerbate the situation.

Treatment may include the use of drugs and specific management programmes in which the physiotherapist may be asked to participate. It is therefore important to have adequate knowledge of the aims and methods employed.

HELPING THE HANDICAPPED CHILD

Before making plans it is necessary to consider the individuals who will be involved in carrying them out.

The child cannot be regarded in isolation; he is part of a family and one of his needs is the knowledge that he 'belongs' and has a part to play. If he suffers from a physical disability it is likely that treatment will be an important part of his life at some stage but it should never over-ride the normal needs of childhood.

Children thrive best in a home of their own. Modern practice provides a wide network of support for parents. Short-term respite care can often be arranged so that the family can have a day out or a holiday without the handicapped member. Some voluntary organisations arrange holidays for handicapped children and their families. Where it is inappropriate for the child to remain at home he may be placed in the care of foster parents, in a hostel, home or special school. Every effort is made to involve parents in seeking a suitable placement and to support them through this decision. Where desirable, regular contact is maintained between child and family.

It is inevitable that parents will spend extra time and effort on their disabled child but over-indulgence and spoiling are not in the child's best interest and will make it more difficult for him to adjust to competition with his peers at school or later in the world outside.

The family

On learning the news that their child will be permanently disabled parents are in a state of shock. This may last many months or even years during which time they will need all possible help and understanding as they enter a life of new and unforeseen difficulties. One effect of shock is the inability to absorb information: this means that details of diagnosis and treatment may have to be repeated many times. Parents may suffer from feelings of loss, disappointment and helplessness; they may also feel guilt, rejection and anger; the latter may be directed towards members of the care team. These are normal reactions and should be respected and treated with sympathy and reassurance.

Because of the extra time required for looking after the disabled child brothers and sisters may be almost forgotten and be deprived not only of material needs but of the care and attention to which they were accustomed. It is important that this should be prevented as far as possible and ways found, perhaps by a baby-minding service, for the rest of the family to enjoy itself together.

Grandparents are also part of the family. They may be able to offer valuable assistance to the family by giving either physical or moral support. If they show interest they should be given the opportunity to learn about the condition and/or treatment.

There is evidence to show that it is better for parents to be told the diagnosis as early as possible, that is, as soon as it is confirmed. While this is the task of the doctor and not the physiotherapist, she will find her position easier if she knows in exactly what terms the disability has been described (e.g. whether the words 'spastic', 'cerebral palsy', 'fits', 'mental handicap', etc have been used). Once the diagnosis is known the parents may seek further information about the condition, prognosis, treatment and other available services. Educational facilities are often an early subject for discussion even if it is several years in the future. The physiotherapist may be able to answer some of the questions but will need to refer others to more appropriate sources of information, e.g. the paediatrician, social worker or one of the voluntary societies for specific conditions (see p. 451). These societies offer advice and information, often in booklet form, in addition to opportunities to meet parents of similarly affected children. Some parents may wish to join a society at once – others prefer to wait until they feel less disturbed and more adjusted to the realities of their new situation.

The team approach

Helping the disabled child to achieve his greatest potential and to lead as full a life as possible is likely to involve a large number of people. It requires a team approach, the most important members of the team being the child himself together with his parents. Other members may include health visitors, the family practitioner, hospital doctors, physiotherapists, occupational therapists, speech therapists, orthoptists, community health doctors, social workers, psychologists, nursery staff, teachers and representatives of voluntary organisations; the list seems endless! It is not hard to see how easily parents could be swamped by information, instruction and advice. In practice only a few people are closely involved with the family at any one time.

A named person may be delegated to act as the family's principal contact; this is usually the person most closely involved with the family, whose job it is to co-ordinate the work of other members of the team. It is important that no one works in isolation; there must be opportunities to discuss plans and share knowledge, otherwise much of the work may be unproductive. Good intentions will not replace good communication.

TREATMENT AND MANAGEMENT

All young handicapped children have much in common; because of their disability they are deprived of the opportunity to learn and develop in the normal way. They need help to do this. Help may be initiated in treatment but success or failure depends on how well it can be translated into daily life. Parents play the major part in this for they are the ones to care for the child and must teach him all those things learnt automatically by a normal baby. It can be a long and difficult task.

Looking after a handicapped baby or child can be time consuming, leaving little time for other essential activities, e.g. housework, cooking, shopping, recreation. With this in mind instructions for therapy should be carefully thought out. Until the routine becomes easier and more established it should include only what is most essential. Parents can usefully reinforce physiotherapy sessions by concentrating on correct handling and positioning in normal daily activities such as feeding, bathing, changing and play; this last includes play on mother's or father's lap and play with toys in the cot or on the floor. This method of working makes no extra demands on time and later may actually save time as parents become more proficient and the child improves. Treatment along these lines should be started as early as possible so that the child has the best chance to achieve his maximum potential. Later as child and parent learn to work together, other activities incorporating more specific therapeutic techniques can be introduced.

Some conditions necessitate regular formal physiotherapy from the start; potential deformities must be prevented, splints checked or applied, tight structures stretched or muscles stimulated. Routine chest care may also be essential in some cases.

One of the most difficult things for parents to accept is the fact that it is often impossible to forecast how far their child will develop. It is also sometimes difficult to explain that although there is no cure for the basic condition it is still possible to help the child develop more fully, by the right sort of stimulation, play and general management. Parents will need help from members of the paediatric team (paediatrician, social worker, therapist) to achieve a realistic approach and to persevere in the training of their child. As members of the team, parents should be encouraged to contribute their own observations which may be remarkably astute; much can be learned from listening to their comments.

One characteristic of mentally handicapped children is their difficulty in initiating any activity; they may have adequate sight, hearing and sensation, they may be able to move, but they cannot link the two. In treatment a way must be found to bridge the gap, to motivate and eventually teach independence. Another factor, following from lack of motivation is resistance to change. This is shared by many physically handicapped children who find it difficult to move and prefer to be left alone. It is essential that they should be moved so as to change their position and activities at regular intervals. It is also important to progress from one activity to the next as soon as the first is becoming established. A list of possible activities may be a useful reminder for those caring for the child, whether at home, nursery or in hospital. This play chart can be made more interesting if it includes photographs of the child 'in action' and a simple description of his problem. This enables anyone with little previous knowledge to understand and to become involved.

As a normal baby learns from the people and things around him, it is important that the handicapped baby should have not less but more opportunities to learn in this way. Mothers (and fathers) are often afraid to disturb their baby because they know there is 'something wrong with him' and need to be reassured that he needs to be picked up and played with like any other baby. It is important to talk to these children even when they are too young to understand so that they become aware of the shades of expression in the voice and in the face. Talking also helps the mother to relax and thus makes a better relationship between her and her child.

Early play

For young babies and the severely retarded it is important to establish eye contact as the first step.

1. Mother should have the baby on her lap, and facing her; she should encourage him to look at her, to hold up his head and to look around. When he can look from side to side, he should learn to look up and then down.

2. The prone position can be introduced early, during bathing and

dressing, when baby can lie across mother's knee for a few minutes; the time should gradually be extended so that he gets used to the position and can enjoy looking at toys, or his brothers and sisters moving round the room.

3. The mother should make the child aware of his limbs by handling and moving his arms and legs; showing him his hands and feet, naming them and other parts of his face and body as she helps him touch them with his hands.

4. Games and rhymes such as Pat-a-cake, Peep-bo, This Little Pig Went To Market, etc teach many things. They may be normal routine in some families but are unknown to others who have been deprived themselves in childhood, or who have a different cultural background.

5. A variety of colourful and different sounding toys, rattles and squeakers will stimulate interest and help to improve eye, head and hand control. Small toys should be placed in the child's hand. He may at first need help to shake a rattle but gradually the help can be withdrawn so that he does it himself. A favourite toy can be held to make him reach for it (Fig. 23/1). Baby balls can be used to hold between his two hands in a similar fashion.

Although 'mother-play' (and 'father-play') are important it is necessary that the child has time and opportunity to play on his own. His cot should be provided with a play bar on which a selection of toys and rattles are suspended (Fig. 23/2). These must be adjusted so they

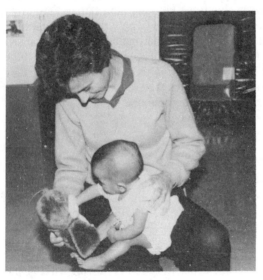

Fig. 23/1   Careful positioning enables the baby to reach and touch a soft, furry toy

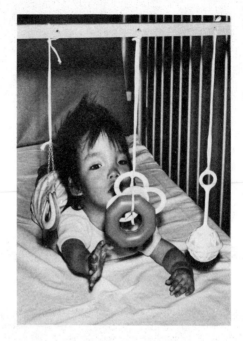

Fig. 23/2   The play bar in use
in a hospital cot

can be seen and touched. They should provide a variation of colour,
shape, sound and texture, and should be changed frequently.

Toys can teach; so the choice of toys for a handicapped child
deprived of many normal opportunities to investigate his surroundings has special significance. Early learning begins with awareness of
the tactile, visual and auditory stimulation which can be provided by
toys. This awareness may progress to knowledge of 'cause and effect'
and the possibility of choice (Figs. 23/3 and 23/4). For toys to be
pleasurable and meaningful the 'reward' (i.e. the feel, movement or
sound produced) must satisfy a need; while the 'task' (what has to be
done – to stroke, poke, pinch) must be within the child's physical and
intellectual ability. To take a simple example: In order to get
eye-tracking the toy must move *slowly* enough for the child to fix and
follow with his eyes, but must be *attractive* enough to retain his
interest and concentration. At all stages of therapy it is necessary to
know how much a child can understand. Where communication is
inhibited by severe physical disability with the chance of only gross
movement, it is necessary to find simple reliable ways in which the
child can respond – eye-pointing has been mentioned and may be used
for this purpose. The physiotherapist should note that effective
eye-pointing relies on postural stability; if the child cannot maintain

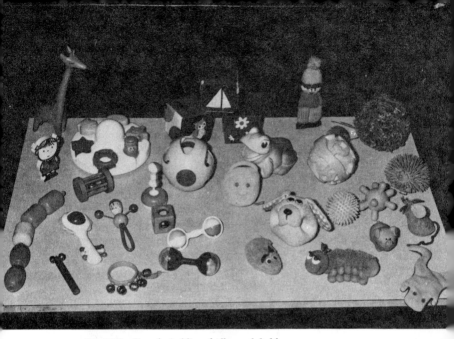

Fig. 23/3 Toys for holding, feeling and shaking

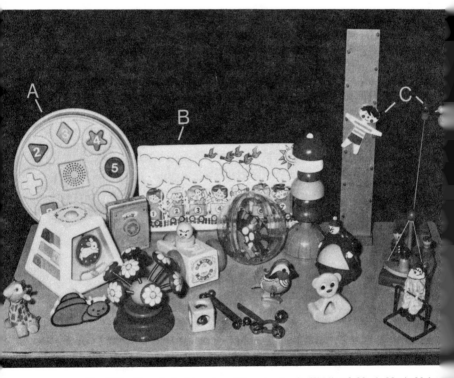

Fig. 23/4 Toys for looking at, and listening to: A. Kiddicraft Magic Music Maker
B. Soft Sounds by Palitoy; C. Tumbledown Boy and Bird

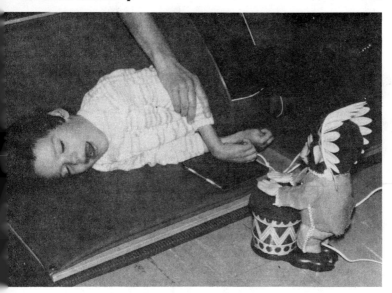

Fig. 23/5   A boy with severe brain damage uses a side-lying board while learning to press the pad linked electronically to the mechanical toy

this for himself he should be provided with adequate seating support. Electronic equipment may be used to enable the child to exercise his choice. In its simplest form this can be an on/off pressure pad, or switch, attached to a mechanical toy so that the child can operate the action at will (Fig. 23/5). At the other end of the scale are sophisticated devices such as Possum, with other less complicated equipment between the two extremes.

Floor play

All babies and physically retarded children should spend several periods each day in the prone position. Older children who have not done so may be quite helpless and miserable in this position which they have never known. These children may find it more tolerable to lie over a foam wedge which makes it easier for them to lift their hands and to play with toys on the floor in front of them (Fig. 23/6).

It may be difficult to convince the parents of the necessity for an older child to play on the floor in this position, when he can appear more socially acceptable propped in a chair. But floor play must continue so as to develop movement and mobility. Rolling is important as an early form of mobility but other means of progression

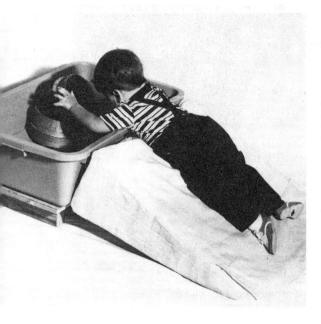

Fig. 23/6   Child lying over a wedge pillow to encourage head control while the hands are free to play

Fig. 23/7   An adapted wooden nursery chair with a large tray and toy frame

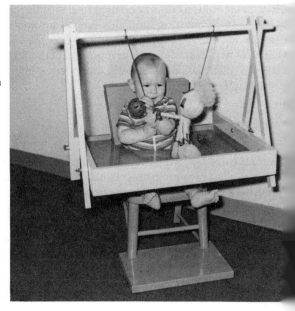

(on knees, seat or feet) must be encouraged as an alternative. A tummy trolley or low hand-propelled trolley (see Fig. 21/5, p. 355) may be appropriate for some children and enable them to explore their surroundings. Once able to move under their own volition they become more interested and better motivated to do so.

Sitting

Sitting up is important for mental development and for the acquisition of head and trunk control. A suitable chair should be found quite early, and used for several short spells during the day. The selection of the chair demands careful assessment of the child's needs and abilities particularly if there is a physical handicap. Consideration must be given to fit, comfort and safety. The chair should be placed so that the child can watch what goes on, as well as being able to play with toys.

A cut-out table with a built-up rim will prevent toys falling off; for younger or more handicapped children a toy frame may be useful to ensure that toys remain accessible (Fig. 23/7).

The type of chair should be reviewed regularly with reference to the child's growth and physical progress. At first he may need full support. As soon as he acquires some head control he should sit for short periods in a chair giving only trunk support. The first chair is then gradually withdrawn. Children who are just beginning to sit but are slow in acquiring sitting balance may do well using a wooden corner seat with a table on which to play. Although designed for use by cerebral palsy children the corner seat is also useful in management of developmental delay. A high corner seat may also be useful occasionally. A selection of chairs is shown in Figure 23/8.

Many new forms of moulded and adaptable seating are being developed, e.g. Matrix. A large variety of chairs are available commercially. A wooden nursery chair can be adapted to many individual needs. Wooden insets made to give support where necessary can be used in conjunction with an ordinary high chair. The Orthokinetic chair provides for accurate and individual adjustment and so gives good and comfortable support precisely where needed (Fig. 23/9B). It can also be used as a pushchair and a car seat. Unfortunately it is not currently available from the Department of Health and Social Security. The Newton 'Avon' chair can be provided with a scoliosis support system similar to that of the Orthokinetic chair and is available from the DHSS (Fig. 23/9A). It is, however, more cumbersome, cannot be used as a car seat and is difficult to transport.

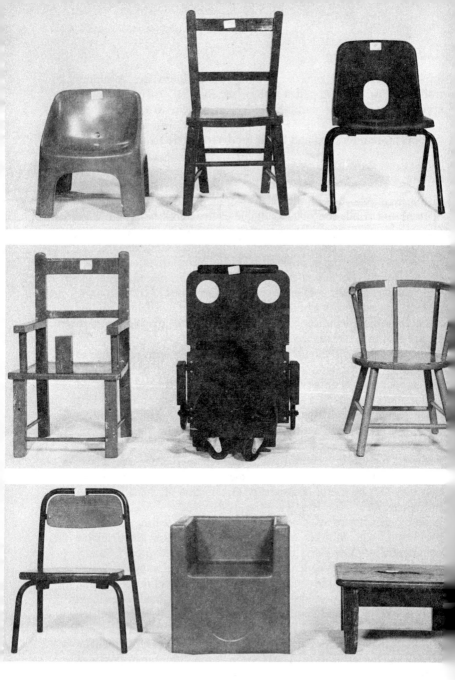

Fig. 23/8 An assortment of seats demonstrating variety of height, width, shape and support. The selection of a seat is important whether the handicap is minimal or severe. In general the feet should rest easily on the floor, and the back or arms of the chair give adequate, but not unnecessary support

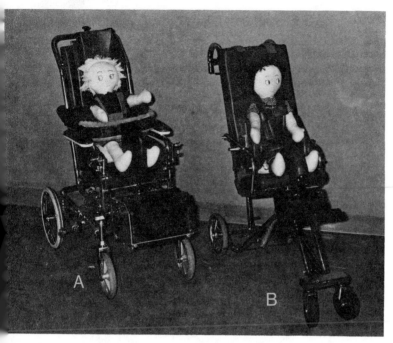

Fig. 23/9   A. The 'Avon' chair with scoliosis support system; B. Orthokinetic chair

Other pushchairs and buggies should not be used as seating as they give insufficient support.

To exclude the danger of the child developing deformities periods of sitting should be restricted and interspersed with time spent in other positions – supine, prone, side lying.

The upright position

Kneeling and standing can be started relatively early so as to provide as much different experience as possible. Help from the physio-therapist or assistant will be necessary at first. Both positions are best introduced with the child playing at a table of a suitable height. If there are sufficient helpers children may benefit from playing together round the table. A prone board is a useful piece of equipment which can be used to prepare for standing. The board is attached to a table and the child placed on it in the prone position. The angle between table and board can be varied from prone to near upright without moving the child who remains fully supported but begins to take

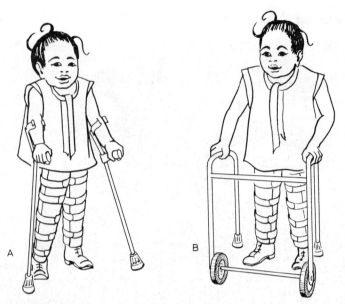

Fig. 23/10 Wearing canvas splints while awaiting calipers: progression to elbow crutches is easily achieved (A), after learning to walk with a Ripmaster walker (B)

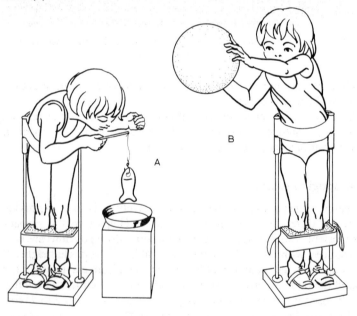

Fig. 23/11 The Flexistand or Newcommen Stander used to control pelvis and legs while the child enjoys games designed to encourage trunk rotation and co-ordination of the upper limbs

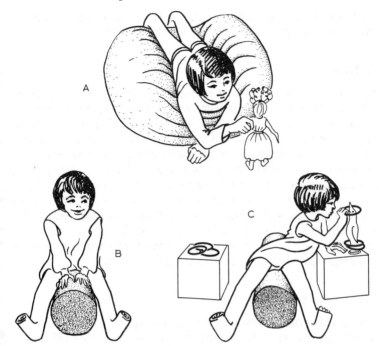

Fig. 23/12   Activities in bilateral above-knee plasters: A. Lying prone over a sagbag is comfortable and fun. It can be started very early and encourages back extension; B. Long sitting on a roll is easier than on the floor; C. In this position balance and rotation are practised

weight through his legs and feet. He feels secure and has his hands free for play.

Standing splints are sometimes useful for children waiting for calipers to be fitted, or for hypotonic or mentally handicapped children, so that they learn to appreciate some independence in the upright position (Fig. 23/10). In the latter case the splints are withdrawn when no longer needed. Splints can be made of Plastazote, Orthoplast, plaster of Paris or of canvas, with steel supports and webbing and Velcro straps. The Flexistand or Newcommen Stander is also useful for some children; it can allow free movement of the upper part of the body (Fig. 23/11).

Treatment in plaster of Paris

Many children require operations and spend long periods in plaster. This time should not be wasted. It can often be used to continue treatment and to make further progress. Much can be done to improve the function of other parts of the body (Fig. 23/12).

Walking

Baby walkers, the Cell Barnes walker and pushing toys are discussed on page 354. Older children who can co-operate and whose arms are relatively unaffected may find the Rollator or the Ripmaster walkers more appropriate to their needs. Each has its advantages and disadvantages. The Ripmaster is less known and although more difficult to manoeuvre in a small space is good preparation for crutch walking as weight is taken through the arms in a similar position (Fig. 23/10).

Some multiply handicapped children will unfortunately never be able to stand and walk alone, but the difficulties of management will be greatly eased if they can be left to stand holding on, and walk with help. Although this appears to be more important when they are older and bigger, it is better to start when they are still young.

Other forms of mobility

Young children and those whose disability prevents them from walking far enough or fast enough for practical purposes will need a buggy pushchair or wheelchair. The DHSS provides a range of buggies for handicapped children from the age of six months. These include the MacLaren Baby Buggy, the MacLaren Lie-back Buggy and the Cindico Lybak Traveller. These are suitable up to the age of three years and are available in a twin version for carrying the sibling of the disabled child. Each buggy has its own specifications and one may be more suited to the needs of a particular child than the other. Other pushchairs can sometimes be provided through the DHSS on special recommendation by a doctor.

For older children the MacLaren Major Buggy is available as a transit chair or for short expeditions. It is useful for children who can walk only short distances as it can easily be taken on public transport. For children who need it for longer periods of time, a child or junior wheelchair is more comfortable, gives better support and is easier to push. The Orthokinetic and Newton 'Avon' chairs have already been mentioned.

Independent mobility

It is important developmentally for all children that they learn not only to move but to *move about* at an early age. A Shasbah type trolley can be manoeuvred by very young children who can progress from this to the Yorkhill wheelchair, quickly becoming independent and able to explore their environment and enjoy activities with their peers. The Yorkhill wheelchair and low self-propelled trolley are available through the DHSS. The decision when to recommend a wheelchair is not easy and deserves careful consideration of all the relevant facts. The lives of very severely physically handicapped children can sometimes be transformed by the provision of an electrically-powered chair (Fig. 23/13). Their particular disability or deformity may

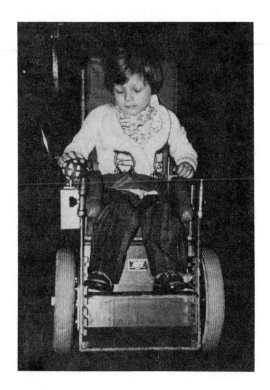

Fig. 23/13 The Bec Bambino electric wheelchair with inset and adapted hand control

require a specially fitted insert to enable them to maintain a sitting position while operating the controls. For some children this is their only independent activity.

If necessary the DHSS will provide a child with several wheelchairs, e.g. one for home and one for school, or one for indoor and one for outdoor use. Electrically-powered chairs supplied by the DHSS are for *indoor* use, and only one of these can be supplied to each child. Sometimes other sources can be found to raise money to purchase a second one if this is desirable. Tricycles are another means of mobility for some children and are sometimes available through the DHSS.

Play and recreation can be common to able and disabled children. Children of all ages and many disabilities like to go swimming. For the very young or severely disabled the water should be comfortably warm, as the children easily become cold and then cease to enjoy or benefit from the session. Pre-swim training is aimed at giving water confidence and teaching safety and independence, and may also involve parents in learning how to handle their child in water.

Horse riding is another sport enjoyed by many physically and mentally handicapped youngsters. Although a great deal of help may be necessary at first many children learn to manage their pony themselves and become independent; for others the ability to sit on a pony with partial control, even though some help is still needed, is sufficient to generate pride and confidence (see Chapter 24). The less disabled enjoy all the normal nursery equipment and apparatus – water play, painting, swings, slides and climbing frames all of which provide an incentive to exercise and exploration. They also like moving to music and action songs; these can be used to help overcome any specific physical difficulty.

Many of the activities mentioned do not come within the training or experience of the physiotherapist, but a broad approach to treatment using every opportunity to learn from other disciplines can add new interest to the task of helping handicapped children.

SUPPLIERS OF GOOD TOYS

Many useful toys can be obtained from toy shops, both large and small. The following represent a selection:

John Adams Toys Limited, Crazies Hill Road, Wargrave, Berkshire RG10 8LT

Combex Toys, Lincoln Road, Peterborough PE4 6LB
  Export and London Showrooms: 117–123 Great Portland Street, London W1N 5FA

Community Playthings, Rifton Equipment, Robertsbridge, East Sussex TN32 5DR

ESA Creative Learning Limited, PO Box 22, The Pinnacles, Harlow CM19 5AY

Fisher Price Toys, PO Box 47, Northampton NN4 0HT (Also from many large stores)

Four to Eight, PO Box 38, Medway House, Northgates, Leicester
  LE1 9BU
James Galt and Company Ltd, Brookfield Road, Cheadle, Cheshire
  SKE 2PN
  (Branches in London, Edinburgh, Bradford and York)
Kiddicraft Limited, Goldstone Road, Kenley, Surrey CR2 5YS
Susan Wynter Toys, Toy Trumpet Workshops Limited,
Church Road, Brightlingsea CO7 0RZ
  (Also from good toy shops)
Mothercare Shops in most towns
Learning Developmental Aids, Aware House, Duke Street, Wisbech
  PE13 7AE
Hestair Hope Ltd, St Philip's Drive, Royton, Oldham OL7 6AG

REFERENCES

Downie, P. A. (ed) (1982). *Cash's Textbook of Neurology for Physiotherapists*,
  3rd edition. Chapter 19, *Spina Bifida and Hydrocephalus*. Chapter 20,
  Cerebral Palsy. Chapter 21, *Muscular Dystrophy*. Faber and Faber,
  London.
Younghusband, E., Birchall, D., Davie, R. and Kellmer Pringle, M. L.
  (1970). *Living with Handicap*. National Bureau for Co-operation in Child
  Care, London.

BIBLIOGRAPY

Bowley, A. H. and Gardner, L. (1980). *The Handicapped Child*, 4th edition.
  Churchill Livingstone, Edinburgh.
Bobath, B. and Bobath, K. (1975). *Motor Development in the Different Types of
  Cerebral Palsy*. William Heinemann Medical Books Limited, London.
Cunningham, C. and Sloper, P. (1979). *Helping Your Handicapped Baby*.
  Human Horizon Series, Souvenir Press, London.
Deich, R. F. and Hodges, P. M. (1977). *Language Without Speech*. Human
  Horizon Series, Souvenir Press, London.
Dubowitz, V. (1969). *The Floppy Infant*. Clinics in Developmental Medicine,
  No 31. William Heinemann Medical Books Limited, London.
The Education Act 1981. HMSO, London.
The Education Act 1981, DES circular 8/81. HMSO, London.
Exley, H. (ed) (1981). *What It's Like To Be Me*. Exley Publications, Watford.
Finnie, N. (1974). *Handling the Young Cerebral Palsied Child at Home*, 2nd
  edition. William Heinemann Medical Books Limited, London.
Gordon, N. and McKinley, I. (1980). *Helping Clumsy Children*. Churchill
  Livingstone, Edinburgh.
Handbook of Wheelchairs and Bicycles and Tricycles, ref MHM 408. Obtainable
  from the DHSS, London.
Hollis, Katy (1977). *Progress to improved movement*.
Hollis, Katy (1977). *Progress to standing*.

Both the above booklets are obtainable from the Institute of Mental Subnormality, Wolverhampton Road, Kidderminster DY10 3PP

Hosking, G. P. (1982). *An Introduction to Paediatric Neurology*. Faber and Faber, London.

Jeffree, D. M. and McConkey, R. (1976). *Let Me Speak*. Human Horizon Series, Souvenir Press, London.

Jeffree, D. M., McConkey, R. and Hewson, S. (1977). *Let Me Play*. Human Horizon Series, Souvenir Press, London.

Kirman, B. and Bicknell, J. (1975). *Mental Handicap*. Churchill Livingstone, Edinburgh.

McCarthy, G. T. (ed) (1984). *The Physically Handicapped Child. An Interdisciplinary Approach to Management*. Faber and Faber. London.

Norris, J. (1974). *Choosing Toys and Activities for Handicapped Children*. Noah's Ark Publications, Toy Library Association, London.

Richardson, A. and Wisbeach, A. (1976). *I Can Use My Hands*. Noah's Ark Publications, Toy Library Association, London.

Sheridan, M. (1977). *Spontaneous Play in Early Childhood*. NFER-Nelson Publishing Company, Windsor.

Simon, G. B. (ed) (1980). *Modern Management of Mental Handicap*. MTP Press Limited, Lancaster.

Stone, J. and Taylor, F. (1977). *Handbook for Parents with a Handicapped Child*. Arrow Books, London.

See also Bibliography on pages 359 and 385.

USEFUL ORGANISATIONS

See page 451.

SPECIFIC INTEREST GROUP

The Association of Paediatric Chartered Physiotherapists is a specific interest group of the Chartered Society of Physiotherapy (CSP). Physiotherapists who wish to know more about the group should write to the group's secretary c/o Chartered Society of Physiotherapy, 14 Bedford Row, London WC1R 4ED.

ACKNOWLEDGEMENTS

The author wishes to thank the following for their help and advice in the revision of these chapters: Dr Richard West MD, MRCP, DCH, consultant paediatrician and Dean of the Medical School, St George's Hospital, London; Professor Joan Bicknell MD, DPM, FRCPsych, Department of the Psychiatry of Mental Handicap, St George's Hospital, London; members of the Child Development Centre, St George's Hospital, London, and in particular Miss Chris Bungay MCSP, peripatetic paediatric physiotherapist, who also provided some of the photographs; and Mr Andrew Rolland, Department of Medical Photography, St George's Hospital, London.

Chapter 24

Riding for the Disabled

by S. SAYWELL, FCSP

Riding for disabled persons whether with physical, mental or mixed disabilities, emerged in the later years of the anterior poliomyelitis epidemic which swept through Great Britain and Scandinavia during the 1940–50 period. Much dedication from physiotherapists, working with the medical profession, was required to maintain clear airways and lung function for those victims of respiratory paralysis. These life-saving efforts demanded and received day and night attention seven days a week. This total involvement of physiotherapists in the field of intensive care left little opportunity for the treatment of sub-clinical and ambulant clinical patients who required advice, supervised exercises and a programme of progressive rehabilitation. It was this group of poliomyelitis victims whose plight alerted certain physiotherapists, who were not free to offer their professional services to hospitals, but whose young children had ponies, to consider riding as an effective treatment programme. The determination and resourcefulness of those early workers created another limb of programmed progressive exercises, mobility and motivation from which have developed international organisations for riding for the disabled in many countries.

This chapter sets out to introduce physiotherapists to this useful form of exercise and recreation for disabled persons. It will show how accepted methods of treatments such as Bobath, Petö and others can be adapted and used with the patient mounted. It will also discuss the need for pony suitability. The application of such techniques in certain conditions is fully described.

PHILOSOPHY

The declared aim of the Riding for the Disabled Association (RDA) is to give an opportunity for any disabled person, who wishes to do so, to ride, as a means of benefiting his general well-being. The range of disabilities among those who are now enjoying this opportunity is remarkable (Figs. 24/1 and 24/2).

The age-range falls mainly between the school-age child and those in the late fifties and above, for whom the benefits are as great as for children. Many of the adults have ridden in all types of equestrian events before becoming victims of accidents or disease. Such riders may require a period in which to assess their riding ability and find, for themselves, local RDA groups. These groups provide the ideal atmosphere for them to make their decisions and, where necessary, the adaptations and alterations which allow for years of enjoyable riding. Other chronically disabled adults and young people, especially school leavers, join riding for the disabled sessions to gain mobility, exercise and a leisure activity in which friendships may be formed among a wide group of both able-bodied and disabled contemporaries.

The structure of RDA groups includes both professional and knowledgeable lay helpers. A *riding instructor*, who may hold professional qualifications, or be a very experienced instructor in the Pony Club, is the acknowledged leader at the riding session. The main element in all groups is the *voluntary helper* who works with the instructor and chartered physiotherapist. The voluntary helper will (1) translate instruction to the rider, allowing each individual to gain as much independence as possible during the riding session; (2) help the rider achieve maximum correct range of movement when special exercises are selected; and (3) report any particular problem arising either from the rider, the saddlery or unexpected reactions of the pony.

The general turnout and appearance is important for all members of the group; suitable clothing and sturdy shoes are as essential for helpers as the regulation hard hat is for the rider.

All RDA affiliated groups are covered by adequate insurance policies and chartered physiotherapists in full work are protected by their membership. Chartered physiotherapists who offer help and who are not working can enrol with the Chartered Society of Physiotherapy's specific interest section, Riding for the Disabled, when insurance cover at low cost becomes available.

For the physiotherapist to give the maximum benefit of her professional training to riders in RDA groups an ability to ride, or, at least, to experience the movements of the horse, is essential. Group instruction will help in providing basic riding lessons for this purpose, but all physiotherapists working with disabled riders should check, by observation, the instruction and progress of a *normal* rider.

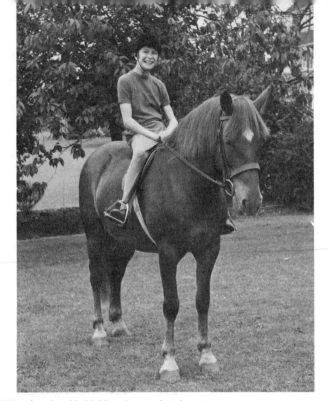

Fig. 24/1   An athetoid girl. Note the use of a safety stirrup

Fig. 24/2   The rider is a spina bifida who is wearing below-knee calipers. This is a perfect example of the right size of pony for its rider

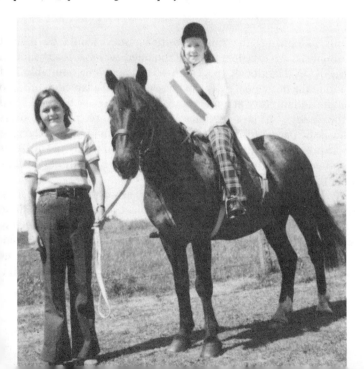

Attendance at ordinary classes of beginners and novice riders, under a good riding instructor, will provide an excellent introduction. The method of suiting rider to the pony/horse can be studied; the placing of each rider and pony in the ride to give maximum benefit to the whole class; the safety procedures; the management of classes of mixed riding skills; and methods of dealing with a variety of temperaments within the class can be observed and understood: all of which is to be recommended strongly.

Parents of disabled children are usually most concerned with sitting balance, standing, and taking some steps; riding can provide the motivation to acquire these skills – although more slowly, as normal chronological progressions are not applicable. Home exercises, an example of which is shown in Figure 24/3a and b, can be taught to

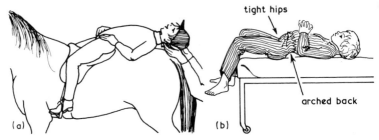

Fig. 24/3   (a) Stretching exercise (only to be used when the pony is accustomed to this type of activity); (b) Home exercise showing the postural difficulties which require attention

parents to enhance the riding positions; they should be revised continuously. An excellent range of mounted exercises is to be found in the RDA Handbook (pages 78–85). Those most suitable and helpful to the individual rider can be selected and adapted in order to maintain and improve at home those skills which have been achieved in the saddle. It is sometimes necessary to restrain the over-enthusiastic parent from a too vigorous approach to home exercises. The acquisition of sitting balance frees the use of hands and arms for more functional activities, and appears to be more readily obtained by riding than any other activity.

Physical activity leads to mental activity even in those who are most severely intellectually impaired. The results of introducing riding to this group of disabled persons are exciting with much encouraging feedback coming spontaneously from parents, teachers and atten-dants who notice the changes in the individual rider. This may be simply a recognition of the riding day by putting on a hard hat, but i may result in greater independence of movement, improved social behaviour and in general health. The physiotherapist will note the build-up of muscle tone (often low in the mentally handicapped person) and improved co-ordination of limbs and body movement. The clumsy child will show the same improvement. Those riders with previous problems of mobility, especially spina bifida or similar conditions, are provided with exercises and incentives to achieve mobility from the pony in stages: beginning with a simple walk forward, steering and stopping, to advanced and increasing balancing movements at varied paces with changes of direction within those paces. Class work gives ample opportunity to achieve goals, however simple, by creating a happy encouraging atmosphere, as well as experiencing the enjoyment of working together. This latter is often denied the disabled person who more usually is an individual within a group and rarely is a team member.

One aspect of handling disabled riders that is often overlooked, is the *natural* ability that many possess and which *can* be developed to give such riders opportunities to compete with able-bodied peers; or, alas, stifled by over-protectiveness. The physiotherapist can instil into group members professional views, give encouragement, create confidence and promote the principle of *keep trying*. The opposite is also true: when a rider who has a progressive disease is no longer able to benefit, the physiotherapist with her professional knowledge can recommend other activities. Such advice expressed with authority tempered by sympathetic understanding can be of great value to members of groups when such problems arise, who otherwise can become confused, worried and feel they have failed.

THE PHYSIOTHERAPIST

The link between the pony/horse and disabled rider presents an exciting challenge for the physiotherapist who is able to select from accepted methods of teaching patterns of movement those most suited to each rider, and adapt them to the individual rider's ability and potential. The opportunities for studying the principles of dynamic balance, co-ordination and acquisition of general agility offers the physiotherapist a series of projects (not as yet fully researched), which may lead to a change of conventional thought and traditional teaching, useful in the management of a variety of disabilities and in the appreciation of basic riding instruction for both able-bodied and disabled persons.

Riding for the Disabled
RECORD CARD

Name..................................

Age................starting riding..................

Disability..................................

△ stiff
O deformed
ⵉ spastic
∥ floppy
□ normal

⌐ curvature
✳ painful
⋰ poor sensation
⬭ appliance
? mental handicap

Points to work on

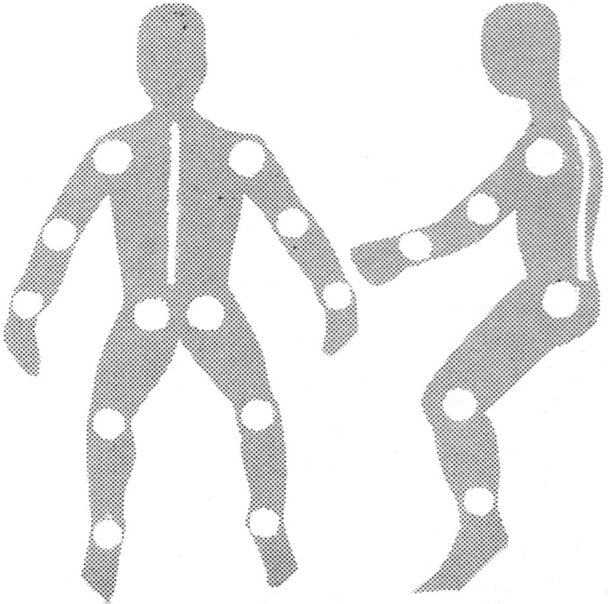

DATE					
Cannot walk					
Walks with — calipers					
crutches					
sticks					
unaided					
Climbs steps					
Wheelchair					
Speech					
Sight					
Hearing					
Social					
RIDING ABILITY					
Wheelchair transfer					
Aided — no. of helpers					
Lifting — one					
two					
three					

TYPE OF PONY

SPECIAL TACK

TESTS PASSED

DATE					
Mounting — unaided					
from block, ramp, pit					
from ground with help					
Walk — led					
free					
no. of helpers					
Trot — led					
free					
sitting					
rising					
no. of helpers					
Canter — led					
free					
no. of helpers					
Jumping — free					
no. of helpers					
Independent — school					
Control — field					

OTHER REMARKS

Fig. 24/4 (a & b) Record card showing both sides. Produced by the CSP special interest group, see p. 440

THE PSYCHOLOGICAL IMPACT OF RIDING IS ALMOST
IMMEASURABLE

The physiotherapist is well adapted to motivating patients, their families or guardians towards achieving seemingly impossible goals. She can therefore develop and encourage these skills through riding, by coaxing the timid to attempt a mobility for which they may lack the necessary mental or physical equipment; dampen the exhausting and unwelcome energies of the hyperactive; give opportunities for character training; enjoy socialising; and assist in the emergence of memory and retained instruction, all of which overflows into the activities of daily living.

RIDING OFFERS A LIFETIME OF OPPORTUNITY TO ACQUIRE THAT
PERFECT PARTNERSHIP WITH A HORSE

This is enriching, not only in the satisfaction of achieving many skills, but also in the friendship formed by mutual affection and respect for horses. Once the basic skills of starting, stopping, steering at walk, trot and, often, canter, are acquired, the pony/horse then becomes the therapist.

Points of observation

AIMS

1. To enable relevant advice to be given to the rider to improve posture and position (when he is able to appreciate this) by the instructor through lay helpers (through the instructor or by arrangement with the instructor).
2. To select possible corrections from application of physiotherapy techniques.
3. To encourage physical and mental targets towards a progressive improvement in riding skills. (Note: All those engaged in the active riding session should appreciate these progressive targets.)
4. Recording progress (Fig. 24/4a and b).

Points	Aim	Suggested Action
Head	Desired control	Steadiness (reflex action through trot work)
Arms	Independent action damping unwanted movement	Bobath/proprioceptive neuromuscular facilitation (PNF) techniques (Fig. 24/5)
Hands	Control of spasticity	Teach helpers correct grasps to hold fingers and wrist. Where to place hand slightly behind saddle and in what position
Seat	Central position and upright. Observe from in front, from the side and most importantly from behind the pony (Fig. 24/6) (Describe and illustrate normal result of sitting to one side)	Accept flexion of hip and shorter stirrup-leather length to gain upright position. Then reduce hip flexion and gain leg length
	Avoid pressure areas	Rising trot helps; or allow push-ups from saddle at appropriate intervals. Pressure changes occur naturally when instructor orders seat corrections
Hips	Relaxed, and angle with body as open as possible. Note: Leg length should come from hip	Exercises to reduce hip flexion contractures
Leg	↓ Extensor spasm	Reduce by appropriate physiotherapy
	↓ Adductor spasm	Riding without stirrups. Choice of pony/saddle by instructor. Note: Warmth of pony is also beneficial
Knees	Away from saddle	No gripping Helper to steady position

Points	Aim	Suggested Action
Lower leg	Hang from knee lightly against pony's side	Helper involvement. Teach correct holds (RDA Handbook, p. 40)
Heels	Lower than toe when condition will allow	Teach helpers correct physiological holds
Lumbar spine	Loose and supple	Corrections by appropriate exercises in all movement planes (RDA Handbook, pp 78/86). Avoid stiffness and hollowing (Fig. 24/7)
Feet	Pointing forward	Correction from hips and directed by helper
	Avoid clonus	Discuss with instructor position of foot in stirrup iron. Riding for periods without stirrups
Note: Breathing	Asthma and allied conditions	Alert organiser. Rider should bring appropriate medication to the lesson. Remove rider from dusty conditions to recover/remount

Remember: Hidden value of exercises, particularly in non-elimination games, in achieving success with rider's position. Freedom of movement. Avoid clinical assessments. Make exercises enjoyable. **The object is fun!**

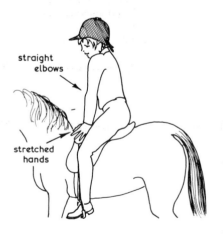

Fig. 24/5   A corrective position; taking weight through the left hemiplegic arm

straight elbows

stretched hands

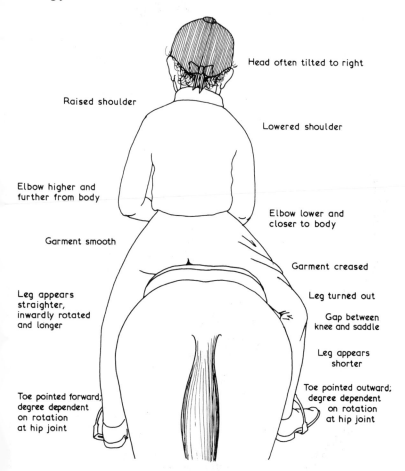

Head often tilted to right

Raised shoulder

Lowered shoulder

Elbow higher and
further from body

Elbow lower and
closer to body

Garment smooth

Garment creased

Leg appears
straighter,
inwardly rotated
and longer

Leg turned out

Gap between
knee and saddle

Leg appears
shorter

Toe pointed forward;
degree dependent
on rotation
at hip joint

Toe pointed outward;
degree dependent
on rotation
at hip joint

Fig. 24/6   Deviation to the left viewed from the rear

CEREBRAL PALSY

The result of a lesion or mal-development of the brain, i.e.
non-progressive in character and existing from early childhood, is one
of the most difficult groups of disability. The motor deficit in
abnormal patterns of movement and posture is enormously varied,
emphasising to professional and lay helpers alike the danger of
classifying disabilities under standard headings (Fig. 24/8).

A good knowledge of normal child development and posture is
required. An alert eye and constant observation will then show the
therapist what is wrong in the movement and posture of riding pupils.

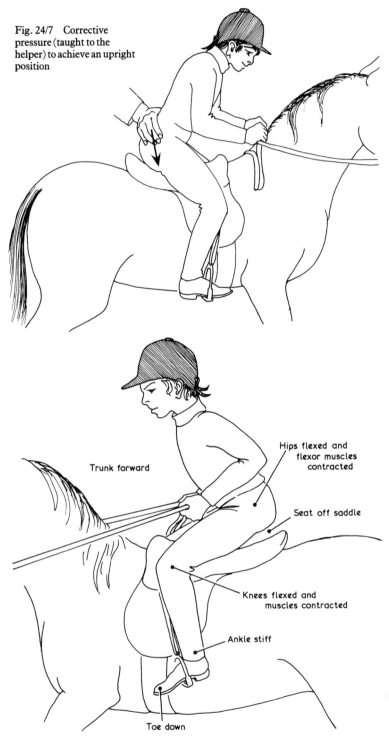

Fig. 24/7 Corrective pressure (taught to the helper) to achieve an upright position

Hips flexed and flexor muscles contracted

Trunk forward

Seat off saddle

Knees flexed and muscles contracted

Ankle stiff

Toe down

Fig. 24/8 The typical riding position of a brain-damaged child

Each rider must be assessed as an individual. The focus of attention is the movement of the pelvis. Only if the pelvis can move freely will the rider be able to follow the movement of the horse – which is the basis of all horsemanship (Podhajsky, 1967: Watjen, 1979).

The work of the Bobaths first drew attention to the manner in which parents and friends could give the child the best opportunities for developing his capabilities, however limited they might be. The advent of the roller, large bouncing ball and the equilibrium board in producing three-dimensional movement in balance, provided an excellent stimulus to both patient and physiotherapist, offering greater input of reflex action by more intensive, continuous and faster repetitions than could formerly be maintained by the physiotherapist or accepted by the patient (Finnie, 1974).

These changing positions provided by roll, ball and board formed an appropriate basis for horse riding and allayed the fears of those solely engaged in Bobath techniques who quite naturally objected in the early years to sports or activities which might negate the desirable movement patterns. Two decades ago this was a real objection, often expressed, which led in some cases to rejection of riding by professionals and parents. Fortunately, by inviting those genuine objectors to riding sessions and demonstrating the incorporation of Bobath techniques into the exercise and riding programme, their fears were proved unfounded.

Problems arising when riding

1. *Unsteady head position, particularly at the trot*: Although this can be a matter of concern to spectators and riding instructors, the physiotherapist can give positive reassurance that only normal postural reflexes are involved and no restriction in the form of collars or splintage should be considered.

2. *Sitting balance*: For the young child, sitting astride the parent's lap is an essential position for acquiring sitting balance, damping out the tendency to straighten the hips and turn legs in. If the base is too broad, however, the position becomes exaggerated, a point to be discussed with the riding instructor who may have the opportunity to acquire a pony of the most suitable size for the rider (Fig. 24/9). This is not always a simple matter – best use has to be made of the availability of ponies which, in most British groups, are supplied voluntarily by their owners. Adjustment to saddlery – or the use of the vaulting pad – may be the answers for the beginner rider.

   Observation by the therapist, and discussion with the instructor will be valuable when such problems arise. From this astride position, the correct riding seat can be encouraged and acquired, the arms and head controlled and a good functional position obtained for progress into achieving forward movement with the pony. The co-operation of parents and friends will be readily obtained once this riding position is explained, and exercises for use at home taught to reinforce and enhance this basic broad base from which balance can be obtained (see Fig. 24/3b).

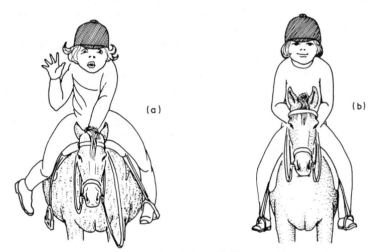

Fig. 24/9   (a) Unhappy rider on too broad a base; (b) The same rider correctly mounted

VAULTING PAD

The vaulting roller or girth has two handles set at an angle – one on either side. The handles stand away from the horse because of the padding underneath the roller. A *thick* piece of foam, approximately 30cm (12in) wide and 1.2m (4ft) long underneath the roller absorbs the pressure. In the centre of the roller is a long strap to help balance beginners. The girth buckles can be covered by a soft leather protector or a short girth used to prevent interference to the vaulter's legs.

CONDUCTIVE EDUCATION AND ITS RELATIONSHIP TO RIDING

Riding instruction for disabled children, particularly the young child, is well adapted to the concept of conductive education which

Professor Andreas Petö of Budapest originated for children affected with cerebral palsy. Such was the success of the Petö method that it was rapidly extended to those with spina bifida, paraplegia and many other neurological disorders.

It is emphasised that conductive education is a method of *education*, not a neurophysiological treatment approach such as Bobath, Kabat, Vojta, Temple-Fay, Rood, etc. All problems are treated as problems of learning. Teaching and medical treatment are inseparable.

Conductive education should be continuous throughout the day and involve all those concerned with the training, upbringing and development of brain damaged children. Therefore the riding session, with its complement of therapist(s), instructor(s) and helpers, offers an exciting challenge to activate and support *symmetrical balanced movements* which increase riding ability and skills. These achievements, in turn, feed back into activities of daily living through the attainment of sitting balance, head control, arm and hand steadiness and independent action; freedom of hip movement, correct position of the legs in sitting and independent action of the lower leg, feet supported in stirrups. School work, feeding and dressing then become easier; independence is achieved and the capacity for increased performance established.

The physiotherapist(s), instructor(s) and helpers should note each little progression, however small, which is important to the individual rider and also the whole group; one child's (rider's) progress assists the performance of others. This constitutes a normal situation in any riding class of able-bodied riders from the beginner to those with considerable riding skill. The physiotherapist must explain to the instructor – and her colleagues – the aim of Rhythmical Intention (that is the use of speech to express intention).
Movement is aimed at a goal and carries a certain motor task.

The sequence of movement must be explained, together with the aims of each progression.

1. The ability to sit in the saddle. This may occur on the pony before sitting balance is achieved in a chair without arms (Fig. 24/10).
2. Ability to keep feet in the stirrups – to give security of position – aided by a helper standing at each side.
3. Ability to move the head independently from body.
4. Ability to keep forearms and hands down – holding the reins (not attached to the bit) or a small stick.
5. Ability to move hands independently from one another – steering the pony through bending poles.
6. Ability to understand the position of the body – up, down, side,

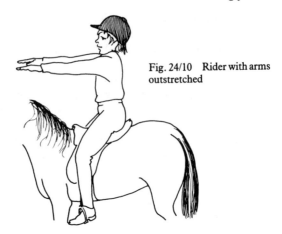

Fig. 24/10   Rider with arms outstretched

middle, left, right, out, in, apart, together, above, below, in front, behind.

7. Ability to understand where the hips are – in relation to the rest of the body – in order to achieve a good sitting position.

Exercises designed to achieve these positions and movements must be accompanied by a stated intention by the rider. As an example:

I pick up the reins.
I sit up tall.
My feet (legs) are hanging down.
I bend forward (Fig. 24/11).

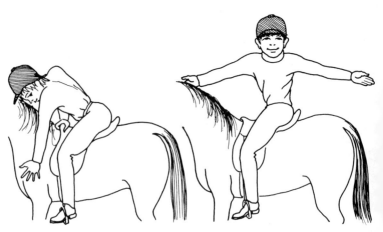

Fig. 24/11   'I bend forward'   Fig. 24/12   'I turn to the left'

I put my head on the pony's neck.
I touch my feet.
I press my elbows to my side.
I turn to the left (Fig. 24/12).
I turn to the right.
I turn to the left and touch my pony's tail.
I turn to the right and touch my pony's tail.

With the whole class using speech and action, the individual rider's attention is drawn to the task. The helpers are also fully involved, interested in the achievements of the rider and therefore will concentrate on the instructor, repeating commands and aiding the intention when necessary.

The physiotherapist must explain that:

(a) These functional movements may take months to acquire; the progress made being scarcely discernible over a period of weeks.
(b) Constant repetition is essential, and therefore the exercise of great patience by the helpers is vital.
(c) Much praise for each small success is important, but praise must not be given if the target is not achieved. The rider will be aware of failure, understand and accept the situation and be ready to make another attempt.

SCOLIOSIS

Since the introduction of screening the school-age child, and the improved philosophy of the management of adolescent scoliosis, there is now an increased demand for riding as an acceptable activity during the developing years. Acceptable, that is, for the orthopaedic surgeon, paediatrician, the parent and family, and, most importantly, the young teenage girl who quite often flatly refuses to wear even the low-profile or Boston brace. *Note*: Young girls with idiopathic scoliosis and no other disabilities may own a pony and ride in ordinary classes or in Pony Club events. These youngsters may need only reassurance, adjustments to the brace (if cut too low), ride with longer stirrups and a little help in mounting.

The carrot of riding is often successful in overcoming this quite understandable resentment at a time of life when ordinary problems of growing up can make the developing years so difficult. The congenitally disabled child has further problems in the same period of development when spinal curvatures may progress rapidly, and bracing becomes a formidable task for surgeon, orthotist, physiotherapist and the wearer.

Exercises can maintain and enhance body tone, and are of value to the patient and family in bringing a positive attitude to the problems of management. The psychological benefits are considerable when riding is introduced, and the activity can be continued with care following surgical stabilisation, including Harrington rod fixation, when the desire to do so is expressed by the child and agreed by the surgeon.

The problems requiring advice from the physiotherapist range from the normal attention to pressure areas (discussion with the orthotist and surgeon being necessary when adjustments are required to the brace itself), to a briefing session with the riding instructor and helpers on the management of brace-wearing riders. The modern materials used in low-profile and Boston braces are *slippery*, and outer garments therefore cannot be grasped securely for balancing support when necessary. It is this situation which demands the use of a firm belt, preferably with hand-holds, used in assisting mounting to steady the rider at moments of imbalance, when riding a circle or turn, or when the pony puts in a surprising sudden stop or turn. Other points to discuss are the restrictions of exercises; the difficulties of turning in the saddle, and therefore awareness of other riders coming from behind; or, if lead file, judging distance from those following.

For the severely scoliotic rider, balancing is achieved through constant small corrective movements especially on circles when centrifugal forces add further difficulties. In the top heavy spina bifida teenage rider (over-weight from limited activity) the percentage of body-weight displaced to one side can be 60 per cent (Fig. 24/13). Such a rider will restrict her type of riding experiences to circumstances which allow instinctive safety with maximum enjoyment. Hacking out, pony trekking and RDA dressage events leading to BHS Riding Club Preliminary and Novice competitions can be within the scope of some of the non-ambulant brace wearers when the curve is a simple one, not exceeding 20 degrees. Cantering is also possible. The adolescent with normal limb function will enjoy these activities and the spirit of competition with her peers.

BALANCE

The related sequence of balance features, from development of head control and sitting balance obtained normally in the seven/eight-month-old infant to the perfection of an athlete, ballet dancer or accomplished educated rider, is well understood. Laboratory investigations of vestibular influence by the brain, eyes, muscle pressure, skin pressure, stretch reflexes, and the effects of drugs on these mechanisms are responsible for our understanding of static and dynamic balance. For the serious student there are textbooks and journals such as *Physiology and Perception* from which to cull further information.

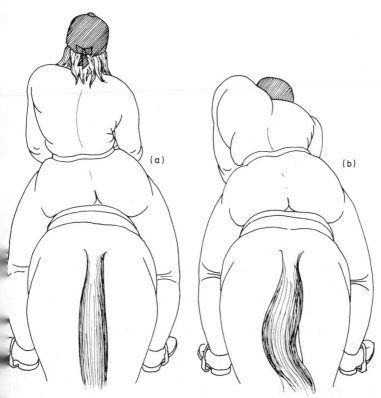

Fig. 24/13 (a) Showing the typical seat position when the body-weight is displaced due to spinal curvature; (b) Showing the grossly distorted position when the rider leans forward

What *is* open to further study is the acquisition of balance despite brain damage and allied disorders on a moving animal, horse or pony with ideas of its own! This is far more challenging for the student to consider than work already undertaken on the balance board, tilting table, roller or large 'bouncing' ball. The horse or pony provides a wide range of progressive balancing skills which should be acquired to give a good position in the saddle for the rider, and an ability to follow the movement of the horse. Apart from work done by the Bobaths, Finnie, Edinburgh Medical School and at Cambridge, an attempt has been made in the gymnasium at Winford Orthopaedic Hospital to simulate the movement of a horse by using a wobble board on a section of the Westminster plinth system. This early experiment showed the effort required by two patients, one recovering from Guillain-Barré disease and one severely scoliotic heavy weight 14-year-old girl. Muscle activity flowed through the spine, accompanied with balancing movements from arms and legs, and, for the rider, gave some indication of the initial instability felt from an early riding lesson. This mock-up could be used with advantage in any group, particularly with the timid wheelchair bound prospective pupil. However, the experiment does not simulate the horse's influence to which the rider must adjust, and needs to be repeated possibly using a system of pulleys, weights and springs.

Mechanical kinaesthesis

Apparatus: Tilt board, mirror, plumb line, flat plinth or broad stool (Fig. 24/14).

The boards: Made of 19mm (¾in) wood, covered by a 6mm (¼in) layer of rubber with a non-slip surface. The essential feature of these boards is the shape of an attachment screwed to the undersurface. In one type of board (Type I) this consisted of two sections of a cylinder placed across the centre of the board so that the board was free to tip in one plane, like a see-saw. In Type II the attachment was shaped as a section of a sphere so that the board was free to tip in all planes.

In Type I boards the cylinder sections rose to a height of 5cm (2in) and were 20cm (8in) in length. In Type II boards the spherical attachment was of the same height and had a circumference of 20cm. The radii of curvature of these two attachments were therefore the same.

Type II boards were made in two overall sizes: 55×55cm (22×22in) and 55×100cm (22×40in). The larger board rocked about an axis parallel with its short side and it therefore gathered more momentum than did the square board. For this reason it was more difficult to control. Type II boards were circular with a diameter of 55cm.

Perception of movement, changes of direction, changes in the riders' posture, proprioception and vestibular inflow all contribute to achieving balance, but key questions about perception, movement

Activation: Pressure from seat bones, body sway.

Observer: Take photographs. Using a plumb line, note and record:
1. Muscle work
2. Curvatures
3. Joint and limb positions
4. Spasm

Use of record card: See Figure 24/4.

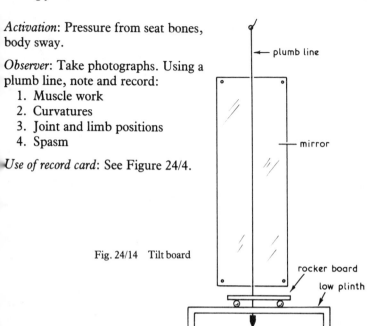

Fig. 24/14 Tilt board

memory, mood, and body image remain unanswered. The pony, by offering such an enormous variety of alteration of pace (from walk, trot or canter, and with variations of speed within those paces), provides the most useful method of acquiring balance; together with constant enjoyment in the struggle for both brain-damaged riders and the clumsy child. Artificial aids could be used as pre-riding exercises, the tilting table or wobble board and the large roller being especially useful and readily available to groups.

Each rider relies heavily on visual kinaesthesis, and is dependent on vision to sense how he is moving in relation to the static or active environment. The blind rider can lose track of how he is moving and requires additional mechanical information (i.e. sound assisted) such as bleepers out of doors, voices, sounding boards indoors (i.e. kicking boards) and a lowered general noise level while acquiring such help.

Apart from the physical aspects of acquiring balance, the visual cortex, perception and behavioural factors all have great influence in normal subjects. The pioneer work of Autrum Jung et al (1978) into the behavioural after-effects of brain injury provided a foundation for contemporary neuropsychology studies in young people, and in the congenitally brain-damaged patient. There are however important gaps in understanding and explanation of everyday perception of motion. At RDA sessions there are many objects, ponies and people all moving in different directions and at different speeds. The brain-damaged rider is receiving many complex stimuli, and may need a moment or two of freedom from too much input to adjust mentally to the task in hand.

The physiotherapist should explain in simple terms to the instructor and helpers the problems that riders suffering from impaired vision have in achieving balance, especially in the confusion of a free-riding session rather than a correctly planned and executed school ride (PC Instructor's Manual). The problem of directional letters, when the standard size cannot be appreciated by some riders with visual disabilities, can be overcome by the addition of a lower case letter, or picture. Pictures must be very clear, and not too artistic with a confusing if visually delightful background. Recognition of colour may be difficult – a point perhaps to be emphasised for those riders with mental handicaps (intellectually disabled).

Physiotherapists can benefit from taking a riding session wearing spectacles designed for a variety of visual handicaps. A selection of spectacles simulating partial vision through its many variations to complete blindness can be obtained from selected county council libraries. The Diamond Riding Centre, Carshalton produced such spectacles for physiotherapists on special interest group courses. The experience was salutary, not only in directional finding but in the confidence in the instructor and with helpers. The bond with these needed to be strong!

Recording balance (balance coding)

Gabell and Simons (1982) described a system of balance coding. It is a simple method of recording functional assessment of ability to cope with different basic types of balance and could be applied to riding. As an example such recording can test the recovery point of leaning forward or sideways from the halt and on the moving pony at different paces and speeds.

REASONS FOR RECORDING

It is essential to learn what the rider can or cannot achieve at any given position and pace: for example:

Numerical Coding 0 = No sitting balance
Therefore support from side helper required
I = Safe when sitting in saddle and being led forward
II = Safe when sitting and being led on 20m circle
III = Safe when sitting and being led on 10m circle
IV = Safe when sitting, being led, on sharp turn.

Variations are equally applicable with the introduction of head, arm and trunk exercises; progressions to independent riding free from the leading rein; more advanced movements at other paces, walk, trot, canter, jumping small spreads at low heights and at varied speeds.

Coding can (1) indicate how the rider should be managed; (2) is a swift compact method of recording, easily translated by helper; (3) indicates progress; and (4) helps in planning individual programmes.

To condense the whole philosophy of riding for the disabled into one chapter is impossible. As an introduction to the subject, the chosen disabilities and the general problems cover those most usually presenting at Group level. Much has been omitted but it is hoped that this outline will stimulate interest and provide a basis for investigating these subjects in greater detail, and widen research into many other aspects of this rewarding and enriching activity.

REFERENCES

Autrum Jung, A., Lowenstein, W. R., Mackay, D. M. and Tewber, H. L. (1978). *Handbook of Sensory Perception*, Vol III. Springer-Verlag, New York.

Finnie, N. R. (1974). *Handling the Young Cerebral Palsied Child at Home*, 2nd edition. William Heinemann Medical Books Limited, London.

Gabell, A. and Simons, M. A. (1982). Balance coding. *Physiotherapy*, **68**, 9, 286–8.

Podhajsky, A. (1967). *The Complete Training of Horse and Rider*. Harrap Limited, London.

Wätjen, R. L. (1979). *Dressage Riding: A Guide for the Horse and Rider*, 2nd edition. J. A. Allen and Co Limited, London.

Handbook of the Riding for the Disabled Association. Regularly updated. Obtainable from Riding for the Disabled Association, National Agricultural Centre (Avenue R), Kenilworth CV8 2LY.

BIBLIOGRAPHY

Keim, H. A. (1976). *The Adolescent Spine.* Gruner and Stratton Inc, New York.

Cotton, E. (1975). *Conductive Education and Cerebral Palsy.* Spastics Society, London.

The Manual of Horsemanship (1981) British Horse Society Pony Club. Obtainable from the British Horse Society, National Agricultural Centre, Kenilworth CV8 2LY.

Pony Club Instructor's Manual obtainable from the British Horse Society, National Agricultural Centre, Kenilworth CV8 2LY.

Vaulting for the Pony Club by Ann Gittins, DipPhysEd, IM Marsh College of Physical Education (published privately). Obtainable from the Pony Club c/o British Horse Society.

ACKNOWLEDGEMENTS

The author thanks Miss A. Smith MCSP at Claremont School, Bristol for her continued support and interest over many years. She also thanks her staff at the Winford Orthopaedic Hospital and the students who spend part of their training in the hospital, for their help and suggestions with this chapter. Dr Alan Irving, MRC Applied Psychology Unit, Cambridge and Dr G. H. Begbie, University of Edinburgh Medical School both provided information, which is gratefully acknowledged.

SPECIFIC INTEREST GROUP

In addition to the Riding for the Disabled Association (address on page 452), there is a Specific Interest Group of the Chartered Society of Physiotherapy. Interested readers should contact the secretary of the Group, c/o The Chartered Society of Physiotherapy, 14 Bedford Row, London WC1R 4ED.

The record card (Fig. 24/14) has been designed by the specific interest group for use by lay helpers after an initial training period. The method discussed on pages 438–9 has yet to be evaluated.

Chapter 25

Terminal Care

by P. A. DOWNIE, FCSP

With the increasing awareness of the needs of patients with progressive illness, and the advocacy of total care for the dying, physiotherapists are becoming more involved in these areas. For this reason it seemed right to include a short general chapter on this aspect and to indicate how physiotherapists may apply their skills for such patients.

We are constantly reminded that death is a taboo subject, but with the increased number of special units being established for the care of the dying, one might feel that the emphasis has now changed. Elizabeth Kubler Ross in the USA has helped considerably in the understanding of dying patients' feelings, as well as in the realisation of the stages in bereavement; the work of Cicely Saunders towards the understanding and alleviation of pain has revolutionised the basic needs of many patients. Much of Kubler Ross's work can be classed as commonsense and this is the prime requirement of the philosophy of approach to the dying patient. While the stages which she describes (Kubler Ross, 1970) are usually discussed in the context of bereavement it is interesting to see how they fit in with the reactions which a person suffers when faced with disagreeable truths, e.g. the patient who is told that he has multiple sclerosis, the mother who is told her baby has spina bifida, the young man who has to be told that his leg needs amputation after an accident. These stages can be summarised as follows: denial of the fact, followed by anger and then the stage of bargaining; depression follows and finally comes the stage of acceptance. Not every patient or family will react in the same way, nor will they all go through each of the stages. If one understands that these reactions are normal it will help the physiotherapist when she comes to treat what to her may be considered 'a difficult patient'.

'Death is not merely an appendix to life in the manner of the ending of a bad play that might turn out anyhow. Death is built into life's structure and issues from its course. It is present long before the conclusion, actually throughout the whole development of life. Life has been defined as a moment directed towards death' (Guardini, 1954). The care of the dying should therefore be seen as a part of the whole treatment plan for a patient.

Care of the dying cannot be neatly slotted into a definite period of time; the actual process of dying may be sudden or it may be a progressive decline, of failing faculties and functions. It is about the latter group that most of the practical comments will be made, since it is these patients who require the encouragement and reassurance to accept their weaknesses and to live. It is of these that the question 'Should the patient be told of his approaching death?', will be asked. In general the answer is probably 'Yes', in as much as they are able to bear it. There is no need to be cold and dogmatic; rather sow the seed and then wait and see what follows. Certainly this telling should be done early in the care of patients so that they are able to assimilate the truth and be helped to come to an understanding. Patients suffering from progressive disease, and particularly those who may have been treated with cytotoxic drugs, become less and less able to respond to the demands of brain and body and consequently, they look always to the familiar things.

Physiotherapy is not prescribed because a patient is dying, but is a continuing part of treatment that was started when the patient was more well. When I use the word physiotherapy I am thinking in the wide term of rehabilitation and total patient care. Some patients with a progressive disease, such as multiple sclerosis, motor neurone disease or severe arthritis, may have been in long-term hospitals for many years and received regular physiotherapy. To withdraw from treating such patients when they rapidly deteriorate would be most unkind, for this is the moment of truth when they require all the help that can be given. When one is privileged to partake in the work of any of the specialist homes for the dying, it becomes patently clear that the goal for each patient must be to live each day as it comes; for the physiotherapist this means adjusting the treatment each day.

Both doctor and physiotherapist, and, indeed, any member of the health care team, need to understand and appreciate the purpose behind treatment for the progressively ill or dying patient. Above all they need to accept that such care is as important as the care which they would bestow upon a young man who receives injuries in an industrial accident. Physiotherapy for the dying should not be regarded as a waste of a scarce professional's time. Death is neither a disaster nor a failure of medicine; but a natural event which terminates people's existence. Physiotherapy that helps the patient to accept his dying and eases his physical discomfort should be prescribed without hesitation.

Complicated treatments are not advocated, but with perception and adroitness it is possible to help many patients up to the point of death. There is no doubt that physiotherapy and occupational therapy have much to offer patients who are reaching the end of their lives. Active encouragement to continue to live each day will help the patient to a better adjustment of approaching death, and the mere fact that somebody is interested in a dying patient's whim or fancy can be therapeutic. For the paralysed and bedridden patient, passive and active assisted movements of limbs will help the circulation and ease uncomfortable joints. Massage has the dual advantage of physical help as well as providing an opportunity for the patient to talk. It needs to be continually repeated that the prerequisite in care of the dying is the ability to give time and to be able to listen and support. The role of the physiotherapist is essentially in this area.

Doctors do not prescribe physiotherapy because a patient is dying but if there is a mutual understanding between doctor and physiotherapist then he may well ask her to treat a dying patient that he may be enabled to die more peacefully. Into this category comes the progressively ill patient who develops pneumonia – 'the old man's friend' as Osler described it. Often, simple physiotherapeutic measures can relieve distress, and then it is justified; heroics in such cases are to be abhorred.

Relatives also need support. If the dying patient is being nursed at home, the visiting physiotherapist can help by showing the relatives how to offer unobtrusive help, how to move painful limbs and how to support where necessary as the patient potters round the room. This help with involvement in care will alleviate the feelings of inadequacy and despair which you so often encounter in families who are trying to cope and do not know how.

Dying patients latch on to unexpected things and people. The physiotherapist must be prepared for this and act accordingly. The author remembers a 60-year-old man who had been diagnosed as having a carcinoma of the bronchus for which no treatment was advised. He was admitted with an acute superimposed chest infection for which physiotherapy was requested. When seen he was acutely distressed and ill. Gentle breathing exercises and vibrations to the chest wall were instituted and with continuous oxygen he gradually relaxed and was able to co-operate. Over two or three days he improved, the infection cleared and he was mobilised to the point of going home. Suddenly his condition deteriorated and at the patient's request the physiotherapist was sent for – in his own gasping words to the ward sister he said: 'She's the only one who's done anything for me.' When I reached him it was abundantly obvious that he was dying with no physical treatment being possible or justified; all I could do was to remain with his wife by the bedside. Care and compassion to the point of death must be accepted when one accepts the treatment of a patient with a progressive illness.

I have questioned whether physiotherapy should be prescribed when a patient is dying, but equally I ask the question, when is a patient dying? I remember a lady, aged 45, with disseminated carcinoma from a primary breast tumour. She developed 'pneumonia', and because the family could not cope was admitted to a nursing home for care and comfort. Twelve months later she was still in the nursing home being kept comfortable on opiates. It was decided to seek another opinion and she was re-assessed. Following this she was transferred for rehabilitation with a view to trying at home. She was weaned off drugs, mobilised, and a month later returned home where she remained for 18 months before dying.

Physiotherapy can also be used in helping nurses to handle patients with greater ease and comfort. Often the patient with advanced malignant disease may have bone metastases and nurses are afraid of handling limbs for fear they may fracture. Nothing transmits itself more readily than fear and if a nurse is afraid of handling such limbs, the patient will soon become aware of this. Firm gentle handling is necessary and often the presence of a physiotherapist, used to moving injured limbs, can give the required confidence to both nurse and patient alike.

The yardstick of all care of the dying is to improve the quality of life remaining in the individual patient; it may entail keeping one patient drowsy and thus unaware of pain, while allowing another patient to live more actively and even more dangerously than might normally have been considered (Graeme, 1975). A physiotherapist involved with care for a dying person needs to be able to appreciate the purpose of life as a whole; she must never be surprised by strange requests; she must certainly not attempt to impose her own ideas upon the patient; and her approach must be positive yet sympathetic.

PHILOSOPHICAL QUESTIONS

In these days of shorter working hours and great demands on the skills of physiotherapists, the question 'I have to treat dying patients and I cannot see the point – they won't recover and I could use the time more profitably' is frequently heard. Who are we to accept the truth of such a question? I would suggest that it is not for any one of us to say that a patient will not recover – very remarkable things do happen and I think it is right that we continue modified treatments, particularly for those patients whom we have known for a long time.

What do I say if a patient asks me if she/he is dying? At first sight, how difficult but most patients do not want an answer – that question is often the cry of desperation to be allowed to talk their way through their thoughts. Don't ignore it and don't run away. Rather sit down and listen, or, give some massage and listen, and turn the question to 'why are you asking me that' or 'what is it that makes you think this?' You will almost certainly find at the end that you have said almost nothing or you have been given time to provide the practical help required. Don't lie to such patients; if you don't know the answer, say so with complete frankness, *but* offer either to find out the answer or at least to find someone else who can help. In all these situations remember the hospital chaplain – he is there to help *you* as well as the patients.

'What do I do if I am asked to treat a dying patient for the very first time?' Here is another often asked question – particularly by students and newly qualified physiotherapists. Invariably it is asked in the context of the patient with disseminated cancer or some other progressive chronic disease, who develops a pneumonia. To any who postulate this question, I always say that if by treating such patients they will die more peacefully, then treat them; when in doubt in your own mind, ask yourself if you would allow your own parents to be treated – if you can honestly answer yes, then treat them. BUT, if you are unhappy about giving such treatments then you must say so. No one will think the less of you for so doing.

Euthanasia

In recent times there has been much talk about the desirability to legalise the practice of euthanasia: many respected and responsible people have spoken for it; there have been, over the last 50 years, three bills presented to Parliament – all have failed. Any professional who has dealings with the chronically sick or dying patient may find herself caught up in this debate. For this reason the following paragraphs are offered.

Even today many people equate dying with pain and euthanasia is raised. It is as well for physiotherapists to be aware of this, to understand the implications, and to be prepared to speak out fearlessly against it. Nowadays pain control, both physical and mental, is better understood; pain is more able to be treated adequately and should not therefore present problems. The positive answer to euthanasia is education of this aspect, and reassurance to the public that such treatment is possible.

The word euthanasia is derived from a Greek word meaning 'peaceful death', but the modern connotation implies the deliberate ending of a person's life. In 1973 the late Cardinal Heenan stated the Christian teaching on the care of the incurably ill as follows:

> It is not for me to give medical and legal arguments against euthanasia. Nor shall I discuss the social implications of killing sick people whether with or without their consent. I do not intend to deal with those for whom men are high-grade animals without responsibility to any law not made by man. It is my task to give briefly the Christian teaching on treatment of the incurably sick.
>
> (1) The first principle is that Almighty God as the author of life is also the Lord of life. God alone is Creator. Parents are called pro-creators. That is our way of saying that they are not absolute in their authority over the life they bring into the world. This is a fundamental truth accepted by all civilised societies until our own day.
>
> (2) The second principle is that no private person has the right to destroy life whether his own or another's.
>
> (3) Thirdly, there are legitimate differences of opinion among believers regarding the rights of the State over life. In general terms these concern killing in war and in peace. Not all agree that the State can authorise the killing (a) of aggressors by force of arms and (b) of criminals by execution. Some Christians hold that killing is legitimate in a just war or in self-defence. Pacifists regard no price as too high to pay for peace. They deny the right and duty of the State to maintain military defences. Some Christians, who are not necessarily pacifists, hold that the capital punishment of criminals is immoral.
>
> (4) Direct killing of the incurably sick, disabled or insane is never justified.
>
> (5) The Catholic Church condemns the direct killing of the living fetus although saving the life of the mother may indirectly involve the death of the fetus.
>
> (6) It is not permissible to withold nourishment or normal medical aids with the object of hastening a patient's death.
>
> It is not for the theologian to define in detail what is meant by normal medical aids. The kiss-of-life or mechanical resuscitation of a patient suffering from shock would now be regarded as normal. The prolonged use of machines to maintain the action of heart or

lungs though commonplace would be regarded as extra-ordinary means of preserving life. In certain circumstances such means might and perhaps ought to be discontinued on ethical grounds.

The patient and the doctor have different responsibilities. It may be the duty of doctor and relatives to provide the opportunity of treatment to save or prolong life. It may be their duty in the old phrase 'to allow nature to take its course'. It is not the duty of the patient to accept treatment which will purchase a further lease of life at the cost of great suffering or discomfort. Thus it would be unethical for the surgeon merely for the sake of research to persuade a patient to submit to an operation which might save the patient from death only to survive in misery.

For the Christian there are many fates worse than death. Often death is the last friend rather than the last enemy. In the *Canterbury Tales* Chaucer says, 'Death is an end of every worldly sore.' Shelley also pays tribute to death: 'How wonderful is Death, Death and his brother sleep!' Death is not a misfortune to be warded off at all costs. The death of God's friends is precious in His sight because it is a homecoming. That is why we need not hesitate to alleviate pain merely from fear of bringing nearer the hour of death. It is good ethics to ensure the comfort of the dying. It disposes of the chief argument in support of euthanasia.

The moral sense and compassion of doctors and nurses must decide what is for the patient's good. It is not euthanasia to refuse to use extra-ordinary methods to conquer a critical condition in a patient already suffering from a chronic terminal illness. To help patients to die in peace and dignity is part of the art of nursing and medicine.

These are the general principles. If we depart from them either to co-operate in suicide or to execute incurables we trespass on God's province and run the risk of destroying the whole moral law. With the decline of religion people have already begun to confuse legality with morality. Abortion and homosexual practices are regarded by many as morally acceptable because they are now permitted by law. If euthanasia were to become legal no sick or old person would be safe. The law of God is also the law of reason.

These are clear facts which should help all physiotherapists to better understand the very real difficulties which can arise in caring for the dying. It is an issue which cannot be evaded and one with which all right-thinking professionals should be concerned. It is probably true to say that it is not death itself which people fear, it is the process of dying and the very real fear of being subjected to unpleasant treatments with no real purpose save that of satisfying medical science. If this latter fear can be confidently resolved, and the patient and his family convinced and reassured that he will neither be allowed to suffer pain, nor be regarded as useless and a nuisance, then the question of euthanasia should not even be contemplated.

True care for the dying patient does not involve sophisticated medical treatments; it demands care, understanding and compassion of the very highest standards, and for all of us in the caring professions it must ever remain the supreme test. For the physiotherapist it must never be regarded as a waste of time.

This chapter has not attempted to touch upon the problems of patients in intensive care units – it has concentrated on the patient who is dying from long-term illness. It is written to encourage the physiotherapist not to be frightened, put off or embarrassed at the thought of treating a dying person. They are still human beings with all the faults and frailties which we know so well; they require help, and if as physiotherapists we can provide this, then we must do so.

REFERENCES

Graeme, P. D. (1975). *Support for the Dying Patient and his Family*. Included in the proceedings of the Marie Curie Memorial Foundation's symposium; *Cancer, the Patient and the Family*. John Sherratt and Sons Ltd, Altrincham.

Guardini, R. (1954). *The Last Things*. Burns and Oates, London.

Kübler-Ross, E. (1970). *On Death and Dying*. Tavistock Publications, London.

BIBLIOGRAPHY

Albanus (1978). To die or not to die. *Therapy*, May 5.

Corr, C. A. and Corr, D. M. (eds) (1983). *Hospice Care: Principles and Practice*. Faber and Faber, London. Published in the USA by Springer Publishing Co Inc, New York.

Hinton, J. (1972). *Dying*, 2nd edition. Penguin Books, Harmondsworth.

Lamerton, R. (1980). *Care of the Dying*. Penguin Books, Harmondsworth.

Lewis, C. S. (1961). *A Grief Observed*. Faber and Faber, London.

On Dying Well: An Anglican Contribution to the Debate on Euthanasia (1975). Church Information Office, London.

Parkes, C. M. (1975). *Bereavement*. Penguin Books, Harmondsworth.

Raven, R. W. (ed) (1975). *The Dying Patient*. Pitman Books Limited, London.

Wilkes, E. (ed) (1982). *The Dying Patient: The Medical Management of Incurable and Terminal Illness*. MTP Press Limited, Lancaster.

Glossary

SUFFIXES

-ectomy From a Greek word meaning 'a cutting out'. Removal of the whole or part of an organ

-gram From the Greek, *gramma*, meaning a mark. Usually used to describe the radiograph obtained following the outlining of organs or vessels by a radio-opaque substance

-ography The examination of a particular organ or system of the body, and the methods used to do so

-oscopy From the Greek word 'to look'. An inspection of a hollow organ or body cavity by means of instruments specially made for this purpose

-ostomy From the Latin, *ostium*, meaning a mouth. The formation of an artificial opening on to the surface of the body, e.g. colostomy

-otomy From the Greek word meaning 'incision'. A surgical incision

-plasty From the Greek word 'to mould'. A surgical procedure for repair of a defect and restoration of a part

resection From the Latin *re*, 'again' and *secare*, 'to cut'. It indicates the operation of cutting out, e.g. rib resection

SURGICAL TERMS

ablation The removal of a part by surgery, drugs or radioactive means

amputation The surgical removal of part of the body, e.g. a limb, breast, penis

arthrodesis The surgical fixation of a joint

arthroplasty The making of an artificial joint by the surgical introduction of a suitable prothesis; e.g. total hip arthroplasty where both the acetabulum and head of femur are replaced by metal or plastic prostheses

caecostomy An opening into the caecum through the abdominal wall for drainage; it is never permanent

cholecystogram   The radiograph (x-ray) of the gall bladder obtained following the outlining of the gall bladder with a radio-opaque substance

colectomy   The excision of part of the colon, e.g. hemicolectomy

colostomy   The surgical formation of an artificial anus, either temporary or permanent, by making an opening into the colon, from the skin

gastrectomy   The excision of the whole or part of the stomach

gastrostomy   The establishment of an opening into the stomach from the skin, for the purpose of feeding

haematoma   A collection of extravasated blood in the body causing swelling and bruising

ileostomy   The surgical formation of a passage through the abdominal wall into the ileum; it is usually permanent and is performed in cases of ulcerative colitis

laparotomy   An incision through the abdominal wall to allow an exploratory examination

laryngectomy   The surgical removal of the larynx

lymphogram   A radiograph of lymph vessels or nodes

lymphography   The radiographic examination of lymph vessels or nodes which are rendered radio-opaque by the injection of dye

mammaplasty   A plastic surgery procedure for the breasts; either augmentation or reduction.

mastectomy   The surgical removal of the breast

mediastinoscopy   The examination of the mediastinum by the use of a mediastinoscope

pancreatectomy   The excision of the pancreas

prosthesis   The replacement for a limb or organ which has been either removed or is missing, e.g. an artificial limb, breast form or eye

pyloroplasty   An operation to widen a contracted pylorus. The fibres of the pyloric canal are divided longitudinally and closed transversely

splenectomy   The surgical removal of the spleen

thoracoscopy   The examination of the pleural cavity by the use of a thorascope

tracheostomy   The surgical formation of an opening into the windpipe (trachea) through the neck

tracheotomy   The operation of incising the trachea

Useful Organisations

Of necessity this is only a select list of organisations and agencies which can offer help, advice and counselling. Mostly they relate to the conditions mentioned in this book, and they have been divided into two sections, general and children. A useful guide book for extensive information about many organisations is the *Directory for the Disabled* edited by A. Darnborough and D. Kinrade and published by Woodhead-Faulkner, Cambridge CB2 3PF. It is regularly updated.

GENERAL

Colostomy Welfare Group
38/9 Eccleston Square (2nd Floor)
London SW1V 1PB   01-828 5175

Ileostomy Association of Great Britain and Ireland
First Floor, 23 Winchester Road
Basingstoke RG21 1UE   0256 21288

Marie Curie Memorial Foundation
28 Belgrave Square
London SW1X 8QG   01-235 3325

Mastectomy Association of Great Britain
25 Brighton Road
South Croydon CR2 6EA   01-654 8643

National Association of Laryngectomee Clubs
38 Eccleston Square
London SW1V 1PB   01-834 2704

Women's National Cancer Control Campaign
 South Audley Street
London W1Y 5DQ   01-499 7532

Royal Association for Disability and Rehabilitation (RADAR)
25 Mortimer Street
London W1N 8AB   01-637 5400

Disabled Living Foundation
346 Kensington High Street
London W14 2BD   01-602 2491

Riding for the Disabled Association
National Agricultural Centre (Avenue R)
Kenilworth, Warwickshire CV8 2LY   0203 56107

The Psoriasis Association
7 Milton Street
Northampton NN2 7JG   0604 711129

National Eczema Society
5 Tavistock Place
London WC1H 9SR   01-388 4097

The National Childbirth Trust
9 Queensborough Terrace
London W2 3TB   01-229 9319

La Leche League of Great Britain
Box 3424
London WC1 6XX   01-404 5011

CHILDREN

A useful booklet giving details of many organisations, as well as
information about allowances and how to claim them, may be
obtained from the Voluntary Council for Handicapped Children,
National Children's Bureau, 8 Wakley Street, London EC1V 7QE. It
is called *Help Starts Here.*

Association for Spina Bifida and Hydrocephalus (ASBAH)
Tavistock House North
Tavistock Square, London WC1H 9HJ   01-388 1382

British Epilepsy Association
Crowthorne House, New Wokingham Road
Crowthorne, Berkshire RG1 3AY   03446 3122

Cystic Fibrosis Research Trust
5 Blyth Road
Bromley, Kent BR1 3RS   01-464 7211

Down's Children's Association
Quinborne Community Centre, Ridgacre Road
Quinton, Birmingham B32 2TW   021-427 1374

Handicapped Adventure Playground Association
Fulham Palace Playground
Bishop's Avenue, London SW6 6EE   01-731 2753

Muscular Dystrophy Group of Great Britain
Nattrass House, 35 Macaulay Road
London SW4 0QP   01-720 8055

National Association for the Welfare of Children In Hospital
(NAWCH)
7 Exton Street
London SE1 8UE   01-261 1738

National Society for Mentally Handicapped Children (MENCAP)
117–123 Golden Lane
London EC1Y 0RF   01-253 9433

Spastics Society
12 Park Crescent
London W1N 4EQ   01-636 5020

Toy Libraries Association
Seabrook House, Wyllyotts Manor
Darkes Lane, Potters Bar EN6 5HL   0707 44571

Index